Small Cell Lung Cancer

CLINICAL ONCOLOGY MONOGRAPHS

Series Editors

John W. Yarbro, M.D., Ph.D.
Richard S. Bornstein, M.D.
Michael J. Mastrangelo, M.D.

HUMAN MALIGNANT MELANOMA
edited by Wallace H. Clark, Jr., M.D., Leonard I. Goldman, M.D., and Michael J. Mastrangelo, M.D.

ONCOLOGIC EMERGENCIES
edited by John W. Yarbro, M.D., and Richard S. Bornstein, M.D.

SMALL CELL LUNG CANCER
edited by F. Anthony Greco, M.D., Robert K. Oldham, M.D., and Paul A. Bunn, Jr., M.D.

Small Cell Lung Cancer

Edited by F. Anthony Greco, M.D.

Associate Professor of Medicine
Division of Oncology
Department of Medicine
Vanderbilt University Medical Center
Nashville, Tennessee

Robert K. Oldham, M.D.

Director, Biological Response Modifier Program
National Cancer Institute
Frederick Cancer Research Center
Frederick, Maryland

Paul A. Bunn, Jr., M.D.

Senior Investigator
National Cancer Institute—Veterans Administration
    Medical Oncology Branch
Veterans Administration Medical Center
Washington, D.C.

GRUNE & STRATTON
A Subsidiary of Harcourt Brace Jovanovich, Publishers
New York   London   Toronto   Sydney   San Francisco

Library of Congress Cataloging in Publication Data

Main entry under title:

Small cell lung cancer.

   (Clinical oncology monographs)
   Includes index and bibliography.
   Contents: Small cell carcinoma of the lung / William
Weiss—Problems in the diagnosis of small cell carci-
noma of the lung / Mary J. Matthews and Fred R. Hirsch—
Tissue culture and in vitro characteristics / Olive
S. Pettengill and George D. Sorenson—[etc.]
   1. Lungs—Cancer. I. Greco, F. Anthony (Frank
Anthony), 1947– . II. Oldham, Robert K. III. Bunn,
Paul A. IV. Series. [DNLM: 1. Lung neoplasms. WF 658
S635]
RC280.L8S62   616.99'424   81-4370
ISBN 0-8089-1345-X   AACR2

Grune & Stratton, Inc.
111 Fifth Avenue
New York, New York 10003

Distributed in the United Kingdom by
Academic Press Inc. (London) Ltd.
24/28 Oval Road, London NW 1

Library of Congress Catalog Number 81-4370
International Standard Book Number 0-8089-1345-X
Printed in the United States of America

Contents

Contents

Foreword

Lung cancer is at one and the same time the most common, the least treatable, and the most easily prevented cancer in this country.

The incidence of lung cancer has steadily increased, first in males and then in females, lagging about two decades behind the altered cigarette-smoking behavior patterns that developed at about the time of World War I in males and World War II in females. Low-tar cigarettes have had a measurable, but far from substantial, impact on this incidence.

No technique for early detection has been developed that substantially reduces mortality rates in a screened population in comparison to patients who present in the conventional manner.

In recent years, diagnostic and staging procedures have improved. Gradually increasing 5-year-survival rates have been reported in surgically resected patients. The rates reported for all patients with lung cancer are approximately 10%, however, and have not changed substantially in four decades. This suggests that reports of improved survival are more likely the result of case selection than of improved therapy. For non–small cell lung cancer with inoperable or unresectable tumor, survival is not substantially prolonged by the routine use of radiation, chemotherapy, or both, and the routine addition of such modalities to surgical resection has not improved survival. It would appear, therefore, that lung cancer is a systemic disease at the time of diagnosis in as many as 90% of the patients.

Small cell carcinoma of the lung (SCC), a histologic type of bronchogenic cancer which comprises about one-fifth of all cases, is biologically distinct from other forms of lung cancer. It has long been recognized that SCC is the most rapidly progressing form of lung cancer, having the highest growth fraction and shortest doubling time. From the earliest years of chemotherapy, it was this cell type that was noted to be the most responsive to treatment. Occasionally, even complete remissions were seen. Experience in many neoplasms has shown that tumors that can be cured by combination chemotherapy share certain characteristics: rapid progression; short doubling time; high growth fraction; frequent response to multiple chemotherapeutic agents, used singly or in combination; and a high incidence of complete remissions, regardless of duration. SCC demonstrates all of these characteristics.

The earliest complete remissions of SCC following combination chemotherapy were of short duration and were followed by recurrent disease, either at the site of the original primary tumor or in the brain. This led to the use of prophylactic central nervous system radiation, as in acute lymphocytic leukemia, and radiation of the site of the primary tumor as a debulking procedure. Central nervous system recurrence was reduced substantially by radiation, but the recurrence at the site of the primary tumor, though reduced, remains a problem. Some patients are now surviving long enough to show other sites of recurrence, such as the liver, that may require attention in future protocols.

It is clear that a "cure" plateau can be seen on survival curves, and some studies suggest that we are presently curing as many as one-fourth of the patients with limited-stage disease. This is a field characterized by rapid change as attempts are made to deal with such questions as the selection of optimal combination chemotherapy regimens, the development of alternate non–cross-resistant regimens, the development of new active drugs, the determination of the optimal dose and schedule for radiation directed at the primary tumor, the reduction of combined radiation-drug toxicity, the identification of the duration of treatment required for cure, and the assessment of the role of consolidation and maintenance strategies in the overall treatment. The contents of this volume represent a major contribution to the clarification of these complex clinical questions.

In addition, this volume deals with several other important issues, including: epidemiologic and etiologic factors, pathology, tissue-culture growth and characteristics, the nude-mouse model, the cellular origin, tumor-associated products and paraneoplastic syndromes, cytokinetics, the biochemical and morphologic heterogeneity before and after therapy, immunologic aspects, primary extrapulmonary tumors, and complications of therapy. A considerable amount of basic and clinical research concerning SCC is in process, and it is likely that the management of patients with this common neoplasm will continue to improve as more information becomes available.

John W. Yarbro, M.D., Ph.D

Contributors

MARTIN D. ABELOFF, M.D., *Associate Professor of Oncology and Medicine, The John Hopkins University School of Medicine, Baltimore, Maryland*

JOSEPH AISNER, M.D., *Chief, Section of Medical Oncology, Baltimore Cancer Research Program, Division of Cancer Treatment, National Cancer Institute, Baltimore, Maryland; Associate Professor of Medicine, University of Maryland School of Medicine, Baltimore, Maryland*

STEPHEN B. BAYLIN, M.D., *Associate Professor of Oncology and Medicine, The Johns Hopkins University School of Medicine, Baltimore, Maryland*

PAUL A. BUNN, JR., M.D., *Senior Investigator, National Cancer Institute—Veterans Administration Medical Oncology Branch, Veterans Administration Medical Center, Washington, D.C.*

DESMOND N. CARNEY, M.D., M.R.C.P.I., *Senior Investigator, National Cancer Institute—Veterans Administration Medical Oncology Branch, Veterans Administration Medical Center, Washington, D.C.*

CHARLES C. CATE, PH.D., *Research Assistant Professor of Pathology, Department of Pathology, Dartmouth Medical School, Hanover, New Hampshire*

MARTIN H. COHEN, M.D., *Senior Investigator, National Cancer Institute—Veterans Administration Medical Oncology Branch, Veterans Administration Medical Center, Washington, D.C.*

JOSEPH C. EGGLESTON, M.D., *Associate Professor of Pathology and Oncology, The Johns Hopkins University School of Medicine, Baltimore, Maryland*

MEHMET F. FER, M.D., *Instructor in Medicine, Division of Oncology, Department of Medicine, Vanderbilt University Medical Center, Nashville, Tennessee*

JAMES T. FORBES, PH.D., *Research Assistant Professor of Medicine, Division of Oncology, Department of Medicine, Vanderbilt Medical Center, Nashville, Tennessee*

ADI F. GAZDAR, M.D., B.S., *Senior Investigator, National Cancer Institute—Veterans Administration Medical Oncology Branch, Veterans Administration Medical Center, Washington, D.C.*

ELI GLATSTEIN, M.D., *Chief, Radiation Oncology Branch, National Cancer Institute, Bethesda, Maryland*

F. ANTHONY GRECO, M.D., *Associate Professor of Medicine, Division of Oncology, Department of Medicine, Vanderbilt University Medical Center, Nashville, Tennessee*

RICHARD L. GREENSTREET, PH.D., *Department of Biostatistics, Cleveland Clinic Foundation, Cleveland, Ohio*

JOHN G. GUCCION, M.D., *Pathologist, Laboratory Service, Veterans Administration Medical Center, Washington, D.C.; Associate Professor, Department of Pathology, George Washington University School of Medicine, Washington, D.C.*

JOHN HAINSWORTH, M.D., *Instructor in Medicine, Division of Oncology, Department of Medicine, Vanderbilt University Medical Center, Nashville, Tennessee*

KENNETH R. HANDE, M.D., *Assistant Professor of Medicine and Pharmacology, Division of Oncology, Department of Medicine, Vanderbilt University Medical Center, Nashville, Tennessee*

HEINE H. HANSEN, M.D., *Chief, Department of Chemotherapy, Finsen Institute, Copenhagen, Denmark*

FRED R. HIRSCH, M.D., *Research Fellow, University of Copenhagen, Copenhagen, Denmark; Departments of Chemotherapy and Pathology, Finsen Institute, Copenhagen, Denmark*

DANIEL C. IHDE, M.D., *Senior Investigator, National Cancer Institute—Veterans Administration Medical Oncology Branch, Veterans Administration Medical Center, Washington, D.C.*

JOHN Y. KILLEN, JR., M.D., *Senior Investigator, Cancer Therapy Evaluation Program, Division of Cancer Treatment, National Cancer Institute, Bethesda, Maryland*

ROBERT M. LEVENSON, JR., M.D., *Clinical Associate, National Cancer Institute—Veterans Administration Medical Oncology Branch, Veterans Administration Medical Center, Washington, D.C.*

ALLEN S. LICHTER, M.D., *Head, Radiation Therapy Section, Radiation Oncology Branch, National Cancer Institute, Bethesda, Maryland*

ROBERT B. LIVINGSTON, M.D., *Chairman, Department of Hematology and Medical Oncology, Cleveland Clinic Foundation, Cleveland, Ohio*

JOHN S. MACDONALD, M.D., *Associate Director, Cancer Therapy Evaluation Program, Division of Cancer Treatment, National Cancer Institute, Bethesda, Maryland*

MARY J. MATTHEWS, M.D., *Senior Investigator, National Cancer Institute—Veterans Administration Medical Oncology Branch, Veterans Administration Medical Center, Washington, D.C.; Professor of Pathology, George Washington University School of Medicine, Washington, D.C.*

JOHN D. MINNA, M.D., *Chief, National Cancer Institute—Veterans Administration Medical Oncology Branch, Veterans Administration Medical Center, Washington, D.C.*

ROBERT K. OLDHAM, M.D., *Director, Biological Response Modifier Program, National Cancer Institute, Frederick Cancer Research Center, Frederick, Maryland*

OLIVE S. PETTENGILL, PH.D., *Research Associate Professor of Pathology, Department of Pathology, Dartmouth Medical School, Hanover, New Hampshire*

RONALD L. RICHARDSON, M.D., *Assistant Professor of Medicine, Division of Oncology, Department of Medicine, Vanderbilt University Medical Center, Nashville, Tennessee*

STANLEY E. SHACKNEY, M.D., *Senior Investigator, Clinical Pharmacology Branch, Division of Cancer Treatment, National Cancer Institute, Bethesda, Maryland*

ANNA SISMANI, M.D., *Division of Oncology, Department of Medicine, Vanderbilt University Medical Center, Nashville, Tennessee*

GEORGE D. SORENSON, M.D., *Professor of Pathology, Department of Pathology, Dartmouth Medical School, Hanover, New Hampshire*

MARC J. STRAUS, M.D., *Chief, Division of Neoplastic Diseases, Section of Oncology, Department of Medicine, New York Medical College, Valhalla, New York*

CHRISTOPHER J. TRAUTH, M.D., *Section of Oncology, Department of Medicine, University of Texas Health Sciences Center, San Antonio, Texas*

WILLIAM WEISS, M.D., *Professor of Medicine and Director, Division of Occupational Medicine, Hahnemann Medical College and Hospital, Philadelphia, Pennsylvania*

PETER H. WIERNICK, M.D., *Chief, Clinical Oncology Branch, Baltimore Cancer Research Program, Division of Cancer Treatment, National Cancer Institute, University of Maryland Hospital, Baltimore, Maryland*

Small Cell Lung Cancer

1

SMALL CELL CARCINOMA OF THE LUNG: EPIDEMIOLOGY AND ETIOLOGY

William Weiss

Epidemiology is defined as the study of the distribution of disease and of its determinants in whole populations. In the absence of human experimentation, the etiology of disease in mankind must be investigated epidemiologically, and we are interested in etiology because it often provides a mechanism for the prevention of disease. For a disease such as lung cancer, the current therapy for which is disappointing, prevention is of considerable importance; this is particularly true of small cell carcinoma (SCC).

Etiological purists insist that cause-and-effect relationships can be proved only by direct experimentation. Because proof of causation of a disease as serious as lung cancer cannot be obtained in humans for ethical reasons, the search for causality depends on circumstantial evidence. Decisions must be made on the basis of judgment, and for this purpose we need a set of criteria. Sir Bradford Hill described such a set in 1965.[1] It includes the following:

1. Strength of the association: the disease is more common after exposure to the agent than in its absence—the bigger the difference, the stronger the association.
2. Consistency of the association: repeated studies, especially those that use different methods, arrive at the same conclusion.
3. Specificity of the association: the agent is associated specifically with

that disease; thus, an agent that is associated with only one disease is highly specific.

4. Temporality: exposure to the agent precedes the occurrence of disease.
5. Dose–response relationship: increasing response occurs with increasing exposure.
6. Plausibility: a criterion that depends on the current state of biologic knowledge.
7. Coherence: agreement exists between the association and other information about the disease.
8. Experiment of an ethical nature: prevention of disease follows cessation of exposure.
9. Analogy: the association is similar to others in which cause-and-effect relationships are accepted.

During the past three decades the study of cause-and-effect relationships has been particularly productive in lung cancer, perhaps because it is the single cancer that has endowed the twentieth century with a major epidemic. The various histologic types of lung cancer show enough epidemiological differences to suggest that this illness is a group of diseases rather than a single entity. Unfortunately, interest in the individual types has developed only recently, and the data are rather limited. In this chapter the epidemiology and etiology of SCC are examined in the light of available information. Whenever it seems reasonable to do so, the gaps are filled in by assuming that SCC has the same characteristics as lung cancer in general.

Descriptive Epidemiology

There are several difficulties in any attempt to describe the epidemiology of SCC with respect to the basic variables of place, time, age, race, and sex. Firstly, an important problem has been the lack of histological standardization. It was not until 1967 that the World Health Organization (WHO) published an international classification of lung tumors.[2]

Secondly, although Kreyberg was the head of the WHO International Reference Center and was instrumental in developing the details of the classification, he had previously published a number of papers in which he lumped types into two broad categories—Group I, which included epidermoid and small cell carcinomas, and Group II, which included all other types (predominantly adenocarcinomas)—on the hypothesis that Group I tumors accounted for most of the increase in lung cancer in large areas of the

Table 1-1
Mean Annual Male Incidence of Lung Cancer in
Olmstead County, Minnesota, by Histologic Type
and Period

Type	1935–1954		1955–1964		1965–1974	
	No.	Rate*	No.	Rate*	No.	Rate*
Squamous cell	13	3.5	25	10.3	58	19.4
Adenocarcinoma	8	2.2	15	6.1	27	9.2
Small cell	8	2.2	15	6.1	17	6.0
Large cell	5	1.4	14	5.8	25	8.4

Adapted from Annegers et al.[7]
*Number per 100,000/yr.

world.[3] Unfortunately, many investigators have since followed suit, so that information on SCC has been lost within a larger category.

Thirdly, tumor typing is not an exact science. Pathologists disagree with each other,[4] and the effect of such disagreement on the limited epidemiologic data available has not been adequately studied.

Fourthly, there has been some suggestion that, just as the incidence of all lung cancer has been changing, so has the distribution of types.[5] However, there is no agreement on this.[6,7] Differences in method and material may account for the disagreement.

Fifthly, not all cases of lung cancer are confirmed histologically. The proportion may be less than 75 percent in some series, especially in elderly people, who often refuse investigation. This may introduce some bias into the statistics.[8]

Lastly, but perhaps most importantly, the information may lack a population base. Risks can only be evaluated reliably by incidence, defined as the number of new cases per unit population per unit time. Thus, incidence is described by a fraction—the numerator being the number of cases and the denominator the population at risk—so that rates or probabilities can be calculated. To assess the determinants of risk, i.e., etiologic factors, both the numerator and denominator must be broken down into various categories. Even the few population-based studies of lung cancer with information on histologic types do not provide all the desired data.

Annegers et al.[7] reported the incidence of lung cancer by histologic type in Olmstead County, Minnesota, over the period 1935–1974. Only in men was the number of cases large enough to establish rates with some stability. The results are shown in Table 1-1. Small cell carcinoma and adenocarcinoma rates were equal and second only to that of squamous cell carcinoma in the first 30 yr, but during the most recent decade, SCC had the lowest rate of the four types studied. Unfortunately the rates are not age adjusted, and age-specific rates are not provided. The area is largely rural.

In the metropolitan area of Portland, Oregon, unpublished data for 1968–1972 (W. E. Morton, personal communication) showed mean annual rates per 100,000 for SCC, age-adjusted to the U.S. 1970 census, of 13 in males and 4 in females. The rates were higher in the urban than in the rural part of the area studied, and tended to be higher among males in the lower socioeconomic areas.

SCC rates among Singapore Chinese in 1968–1972 were 16.9 in males and 2.6 in females.[9] These rates were age adjusted to the 1970 world population and were inflated to approximate the actual figures (since only one-third of the cases were typed) by assuming that distributions by cell type were the same in unproven cases as in those with histologic proof.

In the Philadelphia Pulmonary Neoplasm Research Project (PNRP),[8] a semiannual screening study of 6027 urban males aged 45 yr and over that was conducted during the period 1951–1965, each man was observed for 10 yr. Lung cancer developed after the start of observation in 121, and histologic confirmation was obtained in 90 (74 percent).[10] The cancers were classified by a panel of pathologists according to a slight modification of the WHO schema. There were 17 SCC in 52,487.9 man-years, so the rate was 32.4/100,000 man-years. In the Olmstead County study, the rate was based on males of all ages, whereas the PNRP rate was based on males aged 45 and over. Although the PNRP study group was not a random sample of all Philadelphia males aged 45 and over, the age and race distributions were quite similar.[10] Based on the proportion of males younger than 45 in Philadelphia in 1955 (69.9 percent), the estimated size of the total population of males from which the study group was recruited is 20,000. Using this estimate and assuming that neither deaths nor lung cancers occurred during the 10-yr period among the younger males, 17 cases would have occurred in 192,228 man-years, for a rate of 8.8/100,000 man-years. This is similar to the rate of 6.1/100,000/yr in Olmstead County during approximately the same period.[7] The assumptions, of course, make the PNRP figure an underestimate. The higher rate of 13 in Portland is probably attributable to the later period in which the data were collected (1968–1972), since lung cancer incidence has been increasing steadily. The higher rate in Philadelphia compared with that in Olmstead County may also be partially attributable to the well-known urban–rural gradient seen in studies of lung cancer incidence.

The SCC rates by age found in the PNRP are shown in Table 1-2 (unpublished data). The rate increased with age up to the ages of 55–64 (age being the age at the start of the 10-yr observation period) and then fell.

Table 1-2
Ten-Year Incidence of Small Cell Carcinoma by Age
in Older Males in 1951–1965

Age at Start of Observation	No. of Men	No. of Man-years	Incidence No.	Incidence Rate*
45–54	2804	26,418.6	6	22.7
55–64	2169	18,530.9	9	48.6
65–74	881	6,526.5	2	30.6
75+	173	1,011.9	0	—
Total	6,027	52,487.9	17	32.4

Unpublished data from the Philadelphia Pulmonary Neoplasm Research Project.[8]
*Number per 100,000 man-years.

This decline in the incidence of SCC in men 65 and over is of uncertain significance because of the small number of subjects in this age group, but it is consistent with observations on a period basis for all lung cancers. It is probably attributable to a cohort effect: older people were born into earlier birth cohorts which may have been subjected to less carcinogenic exposure than were younger people born into later cohorts.[11] A similar pattern may be demonstrated in age-specific rates for Portland, Oregon, during 1968–1972 (W. E. Morton, personal communication).

The annual incidence in Iceland for SCC by age, sex, and period can be calculated from data provided by Hallgrimsson (Table 1-3).[12] Lung can-

Table 1-3
Annual Incidence of Small Cell Carcinoma in Iceland
by Sex, Age, and Period

Age	1955–1961 No. of Cases	1955–1961 Rate*	1962–1968 No. of Cases	1962–1968 Rate*
Males				
35–44	2	19.8	0	—
45–54	7	84.9	9	98.6
55–64	7	109.0	11	153.6
65–74	0	—	7	141.6
75+	3	153.4	2	81.9
Females				
35–44	2	20.6	0	—
45–54	0	—	4	44.4
55–64	3	45.4	5	69.2
65–74	3	67.1	2	36.4
75+	3	105.4	1	30.4

From Hallgrimsson.[12]
*Number per 100,000/yr.

cers were typed according to the WHO classification. Because of the small number of cases, interpretation is somewhat restricted but, in general, the age-specific rates showed an increase with time in males, an increase with age in both sexes (with a decline in the oldest age groups during the more recent period), and higher rates in males than in females during both periods. These rates for SCC were considerably higher in Iceland than in U.S. studies cited above, and this is reflected in the fact that SCC contributed a much larger proportion of the lung cancers in Iceland (31–40 percent) than in the United States (9–19 percent). The distribution of histologic types varies with the source of tissue, SCC being more frequent in autopsy than in surgical material,[13,14] and this may account for some of the geographic difference.

Relative Frequency of SCC

There is additional information on the frequency of SCC relative to all lung cancers, information that describes some of its predilections. It should be understood, however, that these data are not an adequate substitute for epidemiologic observations, because the populations at risk—the denominators—are not defined. Still, they may provide some insights that will need to be reconciled with epidemiologic and etiologic studies if a coherent picture of the nature of SCC is to be developed.

A group of sources (Table 1-4) were reviewed for the distribution of cell types in various parts of the world by sex. Those reports in which the origin of tissue was restricted (to autopsy material only, for example) were excluded. The percentage SCC contributed to all lung cancers is shown. Unfortunately, there was considerable variation of the time periods during which the cases were collected, and this may confound the data if there has been any significant change in the relative distribution of types over the past four decades.

Table 1-4 shows a marked geographic variation in the percentage of SCC for both sexes. In males, it was particularly high (over 20 percent) in Sweden, Finland, and Iceland, and in one of four U.S. studies—an investigation of lung cancer in veterans. In females the frequency was especially high in Finland, Wales, England, and Iceland. Thus, when SCC is common, it tends to be common in both sexes. This is also true in a report from New Zealand[22] not included in Table 1-4: cases collected from four hospital thoracic units during 1957–1965 showed that 24.2 percent of 2376 male lung cancer cases and 30.2 percent of 301 female cases were SCC (analysis limited to the four major types).

Table 1-4
Frequency of Small Cell Carcinoma as Percent of All Typed Lung Cancers* by Sex and Country

Country	Reference†	Era	Male			Female		
			No. Typed	SCC No.	SCC %	No. Typed	SCC No.	SCC %
Norway	Kreyberg[14]	1950–1964	709	123	17.3	95	9	9.5
Sweden	Berge[15]	1958–1969	561	153	27.3	149	22	14.8
Finland	Kreyberg[3]	1958–1959	545	152	27.9	21	5	23.8
Wales	Harley[16]	1964–1968	—	—	—	103	37	35.9
England	Kennedy[17]	1955–1971	—	—	—	168	75	44.6
England	Doll[18]	1951–1971	124	17	13.7	—	—	—
Iceland	Hallgrimsson[12]	1941–1968	144	57	39.6	79	26	31.3
Hong Kong	Chan[19]	1976–1977	122	21	17.2	93	13	14.0
United States	Weiss[10]	1951–1965	90	17	18.9	—	—	—
United States	Annegers[7]	1935–1974	240	40	16.7	64	6	9.4
United States	Beamis[20]	1957–1972	—	—	—	201	25	12.0
United States	Herrold[21]	1954–1962	1313	368	28.0	—	—	—
United States	W. E. Morton‡	1968–1972	1283	185	14.4	353	63	17.8

*Includes the five major types: squamous cell carcinoma, small cell carcinoma, adenocarcinoma, large cell carcinoma, and mixed squamous cell and adenocarcinoma.
†First author given.
‡Personal communication, 1980.

7

Table 1-5
Distribution of 709 Male Norwegian Lung Cancer Cases,
1950–1964, by Histologic Type and Age

Age	No. in Age Group	Histologic Type		
		Epidermoid (%)*	Small cell (%)*	Adenocarcinoma (%)*
< 50	104	53.8	26.0	20.2
50–59	298	67.4	17.8	14.8
60–69	249	71.1	15.3	13.7
.70+	58	67.2	8.6	24.1

From Kreyberg.[14]
*Percentage of number in each age group.

Some additional data in the United States were provided by the Third National Cancer Survey,[23] 1969–1971. The results were consistent with the majority of the other U.S. studies shown in Table 1-4: SCC was 13.4 percent of all lung cancers in males and 14.5 percent in females. The total tabulation included a large proportion of unspecified and rare types of tumor (32.1 percent of 20,234 cases). If these are excluded, then SCC (specified as oat cell in this survey) formed 19.8 percent of all cases (both sexes combined because the data published do not permit separation).[24]

SCC as percentage of all lung cancers varies by age, being more common in younger patients. Table 1-5 shows this for males in Norway.[14] This could be attributable to a cohort effect, since older men in a particular period of time were born into earlier birth cohorts whose exposure to carcinogens might have differed from that of later birth cohorts. However, a specific age effect cannot be excluded. Supportive data were provided by several other studies. Kennedy[25] in England investigated 40 cases of lung cancer in patients less than 40 yr of age and found that 19 of 29 males and 7 of 11 females had SCC. Kyriakos and Webber[26] reviewed 102 male cases aged 12–45 in St. Louis and found that 24 percent had SCC compared to 13 percent in patients of all ages. However, Putnam[27] discovered only 2 cases of oat cell carcinoma in 24 patients under age 40 at Walter Reed Army Hospital (both among the 16 men).

Male/female ratios derived from data in Table 1-4 are shown in Table 1-6. These vary greatly for SCC, from 1.6 in Hong Kong to 30.4 in Finland, but it should be noted that the low Hong Kong ratio was recorded 18 yr later than the high Finland ratio. Except for the unpublished data of W. E. Morton in Portland, Oregon (personal communication), the male/female ratios for SCC are higher than those for all other types combined. However, the ratios for other types are high where the SCC ratios are high.

Table 1-6
Male/Female Ratios of Small Cell Carcinomas and of
Other Lung Cancer Types by Country

Country	Reference*	Era	SCC		Other Types	
			M/F Nos.	Ratio	M/F Nos.	Ratio
Norway	Kreyberg[14]	1950–1964	123/9	13.7	586/86	6.8
Sweden	Berge[15]	1958–1969	153/22	7.0	408/127	3.2
Finland	Kreyberg[3]	1958–1959	152/5	30.4	393/16	24.6
Iceland	Hallgrimsson[12]	1941–1968	57/26	2.2	87/53	1.6
Hong Kong	Chan[19]	1976–1977	21/13	1.6	101/80	1.3
United States	Annegers[7]	1935–1974	40/6	6.7	200/58	3.4
United States	W. E. Morton[†]	1968–1972	185/63	2.9	1098/290	3.8

*First author given.
†Personal communication, 1980.

An observation that merits consideration in any etiologic schema is that SCC, unlike adenocarcinoma, is not associated with scarred or otherwise diseased lung. Auerbach et al.[28] recently reported the results of a 21-yr autopsy study involving 1186 U.S. veterans with lung cancer; 82 patients had tumors associated with scars, none of which were SCC, whereas 22.3 percent of the 1104 cases without scars were SCC. Yoneyama et al.[29] studied 1425 patients with lung cancer in Japan; 46 had severe unilateral pulmonary disease and all of 5 SCC occurred in the healthy lung, compared with 19 of 20 squamous cell carcinomas, 4 of 5 large cell carcinomas, and only 9 of 16 adenocarcinomas. These findings suggest that SCC, as well as squamous cell and large cell carcinomas, is characteristically a tumor of well-ventilated lung tissue.

Specific Etiologic Factors

A number of agents have been identified in recent decades as causative factors in lung cancer. Most important is cigarette smoke. Others include ionizing radiation, substances in occupational exposures, and, possibly, ambient air pollution. Unfortunately, the data for SCC in particular are scanty. Wherever there are gaps in the information for SCC, the assumption is made that what is true for all lung cancer probably applies to SCC as well.

The evidence for various agents is evaluated in the light of the criteria for judging an association to be causal, as outlined in the introduction to this chapter. The criteria for temporality, plausibility, and analogy are

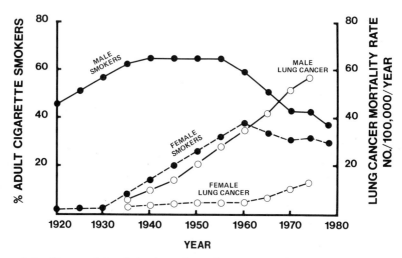

Figure 1-1. *Temporal trends in the estimated percentage of current cigarette smokers in the U.S. adult population by sex[30,31] and trends in the U.S. age-adjusted (to the 1950 population) lung cancer mortality rates by sex.[32]*

taken for granted as long as the agent is inhaled some years before the cancer appears. Thus, we are most concerned with strength, consistency, and specificity of the association, dose–response relationship, coherence, and regression of risk after cessation of exposure (human "experiment"), whenever data are available. The possibility of confounding the effect of one agent by another is considered; for example, because smoking is the most important factor, it must be taken into account in evaluating all other factors.

Smoking

The association between the inhalation of tobacco smoke and lung cancer is a very strong one. This is shown dramatically in Figure 1-1 which assembles data on the proportion of current cigarette smokers by sex in U.S. adults since 1920[30,31] with age-adjusted U.S. lung cancer mortality rates by sex since 1935.[32] Mortality is a good index of incidence for this disease because 90–95 percent of patients die as a result of it.

Cigarette smoking began about the turn of the century in men and reached a peak of 65 percent in about 1940. The lung cancer rate has paralleled the increase in the proportion of cigarette smokers, with a lag of about 40 yr. Women began to smoke in increasing proportions during the 1930s and their lung cancer rate began to rise during the 1960s. A similar

Table 1-7
Crude 10-yr Incidence Rates for Small Cell Carcinoma in
Older Men by Type of Smoking at Start of Observation

Smoking Habit	No. of Men	No. of Man-years	Small Cell Carcinoma No.	Rate*
Cigarettes only	3269	28,153.9	11	39.1
Current	2585	22,176.7	11	49.6
Former	684	5,977.2	0	—
Cigarettes and other	868	7,607.4	6	78.9
Pipe and/or cigars	1032	8,925.5	0	—
Never smoked	830	7,551.1	0	—
Incomplete information	28	250.0	0	—
Total	6,027	52,487.9	17	32.4

From Boucot et al.[8] and unpublished data, 1980.
*Number per 100,000 man-years. Rates are not age adjusted, but differences in age distribution between smoking habit groups are small.

relationship has been described in England and Wales by Cairns,[33] thereby demonstrating the criterion of consistency.

Many epidemiologic studies, both retrospective (case-control) and prospective, have confirmed the strength of the association. Few have provided data on the relationship between smoking and the several histologic types of bronchogenic carcinoma. Table 1-7 shows data from the PNRP. Seventeen of the 121 lung cancer cases were typed as SCC, and all occurred among men who smoked cigarettes at the start of observation. Other types of lung cancer developed in former cigarette smokers and in pure pipe and/or cigar smokers,[8] and the lack of SCC in these groups is interesting. This may be a dose-related effect, as described below.

Data from the prospective study of British male physicians by Doll and Peto[18] showed only 1 case of SCC in 103,383 man-years of observation among those who had never smoked, compared to 14 in 155,708 man-years among cigarette smokers. In this study, only 60 percent of the lung cancers were typed, so the number of SCC cases is undoubtedly underestimated to a greater extent than in the PNRP.

The data from these studies provide evidence of some specificity of the association, in the sense that SCC seldom occurs in the absence of cigarette smoking. However, the converse is not true: cigarette smoking is not associated *only* with SCC. Cigarette smoking has strong associations with other types of lung cancer and weaker associations with certain other diseases. This relative lack of specificity is understandable, however,

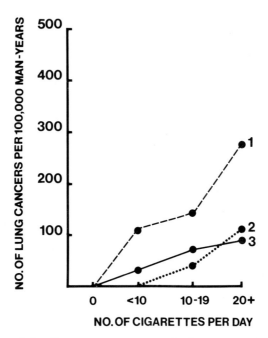

Figure 1-2. *Dose–response curves for lung cancer by cell type in relation to the number of cigarettes smoked per day by males aged 45 and over in the Philadelphia Pulmonary Neoplasm Research Project.*[34] *Cancer types: 1, squamous cell carcinoma; 2, small cell carcinoma; 3, adenocarcinoma. Rates are adjusted for age and race.*

when one considers the many hundreds of substances in cigarette smoke capable of inducing varied toxic effects in protoplasm.

The dose–response relationship between cigarette consumption and lung cancer incidence or mortality has been thoroughly established. This also holds for SCC in both the PNRP[34] (Figure 1-2) and the British physician study[18] (Figure 1-3). In comparing Figures 1-2 and 1-3, it may be noted that the rates are higher in the PNRP than in the British physician study. There are several reasons for this difference: men in the PNRP were screened with chest x-rays every 6 mo, so a higher proportion of cases may have come to attention; additionally, the PNRP men had a higher proportion of smokers, they were older, and a higher proportion of cases of lung cancer were histologically confirmed. Both sets of curves suggest that SCC occurs more frequently in heavier cigarette smokers, and, in contrast to other types of lung cancer, SCC did not occur in men who smoked less

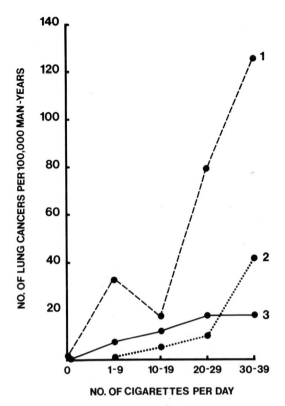

Figure 1-3. *Dose–response curves for lung cancer by cell type in relation to the number of cigarettes smoked per day by British male physicians aged 40–79.*[18] *Cancer types: 1, squamous cell carcinoma; 2, oat cell carcinoma; 3, adenocarcinoma. Rates are not age adjusted, but the distribution of man-years by age does not differ much between smoking habit groups. Age-adjusted rates were calculated from the raw data and showed only slightly smaller values in the heaviest smoking group.*

than 10 cigarettes/day. Table 1-8 shows that the ratio of SCC to all classified lung cancers in the British physician study increases with increasing cigarette dosage. The differences are small, but this relative increase is supported by data from a number of investigations without information on the populations at risk. Yesner et al.[35] recorded an increase from 16 to 29 percent and Auerbach et al.[6] observed an increase from 21 to 39 percent with increasing consumption of cigarettes. Although agreement is not

Table 1-8
Ratio of Oat Cell Carcinoma to Total Histologically
Classified Lung Cancer by Daily Cigarette Dose in
British Male Physicians

No. of Cigarettes Smoked per Day	No. of Oat Cell Carcinomas	No. of Cancers Classified	Ratio
1–9	0	6	0
10–19	2	18	0.11
20–29	4	52	0.08
30–39	7	39	0.18

From Doll and Peto.[18]

complete on this in the limited literature,[36] Table 1-9 shows that, among Norwegian cases of lung cancer, the mean daily cigarette consumption was higher in patients of both sexes with SCC than it was in patients with epidermoid carcinoma or adenocarcinoma, especially women.

Coherence of the association between smoking and lung cancer with other facts known about the disease is illustrated by several observations. In 1961 Auerbach et al.[37] reported on an extensive and meticulous study of epithelial abnormalities in the human bronchial tree at autopsy and showed a close association between cellular atypia and smoking, with a dose–response relationship evident. Recently, Schlesinger and Lippmann[38] showed a striking correlation between particle deposition in hollow casts of the human tracheobronchial tree and lobar localization of lung cancers: both have predilections for the same parts—primarily the upper lobes and the right upper lobe in particular. It has also been shown that, in animals, the length of the induction-latent period from first exposure to a carcinogen to the appearance of tumor tends to decrease as the dose of carcinogen increases,[39] and, finally, there is some evidence that, consistent with the experimental phenomenon, the mean age at diagnosis of lung cancer in humans decreases with increasing cigarette consumption.[40,41]

Table 1-9
Mean Daily Number of Cigarettes Smoked by Patients
with Various Types of Lung Cancer by Sex

Tumor Type	Number of Cigarettes	
	Males	Females
Epidermoid	20.9	14.0
Small cell	22.4	21.0
Adenocarcinoma	16.7	10.0

From Kreyberg,[14] p. 41.

The ultimate evidence that cigarettes cause lung cancer would come from a controlled, concurrent, randomized clinical trial. As this is neither ethical nor feasible, we must consider uncontrolled trials that certain people enter unintentionally. Thus, people who do not smoke rarely develop lung cancer. Likewise, people who belong to groups that espouse opposition to smoking, such as the Seventh-Day Adventists, have a much lower risk of lung cancer than does the general population; careful investigation of the smoking history in those few Adventists in whom lung cancer does develop is likely to yield a positive result.[42]

Smokers who stop smoking gradually experience a decline in the risk of lung cancer, and the risk approaches that of nonsmokers after abstention for 10–15 yr.[43,44] This lowered risk is reflected in a marked reduction of epithelial atypia in the bronchial mucosa and the appearance of cells with disintegrating nuclei.[45]

Support for the causal relationship between smoking and lung cancer has been obtained in animals. The most impressive study is that of Auerbach et al.,[46] who trained beagles to smoke through a tracheostoma with assistance. Invasive bronchiolar–alveolar carcinomas developed in 10 and invasive squamous cell carcinomas in 2 dogs that were heavy smokers of nonfilter cigarettes. The fact that SCC did not occur in these animals may be attributable to a relatively low cumulative exposure to cigarette smoke compared to humans, but this is speculation. SCC rarely occurs in animals, according to Berg.[47] In the discussion published along with Berg's paper, U. Saffiotti confirmed this and suggested that SCC may be the result of carcinogenic events taking place early in life.[47]

Ionizing Radiation

The cause-and-effect relationship between ionizing radiation and lung cancer has been known for many years as a result of occupational studies of miners exposed to the inhalation of radioactive substances.[48–50] External sources of radiation have also increased the incidence of lung cancer, including therapy for ankylosing spondylitis[51] and atomic bomb exposures.[52]

Lung cancers among both the miners and the Japanese exposed to the atom bomb have been studied carefully with respect to cell type. Among the uranium miners of the western United States, as the cumulative dose of radiation increases, not only does the incidence of lung cancer rise, but there seems to be a relative increase in the proportion of SCC, with a particular predilection for type 2b of the WHO classification (slightly larger polygonal cells).[53] However, squamous cell carcinoma and adenocarcinoma also show an increased incidence, and all three major types of tumor show a dose–response relationship (Table 1-10).[54]

Further analysis by Archer et al.[54] suggested that the apparent increase in the proportion of SCC with increasing radiation dose was an artifact caused by dilution of the radiogenic cancers by nonradiogenic cancers at lower dose levels. At *all* dose levels SCC accounted for approximately 70 percent of the excess cases. Thus, SCC is characteristic of this carcinogen, regardless of dose in U.S. uranium miners.

These findings are not universal. In Czechoslovakian uranium miners[50] the absolute increase in lung cancer involves squamous cell carcinoma and SCC, but not adenocarcinoma, whereas in Newfoundland fluorspar miners, also exposed to radon and radon daughters like the uranium miners,[49] 90 percent of the lung cancers have been squamous cell carcinomas.

The factors of duration of exposure and pattern of exposure in the dose–response relationship of excess risk by cell type were recently studied in the Czechoslovakian uranium miners.[55] The dose–response curve is linear only with prolonged exposure and only with rates of exposure that remain unchanged or that decrease over time. In short exposures and in those with increasing rates of exposure, the high cumulative doses are associated with plateauing or show a decrease in cancer frequency at the expense of SCC. These observations suggest that the SCC response to radiation is partially dependent on continuous prolonged exposure and on the dosage early during the exposure period. The implications may be similar to those of the dose–response observations described in the previous section on smoking.

Periodic cytologic studies of sputum in uranium miners by Saccomanno et al.[56] suggested that the pathogenesis of bronchogenic carcinoma develops through a series of identifiable stages of metaplasia and atypia. The progression appears to be orderly in many cases, but sudden changes in the progression may occur, resulting in the skipping of stages or conversion from squamous cell carcinoma to SCC. Morphologically, these investigators consider squamous cell and small cell carcinomas to be at opposite ends of a continuous spectrum, with no clear separation between poorly differentiated squamous cell carcinoma and SCC. The mean age at diagnosis of these two types was 52 yr in 18 cases of poorly differentiated squamous cell carcinoma and 53 yr in 81 cases of SCC, whereas the mean age was 59 yr in 48 cases of well- and moderately differentiated squamous cell carcinomas. This observation is consistent with the suggestion of skipped stages in the development of SCC.

Auerbach et al.[57] made careful studies of the bronchial epithelium at

Table 1-10
Observed and Expected Lung Cancers Among U.S. Uranium Miners, 1950–1970,
by Radiation Dose and Histologic Type

| | Histologic Type | | | | | | | | |
| | Squamous Cell | | | Small cell | | | Adenocarcinoma | | |
Radiation Dose*	Observed No.	Expected No.	Ratio	Observed No.	Expected No.	Ratio	Observed No.	Expected No.	Ratio
1–359	4	3.06	1.31	9	0.73	12.33	2	0.69	2.90
360–1799	14	3.89	3.60	23	0.93	24.73	1	0.87	1.15
1800–3319	8	1.02	7.84	22	0.24	91.67	2	0.23	8.70
3320+	4	0.30	13.33	12	0.07	171.43	3	0.07	42.86
Total	30	8.27	3.63	66	1.97	33.50	8	1.86	4.30

Adapted from data of Archer et al.[54]
*Cumulative working-level months.

autopsy in uranium miners with lung cancer as compared to nonminers with lung cancer. The two groups were matched by age and smoking habits. They found that carcinoma in situ and early foci of invasive carcinoma outside the main tumor mass were more common in the uranium miners. The degree of disorganization in microscopic sections with carcinoma in situ was considerably greater in the miners. These facts attest to the potency of radiation in the pathogenesis of lung cancer and the widespread effects of radiation on the bronchial mucosa.

Cigarette smoke is an important cofactor in the incidence of lung cancer among uranium miners (Table 1-11).[58] The lung cancer rate in men who were heavy smokers and who had had heavy radiation exposure was 67 times the rate in nonsmokers with light radiation exposure. The induction-latent period was shorter in heavy cigarette smokers than in light smokers, ex-smokers, and nonsmokers, an observation suggesting to the authors that cigarette smoke acts as a promoting agent rather than as a synergist.[59]

The association between atomic bomb radiation and lung cancer is not as strong as that found in uranium miners. In a proportional mortality study based on the frequency of lung cancer among autopsies, all three major lung cancer types showed an elevated relative risk, but only the increase of 3.9 for SCC was statistically significant.[52] The increased risk was found only in those people exposed to 200 or more rads at the time of the bomb. The proportional mortality method is not very reliable.

Using a case-control method, a better approach, the results with respect to cell type were not the same: the relative risks were elevated for all three major types but significantly so only for squamous cell carcinoma and adenocarcinoma, not for SCC.[60] Thus, there is some doubt as to whether radiation from the atomic bomb is particularly associated with SCC. Although smoking was a strong factor in the frequency of lung cancer, no evidence could be adduced that either smoking or occupation confounded the relationship between atomic bomb radiation and lung cancer.

A final point to be made concerning radiation in the etiology of lung cancer stems from the observation by Radford and Hunt in 1964 that tobacco contains an emitter of alpha particles, polonium 210.[61] They suggested that this radioactive substance inhaled in cigarette smoke may act as an initiator in the pathogenesis of bronchogenic carcinoma. This hypothesis is given greater credibility by the recent finding that lead 210, with a radioactive half-life of 22 yr, is also present in mainstream cigarette smoke and is highly concentrated in a small number of insoluble smoke particles,[62] thereby providing a mechanism for prolonged cellular contact.

All the criteria for causality in the relationship between ionizing radi-

Table 1-11
Respiratory Cancer Mortality Among White Uranium Miners 5 yr or More After Start of Mining by Radiation Dose and Cigarette Dose, 1950–1974

	Cumulative Radiation in Working-Level Months								
	1–359			360–1799			1800+		
		Cancer			Cancer			Cancer	
Cigarettes/day	Man-years	No.	Rate*	Man-years	No.	Rate*	Man-years	No.	Rate*
0	4918	1	0.20	3488	3	0.86	1437	2	1.39
1–19	3169	5	1.58	2618	3	1.14	717	6	8.30
20	6907	9	1.30	8237	29	3.52	3176	30	9.40
21+	2944	8	2.72	3635	17	4.68	1127	15	13.30
Total	17,938	23	1.28	17,978	52	2.89	6457	53	8.21

From Auerbach et al.[57]
*Number per 1000 man-years.

ation and lung cancer, especially SCC, may be considered to have been satisfied to a marked degree, except that information is lacking on regression of risk after cessation of exposure, and specificity is not of a high order.

Asbestos

Beginning in the 1930s a number of case reports drew attention to an association between asbestosis and lung cancer, but it was not until 1955 that a sound epidemiological study of a small cohort of asbestos workers by Doll[63] showed the risk to be 14 times that expected. This strong association has since been confirmed many times, although it varies somewhat with the type of asbestos fiber, chrysotile being less dangerous than the amphiboles; it also varies with the type of occupational exposure, mining being less hazardous than manufacturing, which in turn seems less hazardous than insulation work.

Close approximations to a linear dose–response relationship on arithmetic coordinates have been demonstrated among Quebec chrysotile miners and millers by McDonald and Liddell[64] and among retired asbestos manufacturing employees by Henderson and Enterline.[65]

Information on the types of lung cancer associated with asbestos is meager. The only really satisfactory study is that of Kannerstein and Churg.[66] These investigators examined in "blind" fashion 50 cases of lung cancer in people exposed to asbestos and 50 matched control cases with no known exposure or asbestos bodies in the lung tissue. There were no significant differences in histologic type between the two groups. SCC occurred in 11 of the 50 asbestos-associated cases and 14 of the 50 control cases. The only prominent difference noted between the two groups was that lung cancer was most common in the lower lobes among asbestos-associated cases whereas it was most common in the upper lobes among the controls, a localization characteristic of lung cancers in the general population.[67] This predilection of asbestos-associated carcinomas for the lower lobes is coherent with the fact that asbestosis is more pronounced in the lower than in the upper lobes.

Another study, by Whitwell et al.[68] in England, suggested an increase in the relative frequency of adenocarcinomas, but this investigation suffered from the lack of a control group. Nevertheless, the facts that asbestosis is characterized by scarring and that pulmonary adenocarcinomas are associated with scar tissue[28] suggest that the British experience needs further study.

During the past 12 yr cigarette smoking has been recognized as an important cofactor in lung cancer among people exposed to asbestos.[69] The interaction of the two agents is synergistic, but lung cancer is almost as rare in nonsmokers exposed to asbestos as in those not so exposed. This observation raises the question as to whether asbestos is merely a carrier of a carcinogen present in cigarette smoke, rather than a carcinogen in its own right, at least for lung tissue. If, indeed, asbestos-associated lung cancers—which are found almost entirely in smokers—have a distribution of types similar to that of unexposed smokers, then this is consistent with the hypothesis that the primary carcinogen in asbestos workers is cigarette smoke. Furthermore, the risk of lung cancer is much lower in asbestos workers who stop smoking than in those who continue to smoke.[69] There is no evidence as yet that cessation of exposure to asbestos reduces the risk of lung cancer, but perhaps this should not be expected, as asbestos fibers persist in the lung after inhalation.

Thus, most of the criteria for causality in the association between asbestos and lung cancer have been satisfied to a considerable degree, but the data suggest the possibility that asbestos is a synergistic promoting agent rather than a primary carcinogen in the lung.

Chemicals

A number of chemical agents have been recorded as causative agents in lung cancer. These have been described in occupational settings, where exposures have generally been high and more or less continuous. However, there are difficulties in making a decision as to whether a suspected agent is really a human carcinogen when the relative risk is only slightly elevated, i.e., when the observed number of cases is less than twice the expected number. The reasons for these difficulties lie in the shortcomings of epidemiologic methods: (1) studies based on small populations lead to sampling errors, (2) subtle systematic bias may produce misleading results, mainly because of the lack of good control population data, and (3) confounding factors may produce spurious associations, particularly variations in smoking habits.

The chemicals for which there seems to be at least fair evidence of pulmonary carcinogenicity in humans include polycyclic aromatic hydrocarbons (PAH), certain metals or their compounds, and certain simple organic chemicals.

Exposure to PAH occurs to varying degrees in a number of occupations, involving coal, gas, coke, petroleum, coal tar, pitch, etc.[70]

Metals or their compounds implicated in lung cancer etiology include chromium, nickel, arsenic, and cadmium. People working in hematite[71,72]

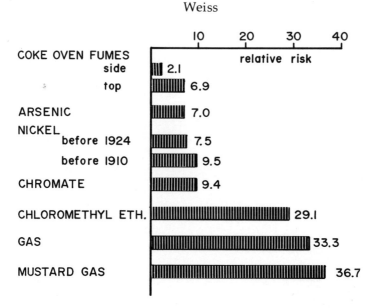

Figure 1-4. *Relative risk of lung cancer, in comparison with unexposed or general population, among workers exposed to chemicals (Weiss[74]). The studies were selected and limited to those with a relative risk in excess of 2.*

and zinc–lead mines[73] are at increased risk, but this appears to be attributable to radiation, so they are mentioned only in passing.

A few simple organic chemicals have been incriminated as lung cancer agents. These include mustard gas, the chloromethyl ethers, vinyl chloride, and recently acrylonitrile.

The relative potency of these various chemicals is difficult to assess because of variations in methods and populations and uncertainty about degrees of exposure—all of which results in variation in the relative risks among published reports. A selected comparison is illustrated in Figure 1-4.[74] This shows that the highest risks occurred among people exposed to chloromethyl ethers, the gas emitted by coal carbonization in Japan, and mustard gas. The data available suggested that the more potent the agent, the shorter the induction-latent period from initial exposure to tumor appearance.

Unfortunately, information in the literature is extremely limited with respect to cell type and is confounded by smoking habits. Many of the reported studies have been based on causes of death and other information gleaned only from death certificates. Particular reports with relevant data are cited.

Lung cancer type-specific rates are generally not available in these studies, but, in some, the relative distribution of lung cancer cases by type is given, albeit the total number of cases is usually quite small. If the relative distribution of types is similar to that among lung cancer cases in the general population, then the elevated risk in occupational groups must signify that the incidences of all major types are increased. But if the relative distribution is distorted, then the increased incidence may be largely limited to the type(s) contributing unusually high proportions to the distribution.

Table 1-12 shows the relative distribution of lung cancer cases by histologic type in recent reports[75-83] that distinguish instances of SCC. Data are given for seven chemical agents and are arranged in order of increasing percentage of total cases due to SCC. The number of typed cases varied from only 6 to 39. With respect to the percentage attributable to SCC, one report at each extreme stands out from all the rest. At one extreme is a small number of cases in workers exposed to vinyl chloride.[75] In this study the relative risk was very low, 1.56 times the expected number, but the types of lung cancer were entirely limited to adenocarcinomas and large cell carcinomas. There is some question as to whether vinyl chloride causes lung cancer, because various reports are inconsistent,[84] but this distribution of cell types is rather unusual.

Reports of lung cancer due to nickel,[76,77] cadmium,[78] arsenic,[79,80] chromate,[81] and acrylonitrile[82] showed percentages attributable to SCC varying from 15 to 33 percent.

At the other extreme is the group of cases in men exposed to chloromethyl ethers (CME) in Philadelphia: 68 percent of 28 cases were SCC.[83] These chemicals—chloromethyl methyl ether (CMME) and bis(chloromethyl) ether (BCME)—are important because, although only a small number of cases have been attributed to them, their relationship to lung cancer has been studied rather thoroughly, because BCME is a very potent carcinogen, and because SCC seems to be a characteristic response. Whereas CMME is a weaker carcinogen than BCME, CMME in the workplace is contaminated with BCME so that workers have been exposed to both chemicals.

For most of the chemicals mentioned above, there are large gaps in the evidence supporting a judgment of causality. However, for CME, all the criteria used to judge whether an association is one of cause and effect have been well satisfied. The association is strong, the overall risk being 5.42 times that expected.[83] There is consistency, since similar elevated risks have been reported in Japan,[85] Germany,[86] and California.[87] The effects are highly specific in that, except for evidence of chronic bronchitis,[88] no disease other than lung cancer has been associated with CME expo-

Table 1-12
Distribution of Lung Cancer Cases by Cell Type and Chemical Agent

Chemical	Total No. of Cases	Cell Type*							
		Squamous Cell		Small Cell		Adeno-carcinoma		Large Cell or Other	
		No.	%	No.	%	No.	%	No.	%
Vinyl chloride[75]	8	—	—	—	—	3	—	5	—
Nickel[76,77]	39	26	67	6	15	7	18	—	—
Cadmium[78]	8	3	—	2	—	3	—	3	—
Arsenic[79]	25	15	60	8	32	—	12	1	4
Arsenic[80]	18	8	44	6	33	2	11	2	11
Chromate[81]	12	8	67	4	33	—	—	—	—
Acrylonitrile[82]	6	4	—	2	—	—	—	—	—
Chloromethyl ethers[83]	28	1	4	19	68	5	18	3	11

*Percent not calculated when denominator is less than 10.

24

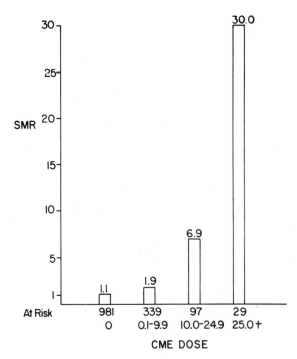

Figure 1-5. *Standardized mortality ratio (SMR) for lung cancer among chemical workers by degree of cumulative exposure to chloromethyl ethers (CME) showing a strong dose–response relationship.*[83]

sure.[89] There is a strong dose–response relationship between cumulative CME exposure and lung cancer incidence (Figure 1-5). SCC is characteristic of workers with moderate to heavy CME exposure, but occurs with the same relative frequency as in lung cancers in the general population among workers with light cumulative exposure to CME (Figure 1-6).

There is coherence between the CME–SCC relationship and what we know about the natural history of SCC. For example, SCC tends to contribute a larger proportion of lung cancers in the young than in the old, as discussed above in the section on relative frequency early in this chapter, and a large proportion of the lung cancers in workers with moderate to heavy CME exposure occur under the age of 50 (Figure 1-7). This tendency may be due to a short induction-latent period associated with potent carcinogens or large carcinogenic doses. It is possible that study of the ante-

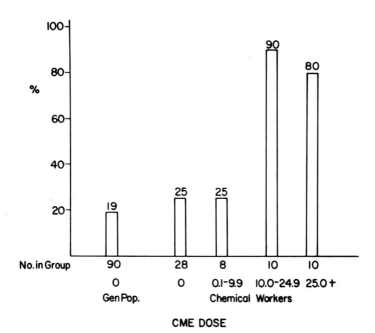

Figure 1-6. *Percentage of small cell carcinomas among lung cancers in the general population (data from the Philadelphia Pulmonary Neoplasm Research Project[10]) and in chemical workers by degree of cumulative exposure to chloromethyl ethers (CME).*[83]

cedents in cases of SCC among young people may reveal previously un-suspected carcinogens.

As for the experimental criterion of causality, while BCME has been shown to be a very potent carcinogen by inhalation in wild rats,[90] there is, as yet, no published evidence of regression of risk after cessation of expo-sure to CME. In Philadelphia, exposure to CME ceased in 1971 after com-plete enclosure and automation of the CME process. Unpublished data suggest that the microepidemic of lung cancer that began in 1960 is begin-ning to subside.

The influence of tobacco smoking on the relationship between chemi-cal carcinogens and lung cancer has seldom been examined in a way that would demonstrate its effect on risk, as has been done in uranium miners and asbestos workers. In these two groups, as described above, the inter-action between cigarette smoke and occupational agent seems to be syner-gistic. The limited data for chemical agents seem to show no effect or ac-tual antagonism. A small case-control study of zinc–lead miners[73] showed

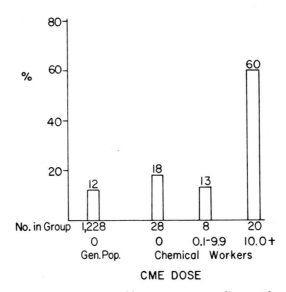

Figure 1-7. *Percentage of lung cancer cases diagnosed under age 50 in the general population (data from the Philadelphia Pulmonary Neoplasm Research Project[10]) and in chemical workers by degree of cumulative exposure to chloromethyl ethers (CME).*[83]

the risk of lung cancer was higher in nonsmokers than in smokers; because the causative agent in these workers is thought to be ionizing radiation rather than metal exposure, this observation contrasts sharply with the synergism noted in uranium miners. Pinto et al.[91] studied mortality in pensioners from a copper smelter, arsenic being postulated as the likely carcinogen, and found that the risk relative to that in U.S. veterans by smoking habits was 5.07 in nonsmokers compared to only 2.45 in ex-smokers and 2.87 in current smokers. The elevated risk in nonsmokers was not statistically different from that in current smokers and ex-smokers combined ($z = 0.75, p > 0.05$), but at least it can be said that there is no positive interaction between smoking and occupational exposure.

In a small 10-yr prospective study of 125 chemical workers in Philadelphia, of whom 88 (later corrected to 91) were exposed to CME, Weiss[88] found that the risk of lung cancer was much lower in current cigarette smokers (3–6 percent) than in nonsmokers (23 percent) and cigar/pipe or ex-smokers of cigarettes (19 percent). The difference between current cigarette smokers and the other two groups combined was statistically significant (chi-square with Yates' correction = 4.86, d.f. = 1, $p < 0.05$). Unpublished data calculating expected numbers of cases by smoking habit from lung cancer rates in U.S. veterans[92] show that, among 51 men with moderate to heavy cumulative CME exposure, 6 cases of lung cancer occurred among 13 men with 112 man-years of observation who were nonsmokers or ex-smokers of cigarettes, when 0.00222 case was expected. In contrast, 5 cases occurred among 38 men with 353 man-years of observation who were current cigarette smokers, when 0.1409 case was expected. The relative risk in nonsmokers and ex-smokers was an astounding 2703 times that expected, and in the current smokers it was only 35 times that expected. The difference between these relative risks was statistically significant, despite the small numbers ($z = 2.40$, $p < 0.02$). This difference could not be accounted for by a small difference in the mean cumulative dose of CME between the two groups.

Air Pollution

Ambient air contains low concentrations of known carcinogens such as PAH, and an association has been reported between air pollution and lung cancer incidence or mortality by geographic area.[93-97] However, the association is weak and inconsistent, specificity is poor, dose–response data are generally lacking, there is lack of coherence because the association does not usually hold for females, there are no reliable data to show a regression of risk after decrease of exposure, and confounding of the association by other causative factors, such as cigarette smoking, is only partially ruled out. Information on lung cancer types is scanty and inconsistent.[93,94]

References

1. Hill AB: The environment and disease: Association or causation. Proc R Soc Med 58:295–300, 1965
2. Kreyberg L, Liebow AA, Uehlinger EA: Histological Typing of Lung Tumours. Geneva, World Health Organization, 1967
3. Kreyberg L, Saxen E: A comparison of lung tumour types in Finland and Norway. Br J Cancer 15:211–214, 1961
4. Yesner R: Histologic typing of lung cancer with clinical implications. Front Radiat Ther Oncol 9:140–150, 1974
5. Vincent RG, Pickren JW, Lane WW, Bross I, Takita H, Houten L, Gutierrez AC, and Rzepka T: The changing histopathology of lung cancer. Cancer 39:1647–1655, 1977

6. Auerbach O, Garfinkel L, Parks VR: Histologic type of lung cancer in relation to smoking habits, year of diagnosis, and sites of metastases. Chest 67:382–387, 1975

7. Annegers JF, Carr DT, Woolner LB, and Kurland LT: Incidence, trend, and outcome of bronchogenic carcinoma in Olmstead County, Minnesota, 1935–1974. Mayo Clin Proc 53:432–436, 1978

8. Boucot KR, Weiss W, Seidman H, Carnahan WJ, and Cooper DA: The Philadelphia Pulmonary Neoplasm Research Project: Basic risk factors of lung cancer in older men. Am J. Epidemiol 95:4–16, 1972

9. Law CH, Day NE, Shanmugaratnam K: Incidence rates of specific histological types of lung cancer in Singapore Chinese dialect groups, and their aetiological significance. Int J Cancer 17:304–309, 1976

10. Weiss W, Boucot KR: The prognosis of lung cancer originating as a round lesion: Data from the Philadelphia Pulmonary Neoplasm Research Project. Am Rev Resp Dis 116:827–836, 1977

11. Weiss W: Predictions of lung cancer mortality; the dangers of extrapolation. Arch Environ Health 28:114–117, 1974

12. Hallgrimsson J: Lung tumours in Iceland. Acta Path Microbiol Scand 81:813–823, 1973

13. Walter JB, Pryce DM: The histology of lung cancer. Thorax 10:107–116, 1955

14. Kreyberg L: Aetiology of Lung Cancer: A Morphological Epidemiological and Experimental Analysis. Universitetsforlaget, Oslo, Norway, 1969

15. Berge T, Toremalm NG: Bronchial Cancer—a clinical and pathological study. II. Frequency according to age and sex during a 12-year period. Scand J Resp Dis 56:120–126, 1975

16. Harley HRS: Cancer of the lung in women. Thorax 31:254–264, 1976

17. Kennedy A: Relationship between cigarette smoking and histological type of lung cancer in women. Thorax 28:204–208, 1973

18. Doll R, Peto R: Cigarette smoking and bronchial carcinoma: Dose and time relationships among regular smokers and lifelong non-smokers. J Epidemiol Community Health 32:303–313, 1978

19. Chan WC, Colbourne MJ, Fung SC, Ho HC: Bronchial cancer in Hong Kong, 1976–1977. Br J Cancer 39:182–192, 1979

20. Beamis JF, Stein A, Andrews JL: Changing epidemiology of lung cancer; increasing incidence in women. Med Clin North Am 59:315–325, 1975

21. Herrold K McD: Survey of histologic types of primary lung cancer in U.S. veterans. Path Annu 7:45–79, 1972

22. Borrie J, Rose RJ, Spears GFS, Holmes GA: Cancer of the Lung in New Zealand. Special Report No. 42. Wellington, New Zealand, National Health Statistics Centre, Department of Health, 1973

23. Third National Cancer Survey: Incidence Data. National Cancer Institute Monograph 41, DHEW Publication No. 75-787. Washington, D.C., National Institute of Health, 1975, p 410

24. Levin DL, Devesa SS, Godwin JD, Silverman DT: Cancer Rates and Risks (ed 2). DHEW Publication No. 76-691, Washington, D.C., National Institute of Health, 1974, p 21

25. Kennedy A: Lung cancer in young adults. Br J Dis Chest 66:147–154, 1972

26. Kyriakos M, Webber B: Cancer of the lung in young men. J Thorac Cardiov Surg 67:634–648, 1974

27. Putnam JS: Lung carcinoma in young adults. JAMA 238:35–36, 1977

28. Auerbach O, Garfinkel L, Parks VR: Scar cancer of the lung: increase over a 21 year period. Cancer 43:636–642, 1979

29. Yoneyama T, Naruke T, Suemasu K, Ishikawa S: Bronchial carcinoma in patients with pre-existing unilateral lung disease. Thorax 31:650–651, 1976

30. Burbank F: U.S. lung cancer death rates begin to rise proportionately more rapidly for females than for males: A dose–response effect? J Chron Dis 25:473–479, 1972

31. Moss AJ: Changes in cigarette smoking and current practices among adults in the United States, 1978. Advance Data From Vital and Health Statistics, DHEW Publication No. 52. Washington, D.C., National Institutes of Health, 1979

32. Devesa SS, Silverman DT: Cancer incidence and mortality trends in the United States: 1935–74. J Natl Cancer Inst 60:545–571, 1978

33. Cairns J: The cancer problem. Sci Am 233(5):64–78, 1975

34. Weiss W, Boucot KR, Seidman H, Carnahan WJ: Risk of lung cancer according to histologic type and cigarette dosage. JAMA 222:799–801, 1972

35. Yesner R, Gelfman NA, Feinstein AR: A reappraisal of histopathology in lung cancer and correlation of cell types with antecedent cigarette smoking. Am Rev Resp Dis 107:790–797, 1973

36. Weiss W, Altan S, Rosenzweig M, Weiss WA: Lung cancer type in relation to cigarette dosage. Cancer 39:2568–2572, 1977

37. Auerbach O, Stout AP, Hammond EC, Garfinkel L: Changes in bronchial epithelium in relation to cigarette smoking and in relation to lung cancer. N Engl J Med 265:253–267, 1961

38. Schlesinger RB, Lippmann M: Particle deposition in casts of the hu-

man upper tracheobronchial tree. Am Ind Hyg Assoc J 33:237–251, 1972

39. Druckrey H: Quantitative aspects in chemical carcinogenesis, in Truhaut R (ed): Potential Carcinogenic Hazards from Drugs, UICC Monograph Series, Vol 7, New York, Springer-Verlag, 1967, pp 60–77

40. Weiss W: Cigarette smoke as a carcinogen. Am Rev Resp Dis 108:364–366, 1973

41. Weiss W: Lung cancer in men: A model for the relationship between age at diagnosis and smoking habits. Am Rev Respir Dis 111:883–886, 1975

42. Lemon FR, Walden RT: Death from respiratory system disease among Seventh-Day Adventist men. JAMA 198:117–126, 1966

43. Doll R, Hill AB: Mortality in relation to smoking: Ten years' observations of British doctors. Br Med J 1:1399–1410; 1460–1467, 1964

44. Doll R, Peto R: Mortality in relation to smoking: 20 years' observations on male British doctors. Br Med J 2:1525–1536, 1976

45. Auerbach O, Stout AP, Hammond EC, Garfinkel L: Bronchial epithelium in former smokers. N Engl J Med 267:119–125, 1962

46. Auerbach O, Hammond EC, Kirman D, Garfinkel L: Effects of cigarette smoking on dogs. II. Pulmonary neoplasms. Arch Environ Health 21:754–768, 1970

47. Berg JW: Epidemiology of the different histologic types of lung cancer, in Nettesheim P, Hanna MG Jr, Deatherage JW Jr (eds): Morphology of Experimental Respiratory Carcinogenesis, Oak Ridge, Tennessee, U.S. Atomic Energy Commission Division of Technical Information Extension, 1970, pp 93–101

48. Lundin FE Jr, Lloyd JW, Smith EM, Archer VE, Holaday DA: Mortality of uranium miners in relation to radiation exposure, hard-rock mining, and cigarette smoking—1950 through September 1967. Health Phys 16:571–578, 1969

49. Wright ES, Couves CM: Radiation-induced carcinoma of the lung—The St. Lawrence tragedy. J Thorac Cardiov Surg 74:495–498, 1977

50. Horacek J, Placek V, Sevc J: Histologic types of bronchogenic cancer in relation to different conditions of radiation exposure. Cancer 40:832–835, 1977

51. Court-Brown WM, Doll R: Mortality from cancer and other causes after radiotherapy for ankylosing spondylitis. Br Med J 2:1327–1332, 1965

52. Cihak RW, Ishimaru T, Steer A, Yamada A: Lung cancer at autopsy in A-bomb survivors and controls, Hiroshima and Nagasaki, 1961–1970. Cancer 33:1580–1588, 1974

53. Saccomanno G, Archer VE, Auerbach O, Kuschner T, Saunders RP, Klein MG: Histologic types of lung cancer among uranium miners. Cancer 27:515–523, 1971

54. Archer VE, Saccomanno G, Jones JH: Frequency of different histologic types of bronchogenic carcinoma as related to radiation exposure. Cancer 34:2056–2060, 1974

55. Kunz E, Sevc J, Placek V, Horacek J: Lung cancer in man in relation to different time distribution of radiation exposure. Health Phys 36:699–706, 1979

56. Saccomanno G, Archer VE, Auerbach O, Saunders RP, Brennan LM: Development of carcinoma of the lung as reflected in exfoliated cells. Cancer 33:256–270, 1974

57. Auerbach O, Saccomanno G, Kuschner M, Brown RD, Garfinkel L: Histologic findings in the tracheobronchial tree of uranium miners and non-miners with lung cancer. Cancer 42:483–489, 1978

58. Archer VE, Gillam JD, Wagoner JK: Respiratory disease mortality among uranium miners. Ann NY Acad Sci 271:280–293, 1976

59. Archer VE, Wagoner JK, Lundin FE Jr: Uranium mining and cigarette smoking effects on man. J Occup Med 15:204–211, 1973

60. Ishimaru T, Cihak RW, Land CE, Steer A, Yamada A: Lung cancer at autopsy in A-bomb survivors and controls, Hiroshima and Nagasaki, 1961–1970. II. Smoking, occupation, and A-bomb exposure. Cancer 36:1723–1728, 1975

61. Radford EP Jr, Hunt VR: Polonium-210: A volatile radioelement in cigarettes. Science 143:247–249, 1964

62. Martell EA: Tobacco radioactivity and cancer in smokers. Am Sci 63:404–412, 1975

63. Doll R: Mortality from lung cancer in asbestos workers. Br J Ind Med 12:81–86, 1955

64. McDonald JC, Liddell FDK: Mortality in Canadian miners and millers exposed to chrysotile. Ann NY Acad Sci 330:1–9, 1979

65. Henderson VL, Enterline PE: Asbestos exposure: factors associated with excess cancer and respiratory disease mortality. Ann NY Acad Sci 330:117–126, 1979

66. Kannerstein M, Churg J: Pathology of carcinoma of the lung associated with asbestos exposure. Cancer 30:14–21, 1972

67. Weiss W, Boucot KR: The Philadelphia Pulmonary Neoplasm Research Project: early roentgenographic appearance of bronchogenic carcinoma. Arch Int Med 134:306–311, 1974

68. Whitwell F, Newhouse ML, Bennett DR: A study of the histological cell types of lung cancer in workers suffering from asbestosis in the United Kingdom. Br J Ind Med 31:298–303, 1974

69. Hammond EC, Selikoff IJ, Seidman H: Asbestos exposure, cigarette smoking, and death rates. Ann NY Acad Sci 330:473–490, 1979

70. Schottenfeld D, Haas JF: The workplace as a cause of cancer. Clin Bull 8:107–119, 1978

71. Boyd JT, Doll R, Faulds JS, Leiper J: Cancer of the lung in iron ore (haematite) miners. Br J Ind Med 27:97–105, 1970

72. Duggan MJ, Soilleux PJ, Strong JC, Howell DM: The exposure of United Kingdom miners to radon. Br J Ind Med 27:106–109, 1970

73. Axelson O, Sundell L: Mining, lung cancer and smoking. Scand J Work Environ Health 4:46–52, 1978

74. Weiss W: Lung cancer due to chemicals. Compr Ther 5:18–23, 1979

75. Waxweiler RJ, Stringer W, Wagoner JK, Jones J: Neoplastic risk among workers exposed to vinyl chloride. Ann NY Acad Sci 271:40–48, 1976

76. Pedersen E, Hogetveit AC, Andersen A: Cancer of respiratory organs among workers at a nickel refinery in Norway. Int J Cancer 12:32–41, 1973

77. Kreyberg L: Lung cancer in workers in a nickel refinery. Br J Ind Med 35:109–116, 1978

78. Lemen RA, Lee JS, Wagoner JK, Blejer HP: Cancer mortality among cadmium production workers. Ann NY Acad Sci 271:273–279, 1976

79. Newman JA, Archer VE, Saccomanno G, Kuschner M, Auerbach O, Grondahl RD, Wilson JC: Histologic types of bronchogenic carcinoma among members of copper-mining and smelting communities. Ann NY Acad Sci 271:260–268, 1976

80. Axelson O, Dahlgren E, Jansson C-D, Rehnlund SO: Arsenic exposure and mortality: a case-referent study from a Swedish copper smelter. Br J Ind Med 35:8–15, 1978

81. Ohsaki Y, Abe S, Kimura K, Tsuneta Y, Mikami H, Murao M: Lung cancer in Japanese chromate workers. Thorax 33:372–374, 1978

82. O'Berg MT: Epidemiologic study of workers exposed to acrylonitrile. J Occup Med 22:245–252, 1980

83. Weiss W, Moser RL, Auerbach O: Lung cancer in chloromethyl ether workers. Am Rev Respir Dis 120:1031–1037, 1979

84. Buffler PA, Wood S, Eifler C, Suarez L, Kilian DJ: Mortality experience of workers in a vinyl chloride monomer production plant. J Occup Med 21:195–203, 1979

85. Sakabe H: Lung cancer due to exposure to bis(chloromethyl)ether. Ind Health 11:145–148, 1973

86. Von Thiess AM, Hey W, Zeller H: Zur toxikologie von dichlordimethylather: Verdacht auf kancerogene wirkung auch beim menschen. Zentralbl Arbeitsmed 23:97–102, 1973

87. Lemen RA, Johnson WM, Wagoner JK, Archer, VE, Saccomanno G: Cytologic observations and cancer incidence following exposure to BCME. Ann NY Acad Sci 271:71–80, 1976

88. Weiss W: Chloromethyl ethers, cigarettes, cough and cancer. J Occup Med 18:194–199, 1976

89. DeFonso LR, Kelton SC Jr: Lung cancer following exposure to chloromethyl methyl ether. Arch Environ Health 31:125–130, 1976

90. Kuschner M, Laskin S, Drew RT, Cappiello V, Nelson N: Inhalation carcinogenicity of alpha halo ethers. III. Lifetime and limited period inhalation studies with bis(chlormethyl)ether at 0.1 ppm. Arch Environ Health 30:73–77, 1975

91. Pinto SS, Henderson V, and Enterline PE: Mortality experience of arsenic-exposed workers. Arch Environ Health 33:325–331, 1978

92. Weiss W: The cigarette factor in lung cancer due to chloromethyl ethers. J Occup Med 22:527–529, 1980

93. Henderson BE, Gordon RJ, Menck H, Soohoo J, Martin SP, Pike MC: Lung cancer and air pollution in southcentral Los Angeles County. Am J Epidemiol 101:477–488, 1975

94. Hirayama T: Epidemiology of lung cancer based on population studies, in Finkel AJ, Duel WC (eds): Clinical Implications of Air Pollution Research. Acton, Massachusetts, Publishing Sciences Group, 1976, pp 69–78

95. Goldsmith JR, Friberg LT: Effects on human health, in Stern A (ed): Air Pollution; A Comprehensive Treatise, Vol 2, (ed 3). New York, Academic Press, 1977, pp 576–577

96. Weiss W: Lung cancer mortality and urban air pollution. Am J Pub Health 68:773–775, 1978

97. Air pollution and cancer: Risk assessment methodology and epidemiologic evidence: Report of a task group. Environ Health Perspect 22:1–12, 1978

2

PROBLEMS IN THE DIAGNOSIS OF SMALL CELL CARCINOMA OF THE LUNG

Mary J. Matthews
Fred R. Hirsch

Small cell carcinoma of the lung (SCC) is one of the few solid tumors in adults that responds with extreme sensitivity to intensive chemotherapy and radiotherapy.[1,2] In the past decade, this tumor has been the subject of numerous clinical trials in the United States and abroad. Objective response rates of over 90 percent are reported.[3] Complete response rates have been attended by prolonged survivals.[4] It has been suggested that patients enjoying a 5-yr disease-free remission may be potentially cured.[5,6] Appropriate pathologic diagnoses are a prerequisite for such results.

The World Health Organization (WHO) classification of lung tumors has been based on light microscopic criteria.[7,8] It is possible to attain consistency and reliability in the diagnosis of SCC in a high percentage of cases when strict criteria are used.[9,10] Although a number of institutions utilize the electron microscope as an adjunct in the diagnosis of SCC, it seems unlikely that this instrument will replace the light microscope for routine diagnostic studies during the next decade. Likewise, experimental tools such as in vitro cultures, nude mice studies, or identification of biochemical markers in tumors are beyond the resources of most institutions at the present time. When uniform diagnostic criteria are not applied, patients may either be deprived of proper treatment modalities or be sub-

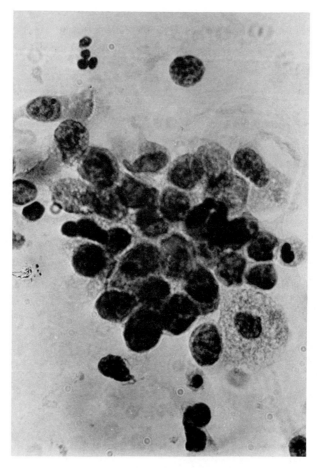

Figure 2-1. *Cytology of SCC. Nuclear chromatin is distributed in a uniform fine and coarse-stippled pattern throughout
the nucleus. Cytoplasm is scanty. Nucleoli are indistinct. Hematoxylin and eosin. Original magnification × 400.*

jected unnecessarily to the morbidity associated with intensive chemo-
therapy/radiotherapy protocols. Moreover, there can be little comparison
of treatment results or responses to clinical trials if wide variations in interpretation of SCC exist from one institution to another.

The histogenesis and pathogenesis of small cell tumors have been discussed elsewhere in this monograph. This chapter focuses on the morphologic features of SCC, as well as technical and interpretative difficulties

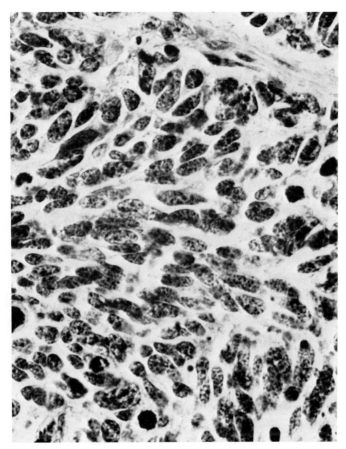

Figure 2-2.   *SCC showing spindled, fusiform pattern. Hematoxylin and eosin. Original magnification × 400.*

which may cause diagnostic problems. Two recent studies of interobserver consistency in the diagnosis of SCC are summarized.

Morphologic Features of SCC

The most diagnostic feature of SCC by light microscopy is its nuclear detail. Nuclear chromatin is distributed in a uniform fine or coarse stippled pattern throughout the entire nucleus (Figure 2-1). Nucleoli are small and indistinct. Rare prominent nucleoli are infrequently observed with

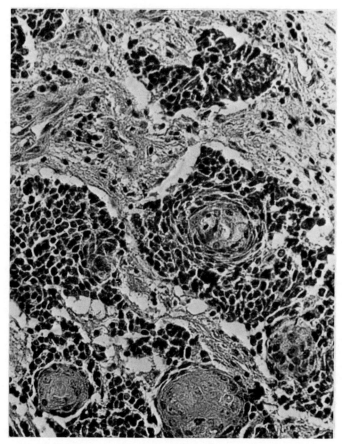

Figure 2-3. *SCC showing foci of squamous differentiation. Hematoxylin and eosin. Original magnification × 400.*

the low-power field. These nuclear features are present regardless of the size or shape of the nucleus or of the cell itself. Mitoses are numerous in well preserved tumors but may be difficult to identify in crushed biopsies. The majority of cells have meager cytoplasm, resulting in molding and contouring of adjoining nuclei. In some tumors, cells may contain a modest amount of cytoplasm. Spindled or fusiform cells are frequently arranged in parallel or in intersecting bundles, trabeculae, or ribbons (Figure 2-2). In some tumors, neoplastic cells cuff thin-walled blood vessels, forming a perivascular mantel (pseudorosettes). In others, classic small cells aggregate to form lumina without sharply demarcated cell borders

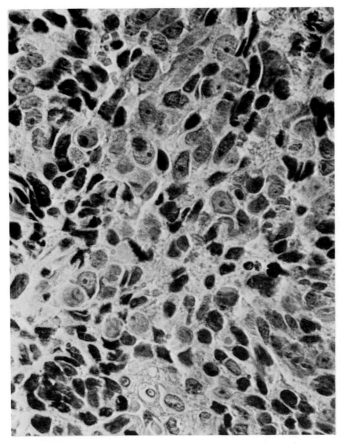

Figure 2-4. *SCC showing foci of anaplastic large cells (discrete clusters of cells with moderate amounts of cytoplasm and distinct prominent nucleoli). Hematoxylin and eosin. Original magnification × 400.*

(rosettes). Occasionally, cuboidal to columnar cells with distinct cytoplasmic margins form distinct lumina (tubules or glands). Rarely, these latter structures may contain mucin, although intracellular mucin is not identified. In a small percentage of SCC, a few discrete foci of squamous differentiation or syncytial multinucleated giant cells may be identified (Figure 2-3). Likewise, in occasional tumors, clusters of enlarged cells with moderate amounts of cytoplasm, condensed nuclear chromatin, and prominent nucleoli may be observed amidst classic small cells (Figure 2-4). This combination has been called a mixed small cell–large cell variant and will be referred to as #22/40 in the remainder of this chapter. In the 1977 WHO lung cancer classification, #22/40 is included as a component of the intermediate subtype of small cell carcinoma.[8]

The supporting stroma of SCC is usually thin, fibrous, vascular, and devoid of significant inflammatory response. In regions of extensive necrosis, elastic fibrils of blood vessels or other preexisting structures may be encrusted by a homogeneous or coarse granular bluish material. Azzopardi[11] has demonstrated that this material is Feulgen positive and DNA in nature.

By electron microscopy, SCC is characterized by round or ovoid nuclei, diffuse fine chromatin, and inconspicuous nucleoli. Membrane-bound secretory granules may be identified, particularly in the pseudopodal processes of some of these cells.[12] It is estimated that these granules measure from 500 to 2000 Å.[13] Hage et al.[14] have suggested that two types of intracytoplasmic granules, distinguished by their size and ultrastructural characteristics, may be associated specifically with SCC.[14] Cytoplasmic organelles in SCC are sparse. Cell membranes of adjacent cells are closely apposed. Desmosomes may be present but are usually small and infrequent.

In cytologic specimens, neoplastic cells are two to four times the size of a lymphocyte. In well preserved specimens, nuclear detail is similar to that described in tissues. The apparent lack of cytoplasm, nuclear molding, and contouring of adjacent cells are characteristic of this tumor. In desquamating and necrotic material, cells may present as "ink dots" without distinct nuclear detail.

Technical Problems in the Diagnosis of SCC

Adequacy of Material

The most frequent sources of diagnostic material for SCC are bronchial biopsies and washings, sputa, and regional lymph nodes (supraclavicular, cervical, mediastinal). The rigid bronchoscope provides the most generous diagnostic material for bronchial biopsies, particularly when gross tumor is evident in major bronchi. Even in the absence of obvious tumor, these biopsies may contain sufficient quantities of identifiable tumor to be diagnostic.[15] When more distal segmental or subsegmental bronchi are involved, rigid bronchial biopsies may be negative. Fiberoptic bronchoscopes permit visualization and biopsy of these more peripheral lesions. The minute particles that are obtained, however, are frequently inadequate for diagnosis. In some instances, only strips of bronchial mucosa are obtained. Instrumentation may cause crushing of bronchial tissues, even in the absence of tumor. Occasionally, overinterpretation of malignancy may be made on the basis of crushed tissues in the presence of a few nondescript darkly staining cells. Bronchial biopsies obtained by either rigid or fiberoptic bronchoscopy may, not infrequently, contain a few cell clusters that are obviously malignant but impossible to adequately type.

Bronchial washings or sputa may be negative or may contain dysplastic cells and/or only rare clusters of malignant cells, even in patients who have well defined radiologic and/or bronchoscopic evidence of tumor. Each pathologist has his/her own threshold for making a diagnosis of malignancy on a minimal number of cells per specimen. In a well differentiated squamous malignancy, it is possible that three to five frankly neoplastic cells in a single specimen may be sufficient to permit some pathologists to make a diagnosis of malignancy and to interpret cell type. More caution and a greater number of neoplastic cells are usually required to diagnose other cell types of lung cancer, particularly SCC. Bronchial washings obtained prior to biopsy and prebronchoscopy sputa may be negative in early stages of SCC because of the predominant submucosal location of the tumor and its minimal tendency to invade the mucosa and exfoliate.[16] Bronchial washings obtained after bronchial biopsy, as well as postbronchoscopy sputa, usually are productive of a higher yield of neoplastic cells, possibly because of biopsy exposure of the submucosal tumor. Bronchial washings and sputa that contain large quantities of inflammatory exudate are difficult to interpret. Neoplastic cells may be masked or lysed by the exudate. Small cohesive clusters of basal cells may be confused with or interpreted as SCC. The nuclei of such cells are smaller than those of SCC. Individual nuclei are separated from each other by distinct cytoplasmic processes, and nuclear molding is not impressive. These basal cell groups contrast with the clusters of malignant small cells, which have larger, denser nuclei with indistinct cytoplasm and which show molding and contouring of adjoining nuclei. Overstained single, stripped and degenerated epithelial cells may also be suggestive of small cell malignancy. It is hazardous to interpret such single cells.

Lymph node biopsies usually provide adequate diagnostic material. However, similar sampling and diagnostic problems may be present in needle biopsies and aspirates from lymph nodes, as well as from aspirates of lung, subcutaneous nodules, liver, or bone marrow. Biopsies of necrotic and poorly preserved tumors may be impossible to interpret or type.

Tissue Processing

Possibly the single most important reason for an inappropriate diagnosis of SCC relates to artifacts caused by improper handling, fixation, sectioning, and staining of specimens. Crushing artifacts are caused by instrumentation at the time of biopsy or during the processing of tissues. In addition to crushing of small bronchial biopsies, crushing may be observed in the absence of tumor in capsular and subcapsular zones of lymph node biopsies and in paratrabecular zones of fragmented bone marrow biopsies. It is tempting to interpret these crushed foci as evidence of tumor, particularly when a patient is known to have small cell carcinoma. A diagnosis of malignancy should be made only after identification of viable neoplastic cells.

Inadequate fixation, particularly of surgically resected specimens such as lung or lymph nodes, causes marked distortion of cellular detail and is a significant deterrent to proper interpretation of materials. In improperly fixed tissues, nuclei of small cell tumors become grossly enlarged and finely or coarsely vacuolated, giving the nuclei a bubbly appearance. The cytoplasm may also appear to be distended with fine vacuoles. The nuclear and cytoplasmic changes may suggest to the unwary observer a non–small cell tumor, usually a large cell carcinoma or poorly differentiated epidermoid carcinoma. The diffuse fine and coarse nuclear chromatin distribution, characteristic of small cell tumors, is lost, as is the tendency to nuclear molding and contouring. At the periphery of the section, where fixation may have penetrated, characteristic small cells may be observed. These often are disregarded for fear of overinterpretation. In such cases, additional material should be obtained for further study. Improper or delayed fixation of bronchial brushings or needle aspirates may cause drying artifacts and loss of nuclear detail, making interpretation difficult.

In thick or overstained tissue sections or cytologic preparations, nuclear detail may be obscured, causing difficulty in identifying tumor type.

Whenever feasible, it seems advisable to obtain material for simultaneous histologic and cytologic examinations. Following needle biopsies of lung, lymph node, liver, or bone marrow, the needle itself may be washed in fixative, and cells submitted for cytologic evaluation. Such materials may confirm the presence and type of tumor or provide diagnostic material when the biopsy or aspirate is inadequate, crushed, and/or negative. Touch preparations can be made of surgically resected materials or bone marrow biopsies. Bone marrow biopsies may be negative for malignancy, although bone marrow aspirates and cell blocks taken immediately adjacent to the biopsy site may be positive.[17] Conversely, dry taps may occur in patients with SCC because of the marked osteoblastic new bone formation and myelofibrosis associated with tumor metastases.[18] Touch preparations of the sclerotic marrow may provide immediate confirmation of the presence of tumor and its histologic type.

Interpretive Problems in the Diagnosis of SCC

SCC and Large Cell Carcinoma of the Lung

Difficulties may be encountered in distinguishing some cases of SCC from large cell carcinoma of the lung. The latter malignancies are characterized by a proliferation of neoplastic cells with moderate to abundant cytoplasm, well defined cell borders, enlarged nuclei with condensed chromatin granules, and prominent nucleoli. SCC tumors that tend to stratify, have a relatively increased amount of cytoplasm, or contain syncytial giant cells may be misinterpreted as large cell carcinoma, even when dense-core granules are identified in the tumor by electron microscopy. Tumors that have lost their nuclear characteristics because of poor fixation may also be interpreted as large cell carcinoma. Neoplasms that combine features of small and large cell carcinoma cause marked disparities in diagnoses even among observers aware of the problem.[9]

Ultrastructurally, large cell carcinoma may show feeble attempts to form microvilli, desmosomes, or tonofilaments. Rarely, dense-core granules have been identified in some true non–small cell tumors.[19]

In cytologic specimens, neoplastic large cells can easily be distinguished from classic small cells. The former have enlarged nuclei, prominent nucleoli, and conspicuous cytoplasm. In cytology specimens of tumors identified as #22/40, classic small cells may be mixed with isolated enlarged neoplastic cells possessing nuclear characteristics as described above. The cytologic distinction of large cell carcinoma from poorly differentiated adenocarcinoma or epidermoid carcinoma may be difficult, if not impossible.

SCC and Adenocarcinoma

The formation of tubular structures with distinct lumina is a morphologic feature of some forms of small cell tumors. Unless this is appreciated, it is possible to misinterpret these structures as evidence of a poorly differentiated adenocarcinoma. A diagnosis of SSC rests, in such cases, on the identification of cells with characteristic small cell nuclear features throughout the remainder of the tumor. In areas of massive necrosis, a single or double layer of neoplastic small cells palisading along the fibrovascular stroma may present as pseudopapillary structures and be misinterpreted as poorly differentiated papillary adenocarcinoma. Holes or "drop-outs" seen in some poorly fixed tissues may also give the impression of gland formation and be interpreted as evidence for adenocarcinoma.

Neoplastic cells in poorly differentiated adenocarcinoma have nuclear features similar to large cell carcinoma. In addition, intracytoplasmic mucin vacuoles may be identified. In many poorly differentiated adenocarcinomas, there may be minimal attempt at acinar formation. In small biopsies, only the large cell component may be identified. Rare tumors composed of combined small cell and adenocarcinoma have been described prior to treatment. These are classified as combined small cell subtype in the 1977 WHO lung cancer classification.[8]

Ultrastructurally, cells of poorly differentiated adenocarcinoma demonstrate microvilli, intracytoplasmic mucin, microacinar formation, abundant organelles and tight junctions adjacent to true acinar spaces.[12] Cytologic characteristics of moderately differentiated adenocarcinoma are distinctive and offer no diagnostic problem. To the contrary, if a diagnosis of adenocarcinoma is made on the basis of tissue biopsy and cytologic diagnosis of small cell carcinoma is made from the same specimen, it is highly likely that the tissue diagnosis is in error and the cytologic diagnosis is correct. The nuclear detail of these "adenocarcinomas" will be of a small cell nature. Additional material should be obtained to confirm the diagnosis.

SCC and Squamous Cell Carcinoma

Minute foci of squamous differentiation may occur in small cell tumors. These nests constitute an insignificant portion of the tumor. Again, the diagnosis of SCC is based on identification of classic small cells throughout the remainder of the tumor. SCC tumors that stratify have, on occasion, been misinterpreted as poorly differentiated epidermoid carcinoma. Such discrepancies can be avoided if strict criteria for epidermoid carcinoma are required, i.e., orderly and distinct intercellular bridge formation with or without some evidence of intracellular keratinization. Special stains for keratin and/or the use of a green filter to enhance the intercellular bridge formation have been recommended by some as aids in the diagnosis of squamous cell malignancies.[7] Rare tumors combining features of SCC and squamous cell tumors occur. These latter tumors have also been placed in a combined subtype of small cell carcinoma in the 1977 WHO lung cancer classification.[8]

Ultrastructurally, cells of poorly differentiated epidermoid carcinoma contain prominent desmosomes, tonofibrils, and other intracytoplasmic organelles. Cytologic features of differentiated epidermoid carcinomas are usually so distinctive that diagnostic problems rarely occur. Degenerated squamous cells with hyperchromatic nuclei and scanty acidophilic cytoplasm have, infrequently, been interpreted as small cell carcinoma. The single nature of the cells, the scanty but distinct cytoplasmic rim, and the lack of nuclear molding should alert one to the non–small cell nature of the tumor.

SCC and Malignant Carcinoids

Carcinoids are usually arranged in a circumscribed trabecular, mosaic, or ribbonlike pattern. Acinar formation and spindle cell variants have been identified.[20] In typical carcinoids, cells have a moderate amount of cytoplasm and relatively uniform vesicular monotonous nuclei and nucleoli. Mitoses are rare, and foci of necrosis are uncommon. On rare occasions, in crushed biopsies, nuclear detail may be poor and the tumor may be interpreted as SCC. In atypical carcinoids, the tumor may be hemorrhagic and necrotic and mitoses may be identified. In some of these latter tumors, there may also be morphologic features of SCC, i.e., lack of circumscription, nuclear molding, and hyperchromasia, making a discriminate diagnosis by light microscopy difficult. Distinction or prediction of clinical behavior and response to therapy of these tumors has not been resolved to date. Classic carcinoids of the lung are argyrophillic, whereas small cell tumors usually are not. The Grimelius silver stain may be of value in identifying carcinoid tumors. It is not known how useful this stain may be in distinguishing atypical carcinoids with small cell features.

Ultrastructurally, carcinoids are characterized by cells with numerous large membrane-bound secretory granules in the cytoplasm of each cell.[21] Hage et al.[22] have suggested that a distinction between SCC and carcinoids may be made on the basis of the morphology of the intracytoplasmic secretory granules.

In cytologic specimens, epithelial cells of carcinoid tumors tend to be monotonous, rounded, and arranged in a linear or single-file pattern. Nuclei are uniform and nucleoli may be present. The diffuse chromatin network and the molding and contouring of small cells are not observed.

Interobserver Studies of Consistency in Diagnosis of
SCC

Two interobserver studies were recently made to identify problems in the diagnosis and reproducibility of typing of SCC.[9,10] A number of observations can be made from these studies:

1. A high degree of unanimity can be achieved in the diagnosis of SCC by pathologists who apply strict criteria for the diagnosis of this tumor. In one study, by 3 pathologists, there was unanimity in over 90 percent of the cases in the diagnosis of SCC. In the second study, by 8 pathologists, there was unanimity in the diagnosis of SCC in 72 percent of the cases and near unanimity (7 of the 8 pathologists) in over 90 percent of the cases.
2. The first of these two studies also made an attempt to assess consistency in the subtyping of SCC. Unanimity in subtyping by the 3 pathologists, using the 1977 WHO classification as a standard, was only 54 percent. This is considered unacceptable. It would suggest that subtyping is subjective, unreliable, and probably without value.
3. Problems identified in the first study chiefly related to the interpretation of mixed small cell–large cell tumors. Lack of strict criteria permitted little or no consistency in diagnosis of this group of tumors. Much additional work is needed to recognize and evaluate this small cell variant.
4. Problems identified in the second study were variable causes for inappropriate diagnoses of SCC. Of a total of 74 cases of proven SCC, 8 pathologists made a diagnosis of non–small tumor in 29 instances (out of a total of 592 observations). It is of interest that more than one-half of these 29 tumors were diagnosed as large cell carcinoma; approximately 25 percent as epidermoid carcinomas; and approximately 20 percent as adenocarcinomas.

Comments and Summary

A number of comments may be made about diagnostic problems of SCC:

1. Diagnostic difficulties in SCC can most frequently be ascribed to inadequacy of material, poor technical quality of tissue or cytologic

processing, and/or failure to apply appropriate criteria in interpreting these tumors.

2. The simultaneous processing of tissue and cytologic material for examination reduces the likelihood of inadequacy of material, provides confirmatory evidence of tumor and its cell type when both specimens are positive, and permits a greater possibility of obtaining identifiable tumor when one of the two specimens is suggestive of malignancy, is negative, or has been subjected to the artifacts of fixation.

3. Diagnostic criteria of SCC are based on nuclear detail. In pretreatment specimens, small cell tumors may assume variable patterns. Only 10 percent of small cell tumors should provide any significant diagnostic difficulty. Tumors that contain squamous nests, tubules, or clusters of cells with large cell features are responsible for most diagnostic problems. It is important that these small cell variants be recognized so that patients can be placed on appropriate chemotherapy/radiotherapy protocols.

4. Patients with these small cell variants respond well to treatment. Little is known, however, concerning the median survival and long-term survival of patients identified as having these elements. In a preliminary study of 18 patients with #22/40 treated on intensive small cell chemotherapy protocols, median survival was 6.6 mo, as compared to median survival of 10.2 mo for patients with classic small cell tumors treated on the same protocol.[23] Objective response of patients with #22/40 was 56 percent, in contrast to an objective response rate of more than 90 percent for patients with pure small cell tumors. In spite of this fact, it is obvious that an objective response rate of 56 percent is much higher than might be expected of non–small cell lung tumors.

5. There is a growing appreciation of the variable histologic patterns of SCC. A high degree of consistency in the light-microscopic diagnosis of this tumor is possible if uniform criteria are accepted by the pathology community.

6. There is also a growing awareness that small cell tumors that recur following intensive therapy may undergo significant morphologic changes in both in vivo and in vitro systems.[24-26] This morphologic change is associated with loss of biochemical markers and hormone production. It is reasonable to suggest that the nonresponsiveness of a recurrent tumor may be caused by its profoundly altered morphology. Post-therapy biopsy and autopsy material may offer even greater problems in diagnosis. It is apparent that these materials should be used with caution in retrospective diagnoses or typing of tumor.

7. It is possible, and ironic, that experimental studies being conducted at present will define the nature of this tumor more sharply, thereby eliminating problems in diagnosis altogether.

References

1. Hansen HH, Dombernowsky P, Hansen M, et al: Chemotherapy of advanced small cell anaplastic carcinoma. Superiority of a four drug combination to a three drug combination. Ann Intern Med 89:177–181, 1978
2. Bunn PA, Cohen MH, Ihde DC, et al: Commentary. Advances in small cell bronchogenic carcinoma. Cancer Treat Rep 61:333–341, 1977
3. Greco FA, Einhorn LH, Richardson RL, et al: Small cell lung cancer: Progress and perspectives, Sem Oncol 3:323–335, 1978
4. Minna JD, Brereton HD, Cohen MH, et al: The treatment of small cell carcinoma of the lung. Prospects for cure, in Muggia F, Rozencweig M (eds): Lung Cancer: Progress in Therapeutic Research. New York, Raven Press, 1979, pp 549–558
5. Brigham BA, Bunn PA, Minna JD, et al: Growth rates of small cell bronchogenic carcinomas. Cancer 42:2880–2886, 1978
6. Matthews MJ, Rozencweig M, Staquet MJ, et al: Long-term survivors with small cell carcinoma of the lung. Eur J Cancer 16:527–531, 1980
7. Kreyberg L: Histological Typing of Lung Tumors. International Histological Classification of Tumors. Geneva, World Health Organization, 1967
8. Sobin LH: The WHO histological classification of lung tumors, in Muggia F, Rozencweig M (eds): Lung Cancer: Progress in Therapeutic Research. New York, Raven Press, 1979, pp 83–90
9. Hirsch F, Matthews MJ, Yesner R: Problems in the histopathologic classification of small cell carcinoma of the lung. An interobservational examination. Abst Int Assoc Study Lung Cancer, Copenhagen, 1980, p 77
10. Janis M, Matthews MJ, Bonfiglio T, et al: Consistency in the diagnosis of small cell carcinoma of the lung. Abst Int Assoc Study Lung Cancer, Copenhagen, 1980, p 79
11. Azzopardi JG: Oat-cell carcinoma of the bronchus. J Pathol Bacteriol 78:513–519, 1960

12. Mackay B, Osborne BM, Wilson RA: Ultrastructure of lung neo-plasms, in Straus MJ (ed): Lung Cancer: Clinical Diagnosis and Treatment. New York, Grune & Stratton, 1977, pp 71–84

13. Hattori S, Matsuda M, Tateishi R, et al: Oat cell carcinoma of the lung. Clinical and morphologic studies in relation to its histogenesis. Cancer 30:1014–1024, 1972

14. Hage E: Ultrastructure of endocrine cells and endocrine tumors of the human lung. Abst Int Assoc Study Lung Cancer, Copenhagen, Denmark, 1980, p 64

15. Kato Y, Ferguson TB, Bennett D, et al: Oat cell carcinoma of the lung. A review of 138 cases. Cancer 23:517–524, 1964

16. Ihde DC, Cohen MH, Bernath AM, et al: Serial fiberoptic bronchoscopy during chemotherapy for small cell carcinoma of the lung. Early detection of Patients at high risk of relapse. Chest: 74: 531–536, 1978

17. Hirsch F, Hansen HH, Dombernowsky P, et al: Bone marrow examination in the staging of small cell carcinoma of the lung, with special reference to subtyping. Cancer 39:2563–2569, 1977

18. Ihde DC, Simms EB, Matthews MJ, et al: Bone marrow metastases in small cell carcinoma of the lung: Frequency, description, and influence on chemotherapeutic toxicity and prognosis. Blood 53:677–686, 1979

19. Geller SA, Toker C: Pulmonary adenomatosis and peripheral adeno-carcinoma of the lung: An ultrastructural demonstration of common morphologic features. Arch Pathol 88:148–154, 1969

20. Gillespie JJ, Luger AM, Callaway LA: Peripheral spindled carcinoid tumor: A review of its ultrastructure, differential diagnosis and bio-logic behavior. Human Pathol 10:601–607, 1979

21. Hage E: Histochemistry and fine structure of bronchial carcinoid tumors. Virchows Arch (Pathol Anat) 361:121–128, 1973

22. Hage E: Ultrastructure of endocrine cells and endocrine tumors of the human lung. Abst Int Assoc Study Lung Cancer, Copenhagen, Denmark, 1980, p 64

23. Matthews MJ, Gazdar AF: Small cell carcinoma of the lung and its variants. A clinicopathologic correlation, in McGuire W, Livingston RB (eds): Lung Cancer: Advances in Research and Treatment. The Hague, Martinus Nijhoff, 1981, pp 283–306

24. Matthews MJ: Effects of therapy on the morphology and behavior of small cell carcinoma of the lung. A clinicopathologic study in: Muggia F, Rozencweig M (eds): Lung Cancer, Progress in Therapeutic Research, New York, Raven Press, 1979, pp 155–164

25. Brereton HD, Matthews MJ, Costa J, et al: Mixed anaplastic small cell carcinoma of the lung. Ann Int Med 88:805–806, 1978
26. Abeloff MD, Eggleston JC, Mendelsohn G, et al: Changes in morphologic and biochemical characteristics of small cell carcinoma of the lung. Am J Med 66:757–764, 1979

3

TISSUE CULTURE AND IN VITRO CHARACTERISTICS

Olive S. Pettengill
George D. Sorenson

The development of a continuous cell culture from human small (oat) cell carcinoma of the lung (SCC) was first described by Oboshi et al.[1] A population of floating cell clumps was established in vitro from a lymph node metastasis. Few neurosecretory-type granules—referred to here as dense-core vesicles (DCV)—were observed ultrastructurally, and there was no evidence of peptide hormone secretion in vitro. Xenografts appeared and then regressed when cultured cells were implanted in the cheek pouch of hamsters preirradiated with a dose of 300 rads.

Ellison et al.[2] have established continuous cell lines from SCC and have given particular attention to the regulation of the secretion of calcitonin and ACTH by tumor cells in vitro. The presence of DCV, thought to be related to intracellular storage of hormones, was observed in all cell lines examined by electron microscopy.

Another continuous cell line derived from SCC grew as a monolayer with a doubling time of 24 hr.[3] Xenografts were readily obtained in cortisonized hamsters as well as in nude athymic mice. Cultured cells stained positively with the argentaffin reaction and for formaldehyde-induced flu-

This work was supported in part by U.S. Public Health Service Grants CA17710, CA04326, and CA25845; National Cancer Institute Contract No. 1 CP65776; General Research Support Grant RR-03592 from the Division of Research Facilities and Resources, National Institutes of Health; and Hitchcock Foundation, Hanover, New Hampshire.

51

orescence (FIF). The presence of 5-hydroxytryptamine derivatives, but not the amine itself, was detected in the medium by fluorospectroscopy. In these cells, DCV were not clearly identified by electron microscopy.

The appearance of phenotypic properties characteristic of neural cells has been induced in a culture of SCC cells.[4] These properties were thought to provide evidence for the neuroendocrine origin of this tumor-cell type. Within a group of 11 cell lines derived from 3 histologic types of lung tumors, only the one derived from small cell carcinoma, which normally grew in suspension, was induced to attach to the substrate and develop neuritelike cellular processes in response to treatment with dibutyryl cyclic adenosine 3'5'-monophosphate (dbcAMP). No catecholamines, ACTH, or serotonin were detected in culture medium of untreated cells, although neurosecretory-type granules were observed by electron microscopy. After exposure to dbcAMP for 1 wk, however, norepinephrine and epinephrine were detected in culture medium.

Further evidence of neuritelike properties of SCC cells was observed in primary cultures of SCC which produced an action potential in response to electrical stimulus.[5]

In our laboratory, we have initiated a study of pathobiology of SCC by establishing a group of continuous cell lines from primary and metastatic tumor tissue obtained from patients with SCC.[6,7] Cultured cells have retained many of the characteristics of the tumor cells from which they were derived. Specific properties such as peptide hormone synthesis have been and are being used for characterization of tumor cells in vitro, where the isolated cancer cell can be studied and compared with tumors arising from the same cells in nude athymic mice in parallel studies in vivo (see Chapter 5, this monograph).

Experimental Studies

Materials and Methods

A variety of types of specimens from patients with SCC were placed in culture (Table 3-1). Material was obtained during diagnostic or therapeutic procedures or at autopsy, and the culturing procedures were carried out with minimum delay. For example, bone marrow aspirates were placed directly into culture medium, immediately transported to the laboratory, and prepared for incubation. All other specimens were handled as expeditiously as possible and were taken directly from the operating room or autopsy room to the laboratory. Most autopsy specimens were obtained within 4 hr postmortem.

Table 3-1
Origin of Small Cell Lines

Specimen (SCC)	Total No. Examined	Tumor Cell Lines (SCC)	Lymphoblastoid Cell Lines
Primary lung tumor			
Biopsy			
Open biopsy	2	1	0
Needle biopsy	1	1	0
Bronchoscopic specimen	1	0	0
Autopsy	8	2	0
Pleural fluid	6	5	2
Bone marrow aspirate	80	8	15
Lymph node			
Biopsy	4	0	1
Autopsy	3	1	0
Liver			
Biopsy	1	1	0
Autopsy	11	3	0
Other tumor metastases			
Biopsy	6	0	0
Autopsy	2	2	0
	125	24	18

From Pettengill et al.[7]

Solid tissue specimens were prepared for incubation with as little manipulation as possible. Usually, tumor was cleaned of necrotic tissue, minced into 1-mm^3 pieces, and incubated in complete medium, although, occasionally, a cytosieve was utilized to obtain a cell suspension. Trypsinization of minced solid tissue was performed in some cases, especially in autopsy specimens, in order to eliminate necrotic tissue. For the most part, specimens containing a large amount of dead tissue did not progress to tumor cell lines in culture, with or without trypsinization.

Pleural fluid specimens contained viable tumor as a suspension of small clumps of cells. Fluids were generally collected without any anticoagulant and were centrifuged, resuspended, and dissociated in culture medium, for plating at a concentration of $1-2 \times 10^6$ tumor cells/ml.

Cultures were established in 25-cm^3 plastic flasks. Tissue culture medium employed for establishing cell lines and maintaining established cell lines was RPMI 1640 and Waymouth's MB 752/1 with the addition of 20 percent heat-inactivated (30 min at 56°C) fetal calf serum (FCS). Both Ham's F-12 and Dulbecco's Modified Eagles Medium were used during the early stages of this work to no significant advantage, and their use was

discontinued. If conditions of collection indicated probable bacterial con-
tamination, the primary specimens were washed in antibiotics, and the
initial feeding contained antibiotics. However, cells were usually established and were always maintained without the use of antibiotics.

Maintenance of Established Cell Lines

Cultures were fed at intervals of 3–4 days, depending on pH change
of the medium. All cell lines required trypsinization for subculture, except
DMS 79, which could be dissociated mechanically. Some cell lines could
be transferred without trypsinization, as cells growing in suspension or
flushed from the surface of the culture vessel. However, the tendency for
dying cells to remain trapped in large clumps of cells, always present in
the culture, made it necessary to trypsinize even DMS 79, periodically, to
remove the dead cells.

Cell lines were maintained in the medium in which they had been
established in culture, and frequently cell lines were established in both
media—RPMI 1640 and Waymouth's MB 752/1 with 20 percent FCS.

Subcultured cells were established at 5×10^5 cells/ml and placed in
plastic disposable culture flasks for incubation at 37°C in 5 percent CO_2
and air. Cell counts were made in a hemacytometer in the presence of
trypan blue.

Establishment of SCC Cell Lines

The most important factors for success in establishing cell lines from
SCC were the source, condition, and amount of tumor tissue that could be
made available for use. Because primary tumors were infrequently treated
surgically, lung tumor tissue was obtained only from biopsy or at autopsy,
and most tumor cell lines were obtained from metastatic tumor tissue.

Bone marrow aspirates, which were the most commonly available
specimens for culture, showed the greatest degree of variability in tumor
cell content. Some contained no visible tumor cells in the aliquot obtained
for cell culture, although the accompanying specimen, examined pathologically, contained many tumor cells. From other specimens, cell lines
were obtained even though tumor cells were not observed in stained preparations of the aspirate cells. One likely reason for the inconsistency observed between the growth of a cell line from a bone marrow aspirate and
the identification of tumor cells cytologically was noted by Wurster-Hill
and Maurer[8] in their observations on specimens harvested for chromosomal analysis. Tumor cells in bone marrow frequently occur as single

cells, which would not be recognized in a specimen prepared for cytological examination. The development of cell lines from bone marrow aspirates often required 2–3 mo longer. In some cases, 2–3 mo elapsed before a recognizable colony of tumor cells was seen, suggesting that it could have originated from a single cell. The establishment of a cell line, then, required several additional months.

A cell line has been defined[9] as the population of cells that grows from a primary culture after the first subculture. This includes a population selected from the primary specimen, which can encompass all cell types found in the primary specimen. In contrast, we have used the term "cell line" to define a culture that can be expanded through subculture by trypsinization or mechanical dissociation on a regular basis. This may follow several subcultures, during which trypsinization was used to stimulate growth and to disperse large clumps of cells in primary cultures. A continuous cell line is defined as one with infinite growth. The time necessary to establish a continuous cell line was variable: it occurred as quickly as 6 wk after explantation and required over a year in several instances.[7] Because of our observation of the apparently high level of cell death in rapidly dividing cultures, the lengthy period of adaptation may be related to the selection of a cell better adapted for in vitro growth. The rate of proliferation exceeded the rate of cell death.

In general, specimens obtained following therapeutic or diagnostic radiation exhibited poor growth; this was especially apparent in bone marrow specimens. Aspirates from untreated patients grew most rapidly, provided tumor cells were present in sufficient numbers.

The development of a continuous cell line from the first specimen obtained—a bone marrow aspirate—provided a basis for monitoring subsequent specimens for similarly growing tumor cells. The first line, DMS 44, appeared after 10 wk as a group of 3–4 cells, which gradually increased in number (Fig. 3-1). This colony was found among the original outgrowth of normal fibroblasts, which were deteriorating by this time. Had there not been an increase in colony size, the culture would probably have been discarded, as the stipled appearance of the cells suggested a state of deterioration rather than of growth. Very shortly thereafter, additional colonies of cells were observed at a distance, seemingly arising by the detachment of cells from the first colony, which had reattached in another area of the culture flask that had been previously preconditioned by the growth of fibroblasts. This pattern in the establishment of cultures has been observed frequently. In all specimens from which a cell line was obtained, the primary growth of tumor cells was attached to the culture vessel. In some cell lines, some colonies of cells that proliferated to form large

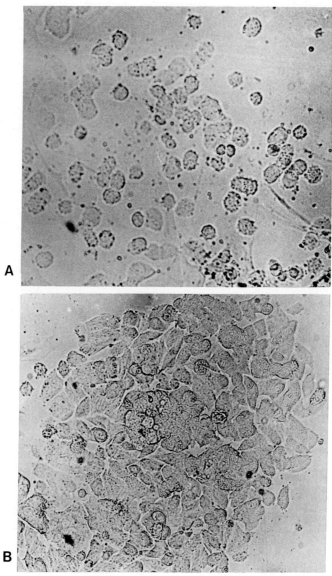

Figure 3-1. *DMS 44. (A) Original colony of cells, 10 wk after initiation of culture. (B) Appearance of a similar colony, 3 mo after initiation of culture, first subculture. Living cultures photographed with bright-field illumination. Original magnification × 110.*

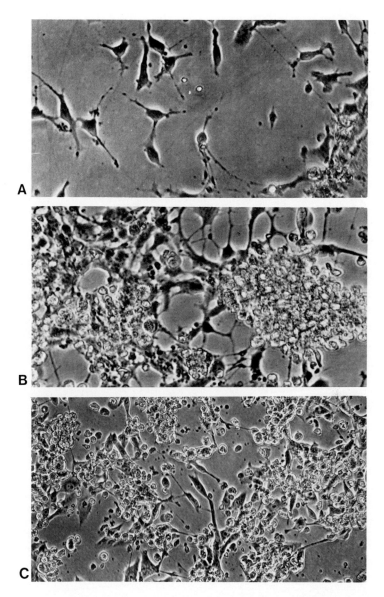

Figure 3-2. *Neuritelike extensions in cultured cells. (A) DMS 106. Tumor cells appearing in culture 4 wk after explantation; note tenuous, beaded processes between cells. (B) DMS 106, 2 wk later, showing large clumps of tumor cells, with processes that now appear thicker. (C) DMS 273. Established cell line which continues to exhibit intercellular processes. Living cultures photographed with phase-contrast illumination. Original magnification × 110.*

57

clumps were observed to detach from the substrate and to remain viable in suspension.

A frequent observation during the early phase of establishment of a cell line was the appearance of cellular processes, very suggestive of neuritelike extensions. In view of the proposed origin of SCC from cells derived from neural crest and of the many similarities of SCC cells with neuroendocrine cells, this was a provocative observation. The processes were intercellular, always connecting one cell with another, and, in a few cases, were extensive enough to form a network (Fig. 3-2). Beadlike protuberances were present on the processes. In attached cell lines, processes connecting cells are still present after several years of in vitro cultivation (DMS 273, Fig. 3-2, panel C). Because they required substrate adhesion, processes did not persist in those cells that developed into cultures that grew primarily in suspension.

Whether the capacity to form these processes under appropriate in vitro conditions is retained must be determined through manipulation of in vitro conditions with agents such as dbcAMP or other inducers of differentiation.

Several different patterns of events occurred in primary cultures, and these bore some relationship to the type of specimen—aspirate, pleural fluid, or solid tumor.

Pleural fluid specimens provided the best source for establishing continuous cell lines. Five SCC cell lines were obtained from the 6 pleural fluid specimens. From the sixth, a lymphoblastoid cell line was isolated instead of an SCC line. Lymphoblastoid cell lines developed for some specimens, and, when this occurred, it precluded continuous growth of tumor cells in any type of tumor specimen owing to the rapid growth of the transformed lymphoblastoid cells. The possibility of inhibition of lymphoblastoid cell growth by addition of glucocorticoids to culture medium has not been tested. A consistent pattern has been observed during the primary growth of pleural fluid specimens, where a pavementlike, more epitheloid (rather than fibroblastic) type of monolayer is formed, on which small clumps of tumor cells subsequently become apparent (Fig. 3-3, panel A). This was in contrast to the pattern seen in bone marrow aspirates and in solid tumor specimens, in which an endogenous population of fibroblasts on which tumor cells seemed to grow preferentially usually appeared (Fig. 3-3, panel B). Fibroblasts never created a problem of overgrowth of tumor cells; they disappeared spontaneously or, on a few occasions, were controlled by the addition of collagenase to growth medium for brief periods.[7]

One pleural fluid specimen (DMS 353) produced a lymphoblastoid cell

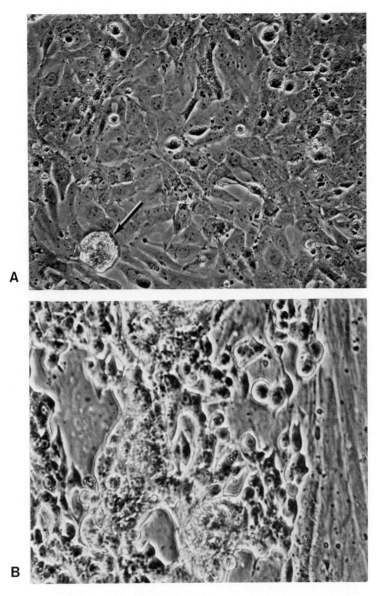

Figure 3-3. *(A) DMS 330. Epitheloid-type cell growth associated with primary cultures of pleural fluids. Note clumps of SCC tumor cells (arrow) growing in association with monolayer. (B) DMS 92. Appearance of tumor cell population arising on endogeneous population of fibroblasts, from bone marrow aspirate. Living cultures photographed with phase-contrast illumination. Original magnification × 110.*

59

line in RPMI 1640/20FCS and a SCC cell line in Way/20FCS. In one other case, it was possible to separate physically, with a capillary pipet, a lymphoblastoid cell line and a SCC cell line (DMS 187) that had appeared simultaneously in the same primary culture of a bone marrow aspirate.

The appearance of a lymphoblastoid cell line was usually associated with a "crisis" or sudden increase in the rate of proliferation. This was observed in nests of attached cells that began to proliferate rapidly, 4–8 wk after initiation of the primary culture, and subsequently grew only in loose clumps in suspension. Because such cell lines probably originated from normal lymphoid cells that had become transformed, this was not an unexpected observation.[10] In contrast, SCC cells never appeared to pass through a crisis, but grew at a more or less regular rate until they became an established cell line. Lymphoblastoid cell lines arose only in specimens that contained lymphoid cells, i.e., bone marrow, lymph node, or pleural fluid. Such cell lines were identified by the presence in growth medium of one or more human immunoglobulins and by their characteristic ultra-structure, as observed by electron microscopy.[7]

From solid tumor specimens, such as those obtained from the lung or liver metastases, a frequent feature of primary cultures was the presence of tumor cell aggregates, attached to the substrate, which divided rapidly at the periphery, but remained stationary in size. New cells escaped into the medium, where their survival was apparently very poor. In 2 such examples, almost 1 yr passed before a cell line was obtained that could be expanded easily on a regular basis.[7] In one of these, DMS 53, a distinctive nuclear morphology that was evident in the very early outgrowth, a few days after the original explantation, is still apparent in living cultures after 5 yr in vitro (Fig. 3-4).

Solid tumors were the only specimens obtained at autopsy. These adapted to in vitro conditions as readily as did the premortem specimens (Table 3-1). Of the specimens obtained from solid tumors (primary and metastatic), 25 percent of those obtained prior to death provided cell lines, whereas 33 percent of those obtained at autopsy developed cell lines. There was no significant difference in the yield of continuous cell lines from primary or metastatic tumors.

Characteristics of Established Cell Lines

Morphology in Cell Culture

Each of the SCC cell lines showed an individual morphology in culture. Cells varied in size from 10 to 20 μ. They rarely grew singly; rather, most grew as clumps of attached or suspended cells with a high refractive

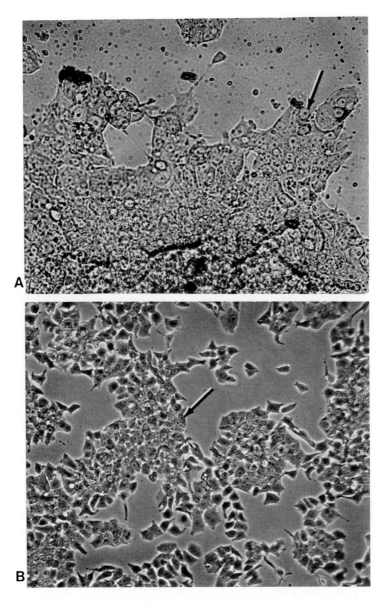

Figure 3-4. *DMS 53 cell culture, illustrating presence of morphologically similar cells in cells at different times. (A) Original outgrowth of tumor cells from explanted material 6 wk after explantation. Bright-field illumination. Original magnification × 110. (B) DMS 53, after 4 yr in vitro passage. Note presence of the same nucleolar morphology in cells in both populations (arrows). Phase-contrast illumination. Original magnification × 110.*

61

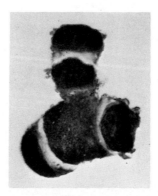

Figure 3-5. *DMS 44. Clump of cells resistant to trypsiniza-tion, showing characteristic molding as observed in SCC cul-tured cells. Giemsa stain of cell smear. Original magnification × 1000.*

index and a glassy appearance. Clumping was also observed as a "chain" of cells, which gave the cells a molded appearance (Fig. 3-5). Some clumps observed microscopically were seen to consist of a central round cell around which other crescent-shaped cells were molded. In most instances, clumps required trypsinization followed by vigorous dissociation for preparation of a single-cell suspension. Only one cell line (DMS 79) could be dissociated physically, but cell death always occurred with either procedure. The fragility of cultured cells may be analogous to the "crushing" artifact described in cytologic examination of clinical specimens.

The three types of growth patterns seen after SCC cell lines had become established are illustrated in Figure 3-6.

1. In the most frequently observed growth pattern, cells attached to the substrate after trypsinization, but, as cell density increased, large clumps detached from the surface of the culture dish and floated. These suspended colonies were viable and could be maintained in this manner with regular feeding for several months. Dead cells that accumulated within the clumps were removed by trypsinization, whereupon the cycle was repeated.

    In one case (DMS 153) clumps in suspension appeared to have the properties of spheroids and presented a tissuelike appearance within the clump. These were completely resistant to dissociation by mechanical means (Fig. 3-7). A spheroid has been likened to a small tu-

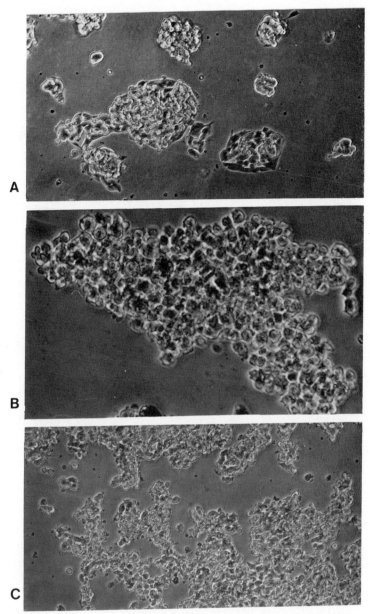

Figure 3-6. *Comparison of three types of morphology seen in established cell cultures. Living cultures photographed with phase-contrast illumination. Original magnification × 110. (A) DMS 44, 47th subculture. Cells grow in attached colonies, which do not become confluent, but contain clumped cells. (B) DMS 79, 1 yr in vitro. Cells grow only in loose clumps in suspension. This morphology has persisted for 5 yr. (C) DMS 153, 47th subculture. Cells attach after trypsinization, but also grow in clumps of cells detached from the substrate. Attached population shown here.*

63

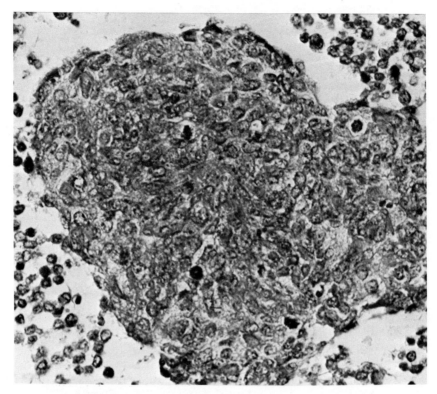

Figure 3-7. *DMS 153. Clumps of cells growing in suspension have properties of spheroids. Suspended cultured cells collected by centrifugation, and fixed prior to paraffin embedding. Hematoxylin and eosin. Original magnification × 500.*

mor growing in suspension, with characteristic hypoxic central areas,[11] and thus provides a useful modified in vitro system for growth studies in carcinomas.

2. In some instances, cell lines grew only as attached populations (DMS 44, 47, 53, 114, 273).

3. Finally in the least commonly observed growth pattern, cells grew only in large clumps in suspension (DMS 79).

There was an increased tendency for cells to attach to the substrate in Waymouth's medium as compared to RPMI 1640. Neither variation of sera—FCS, newborn calf serum, or horse serum—nor variation in concentration of FCS appeared to influence culture morphology or cell attachment. In all cases, SCC cells in vitro grew as clumps of cells. When examined ultrastructurally, the presence of membrane junctions was characteristically seen, which may account for their adhesion to each other.

Histology

The morphology of stained cells is similar to that described for SCC. Cultured cells were controlled in a pellet, fixed, and embedded in paraffin for preparation of sections to be compared with tumors. Cells were small, with a high nucleus-to-cytoplasm ratio. Periodic acid–Schiff stained sections did not exhibit the presence of glycoproteins, nor was mucin (mucicarmine stain) or keratin (hematoxylin and eosin stain) present.

Ultrastructure

All the cell lines described here have been shown to contain dense-core vesicles (DCV), which may be the most reliable hallmark of these cells yet recognized (Fig. 3-8). Compared to DCV in normal endocrine cells, the vesicles are more pleomorphic in their shape and vary considerably in size. They are thought to be related to the storage of peptides and/or biogenic amines known to be associated with this tumor in patients. The nucleus is frequently cleft, and its chromatin is clumped at the periphery as well as dispersed throughout the nucleus. One or more prominent nucleoli are present. Specialized membrane junctions are seen, e.g., tight junctions, desmosomes, and gap junctions, suggesting an epithelial origin for SCC. In one case, intracellular cilia have been observed, but this is a rarity.

Chromosomes and Isoenzymes

Chromosome analysis utilizing Giemsa banding techniques has been carried out on many SCC lines,[7] and all were found to be of human origin. The modal numbers of chromosomes ranged from 40 to 88, some cell lines containing 2, and 1 line containing 3 modal concentrations.

The isoenzyme pattern of all cell lines tested for glucose-6-phosphate dehydrogenase indicated only the presence of the A band,[7] and, on this basis, it was concluded that SCC lines were not contaminated with HeLa cells.

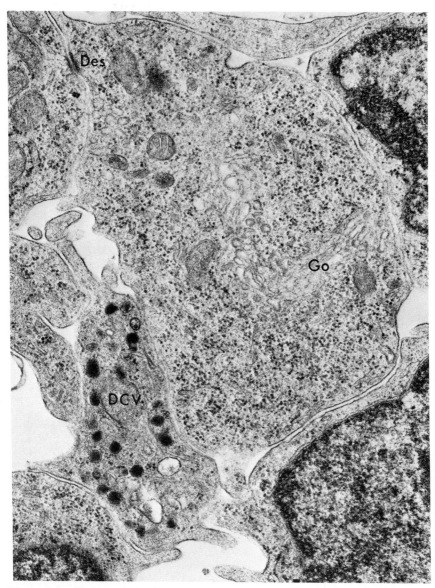

Figure 3-8. *Characteristic ultrastructure of SCC cell lines. Note characteristic dense-core vesicles (DCV), membrane junction, seen here as a desmosome (DES), and active Golgi region (Go). Numerous free ribosomes are present, but rough endoplastic reticulum is scanty. Original magnification × 35,000.*

Growth Rate

Doubling times were found to be relatively long and variable for SCC cell lines (Table 3-2).[7] Even though the growth rate has increased as cell lines were passaged over a period of several years, the most rapidly growing cells require 36 hr for one population doubling, and some require as long as 3–4 wk.

The incorporation of ^{3}H thymidine (TdR) was measured autoradiographically, to evaluate the proportion of cells in the population that were in the S period of the cell cycle, under conditions of pulse labeling (Table 3-2). Cells were labeled for 1 hr in a medium containing 1 μC/ml ^{3}H-TdR and were washed one time to remove excess ^{3}H-TdR before fixation. Labeling indices, when compared to doubling times, illustrate the great variation in growth that exists among cell lines. A cell line such in DMS 55, which has a labeling index of 45.3 percent and a doubling time of 4.8 days, when compared with DMS 53, which has a labeling index of 19.9 percent but also has a doubling time of 4.9 days, illustrates the point. Either the duration of the S period is twice as long in DMS 55, or the death rate of cells is higher than that of DMS 53. Another and perhaps significant difference lies in their growth pattern: DMS 55 grows primarily in suspension, whereas DMS 53 grows only when attached. In general, the attached cell lines have lower labeling indices, and DMS 79, which grows only in suspension, has the highest labeling index. No correlation between labeling indices and doubling times is apparent in these data, indicating the need to investigate other variable factors.

Cell cycle time has been determined for one cell line by the percent labeled mitosis method (PLM).[7] For DMS 79, the estimated cycle time measured by PLM was 28 hr. However, at that time, doubling time of a population of DMS 79 cells was estimated to be 4 days in vitro and 10 days in vivo, as measured in tumors in nude mice. The extended doubling time in vivo was clearly related to cell death, which was apparent in sections of the tumor. Cell death in DMS 79 in vitro was not extensive in cell cultures, as the average cell viability was estimated to be 90 percent by trypan blue dye exclusion techniques. Some cells may persist in a nondividing state for much longer than the measured cycle time. In PLM methods, the analysis was based only on cells undergoing mitosis. When DMS 79 cells were continuously exposed to low levels of ^{3}H-TdR, only 60 percent were labeled at 36 hr, but, after 72 hours, the percentage had increased to 96 percent. The best estimate of the total cycle time was 28 hr (above), during which time slightly more than half the population passed through DNA

Table 3-2
Summary of In Vitro Characteristics of Cell Lines Obtained from Patients with a Pathologic Diagnosis of Small Cell Carcinoma of the Lung

| Cell Line* | Tissue of Origin | Patient Data | | Doubling Time | Labeling Index | Total Months in Culture | Hormones Produced | Oncogenicity in Nude Mice§ |
		Sex	Age (yr)					
DMS 44	Bone marrow aspirate	M	62		22.8%	26	Calc, ACTH, Glu, E-2	+
DMS 47	Liver biopsy	M	40	(4 wk)†	ND‡	15	E-2	ND
DMS 53	Lung biopsy	M	53	4.9 days	19.9	59	Calc, ACTH, PTH, LH, hCG, GH, SRIF, NP, E-2	+
DMS 55	Bone marrow aspirate	F	74	4.8 days	45.3	52	ACTH, LH, NP, E-2	–
DMS 79	Pleural fluid	M	64	5.8 days	56.4	51	Calc, ACTH, PTH, β-end, Lipo, NP, E-2	+
DMS 92	Bone marrow aspirate	M	39	5.5 days	24.3	47	ACTH, N , E-2	+
DMS 106	Bone marrow aspirate	F	61	ND	ND	5		ND
DMS 114	Lung biopsy	M	65	1.6 days	25.3	48	ACTH, TH, Glu, Pro, NP, E-2	+
DMS 139[a]	Bone marrow aspirate	M	57	5 wk	ND	14		ND
DMS 148[a]	Liver (autopsy)	M	57	4–5 wk	20.9	25	ACTH, E-2	ND

DMS 149[a]	Lung (autopsy)	M	57	4–5 wk	18.2	18	ACTH, E-2	ND
DMS 153[b]	Liver (autopsy)	M	44	5.8 days	12.1	42	Calc, ACTH, NP, E-2	+
DMS 154[b]	Lymph node (autopsy)	M	44	5 wk	22.1	25		ND
DMS 187	Bone marrow aspirate	M	52	4.1 days	ND	39	NP, E-2	+
DMS 217	Pericardial mass (autopsy)	M	57	4 wk	ND	15	ACTH, NP, E-2	ND
DMS 235[c]	Bone marrow aspirate	F	44	4.6 days	ND	26	Calc, LH, NP, E-2	ND
DMS 240[c]	Liver (autopsy)	F	4	7.4 days	ND	26		ND
DMS 273	Pleural fluid	F	50	6.2 days	ND	16		+
DMS 319[d]	Pleural fluid	M	62		ND	8		ND
DMS 329[d]	Bone marrow aspirate	M	62		ND	7		ND
DMS 330[d]	Pleural fluid	M	62		ND	5	ACTH	ND
DMS 333[d]	Lung (autopsy)	M	62		ND	9		ND
DMS 353	Pleural fluid	M	71		ND	8		ND

From Pettengill et al.[7]

*(a)–(d), multiple specimens on 4 patients.

†Figures in parentheses indicate subculture interval, approximately equal to one doubling time.

‡ND, not done.

§From Pettengill et al.[26]

69

synthesis (S) and thus contributed to these calculations. It appears, then, that a portion of cells in the DMS 79 population (i.e., 40 percent) persist in the nondividing state for longer than the estimated 28-hr cycle time.

APUD Characteristics of SCC Lines

SCC has been categorized as having "amine precursor uptake and decarboxylation" (APUD) characteristics. This concept originated with Pearse,[13] and Tischler[12] has summarized these characteristics, especially with reference to the origin of neuroendocrine tumors. APUD cells were originally grouped together because of their common histochemical similarities, which include (1) the uptake and decarboxylation of amines that can be detected by FIF, (2) the ability to synthesize biogenic amines and/or peptide hormones, and (3) the presence of acetylcholinesterase and other enzymes. Because some cells within this group were shown to be derived embryologically from the neural crest, the supposition was made that all neuroendocrinelike cells that have APUD characteristics might share the same embryologic origin. However, no evidence is available as yet for the neural-crest origin of bronchial epithelial cells.

K-type cells of the bronchial epithelium possess some of these characteristics, i.e., presence of neurosecretorylike granules (DCV), a high content of serotonin, which may be associated with one type of DCV, and a high level of acetylcholinesterase activity.[14] The concept of K cells as the putative cell of origin of SCC is based on their common possession of these characteristics. Table 3-3 summarizes the appearance of these properties in those cell lines that have been examined thus far.

None of these cell lines store biogenic amines at sufficient levels to fluoresce when exposed to formaldehyde vapors.[15] This is a general characteristic of APUD cells.[12] However, most cell lines can accumulate L-dopa added to the medium and then become highly fluorescent, as illustrated in Figure 3-9 and Table 3-3.

Acetylcholinesterase was demonstrated histochemically in some cell lines, but not in others (Table 3-3). For these studies, mouse neuroblastoma N18 was used as a positive control. In addition to acetylthiocholine, butyrylthiocholine was also utilized as a substrate, to indicate the presence of nonspecific cholinesterases.

Of those examined, only DMS 79 did not contain acetylcholinesterase or butyrylcholinesterase activity. It also did not exhibit formaldehyde-induced fluorescence after incubation with L-dopa.

Staining of dissociated cells from several cell lines for demonstration of argyrophilia[17] showed that silver grains were present in some cell lines,

Table 3-3
APUD-like Characteristics

Cell line	Formaldehyde-Induced Fluorescence*		Acetyl-cholinesterase[t] Activity	Argyrophilia[‡]
	Endogenous	After Pre-incubation in L-dopa		
DMS 53	−	+ + + +	+	+ + +
DMS 55	−	+ + +		−
DMS 79	−	−	−	+ +
DMS 114	−	+ +	+	−
DMS 153	−	+ + + +		−
DMS 187	−	+ + + +	+	
DMS 235				−
DMS 240	−	+ + +		
DMS 273	−	+ +	+	+

*Formaldehyde-induced fluorescence, after method of Falck and Owman.[15] Cells were examined before and after incubation in 50 μg/ml L-dopa for 1 hr.
[t]Acetylcholinesterase, examined histochemically by method of El Badawi and Schenck,[16] using acetylthiocholine and butyrylthiocholine as substrates.
[‡]Argyrophil staining, after method of Pascual.[17] Cells were trypsinized, collected on slides by cytocentrifuge, and fixed in 4 percent Formalin prior to staining.

but other cell lines were essentially negative (Table 3-3 and Fig. 3-10). There was no correlation between FIF and argyrophilia. The most striking difference was seen in DMS 153, in which cells fluoresce intensely (FIF) after preincubation with L-dopa, but contain no argyrophilia. DMS 53 reacted strongly with both staining techniques. Although this is an interesting difference, neither method is specific for any of the amines, and this observation emphasizes the need for further specific characterization of these cell lines by other methods.

Hormone Synthesis and Secretion

A variety of peptide hormones have been identified by radioimmunoassay (RIA) in the culture medium from SCC cell lines (Table 3-2).[18] Not all cell lines have been assayed for each peptide. A summary of the peptides known to be found in the medium indicates the wide spectrum synthesized by some cell lines, such as DMS 53. The question of whether or not a single cell is producing more than one hormone is being examined in two ways: isolation of cloned populations and immunocytochemical localization.

Clones have been isolated from several cell lines. Preliminary data

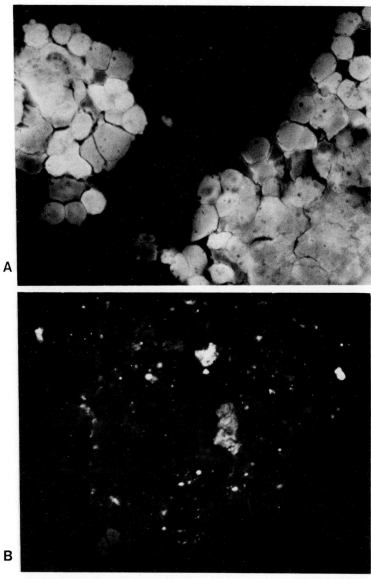

Figure 3-9. *Formaldehyde-induced fluorescence (FIF). DMS 55 cells, incubated 1 hr with 50 μg/ml L-dopa. Cell smears prepared by cytocentrifugation, and cells exposed to formaldehyde vapor according to Falck and Owman.[15] Original magnification × 500. (A) Test preparation, with positive fluorescence. (B) Control preparation, lacking incubation with formaldehyde. Bright spots represent artefactual fluorescence, of a bright yellow color, probably caused by presence of some dead cells. Green fluorescence is present in positive preparations. Original magnification × 500.*

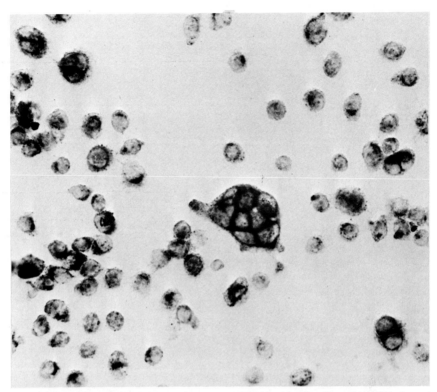

Figure 3-10. *Argyrophilia. DMS 53 cells, trypsinized, and collected on slide by cyto-centrifugation. Silver stain[17] to demonstrate argyrophilia. Original magnification* × *500.*

indicate the production of ACTH, calcitonin, and somatostatin by all five clones isolated from DMS 53, which secretes all three of these peptides. In no clone is there complete deletion of any of these peptides, nor is there a greater level in any clone than that observed in the parent cell line. These data suggest that a single cell can synthesize more than a single hormone. Further investigation is required for complete understanding of this characteristic.

With an additional cell line (DMS 114), segregation of a parental characteristic was observed among clones. The presence of gap junctions observed in the parent cell line was noted in one clone, but not in a second clone isolated at the same time, suggesting the presence of at least two different cell types in the parent population.

The relatively consistent levels at which different cell lines continue to produce their particular peptides over time has been observed repeatedly. This has been notably true of ACTH production, both in vitro and in vivo in tumors arising in nude mice from inoculated cultured cells. Cell lines known to be high, moderate, or low producers of immunoreactive ACTH in culture repeatedly give rise to tumors that contain extractable ACTH in the same relative quantities (C. C. Cate, O. S. Pettengill, and G. D. Sorenson, manuscript in preparation).

In addition to peptide hormones, the secretion of estradiol into culture medium appears in most cell lines that have been assayed, and, in all but one cell line, higher levels were found in cell lines from female patients than in those from males.[18] The presence of estradiol in medium was a surprising finding. The first steps in determining the extent to which estradiol biosynthesis can be carried out by SCC in vitro, and the precursors required, have been described with DMS 44 cells; these were found to be capable of aromatizing testosterone, converting it to estradiol.[19]

With the use of DMS 79 cells, which synthesize a number of related peptides, information concerning their relative rates of synthesis and their relationship to a high-molecular-weight precursor molecule, has been investigated. ACTH, β-lipotropin, γ-lipotropin, and β-endorphin were secreted simultaneously into the medium and appeared to be derived from a common high-molecular-weight precursor molecule also present in the culture medium.[20,21]

Using the media from the same cell line and immune affinity chromatography, it was possible to distinguish immunoreactive calcitonin from ACTH and its related peptides.[22] These data strongly suggest the lack of a common precursor molecule for human ACTH and calcitonin.

Somatostatin is secreted in varying amounts by SCC cell lines (Table 3-2). Its synthesis by DMS 53 cells has been examined with both immunoreactivity and biological activity.[23] The secretion of a high-molecular-weight form as well as the low-molecular-weight form were described, and the larger molecule may be a precursor of the biologically active smaller form.

Discussion

The adaptation of tumor cells from SCC to in vitro conditions has permitted a closer examination of the biological properties of this histologic type of lung tumor. The putative cell of origin of SCC is currently thought to be the Kulchitsky or K-type cell of the bronchial epithelium. An argyrophil cell, classified as a member of the APUD system, the K-type cell is circumstantially thought to arise from the neural crest region of the embryo because of its similarities to neuroendocrine cells known to be derived from the neural crest. SCC cells likewise have many properties similar to those of neuroendocrine cells. This has led to a search for specific properties that might permit positive identification of the cell of origin. In the normal lung, K cells are thought to function as chemoreceptors, responding to ambient alveolar oxygen tension.[14,24] They are characterized by the presence of acetylcholinesterase and high levels of serotonin, the latter thought to be the mediator of vasoregulator effects. The presence of DCV in the cytoplasm of K cells observed by electron microscopy is considered to be the critical mark of identification for SCC.[12] These properties have been used to characterize SCC in vitro cell lines.

With one exception, synthesis of peptide hormones, which has frequently been associated with the tumor in patients, is not known to be associated with the bronchial K cell. The only peptide that has as yet been recognized in a lung cell, by immunohistochemical techniques, is bombesin, which exhibits vasoactive properties.[25] Bombesin has been found in fetal and neonatal human lung cells of bronchial and bronchiolar epithelium, both in single cells and in small clumps of cells that were variable in shape and located close to the basement membrane. No bombesin has been found in adult lung, although endocrine cells are known to be present.[25]

It has generally been assumed that synthesis of hormones by SCC cells is related to the level of gene derepression that has occurred in their transformation to tumor cells, as, with the possible exception of bombesin, peptide synthesis is not known to be a function of normal lung cells. The wide variation in properties among the SCC cell lines that have been described here suggests that each tumor cell line may consist of a population of cells that express a phenotype associated with the particular level of the developmental pathway achieved by the cell of origin of this tumor. The ability to synthesize and secrete hormones is not uniformly present (on the basis of current data) in all cell lines, nor is their expression of properties associated with APUD cells in general, and K-type cells specifically.

Common properties expressed by all continuous SCC cell lines that have been described here are presence of DCV, membrane junctions characteristic of epithelial cells, and the growth of tumors in nude athymic mice inoculated with cultured cells[26] (see also Chapter 5, this monograph).

References

1. Oboshi S, Tsugawa S, Seido T, et al: A new floating cell line derived from human pulmonary carcinoma of oat cell type. Gan 62:505–516, 1971

2. Ellison ML, Hillyard CJ, Bloomfield GA, et al: Ectopic hormone production by bronchial carcinomas in culture. Clin Endocrinol (Suppl) 5:397S–406S, 1976

3. Ohara H, Okamoto T: A new in vitro cell line established from human oat cell carcinoma of the lung. Cancer Res 37:3088–3095, 1977

4. Tsuji K, Hayata Y, Sato M: Neuronal differentiation of oat cell carcinoma in vitro by dibutyryl cyclic adenosine 3′,5′-monophosphate. Cancer Lett 1:311–318, 1976

5. Tischler AS, Dichter M, Biales B: Electrical excitability of oat cell carcinoma. J Pathol 122:153–157, 1977

6. Pettengill OS, Faulkner CS, Wurster-Hill DH, et al: Isolation and characterization of a hormone-producing cell line from human small cell anaplastic carcinoma of the lung. J Natl Cancer Inst 58:511–518, 1977

7. Pettengill OS, Sorenson GD, Wurster-Hill DH, et al: Isolation and growth characteristics of continuous cell lines from small-cell carcinoma of the lung. Cancer 45:906–918, 1980

8. Wurster-Hill DH, Maurer LH: Cytogenetic diagnosis of cancer: Abnormalities of chromosomes and polyploid levels in the bone marrow of patients with small cell anaplastic carcinoma of the lung. J Natl Cancer Inst 61:1065–1070, 1978

9. Usage of vertebrate cell culture terminology, TCA Newsl 10:1–4, 1976

10. Ponten J: Spontaneous and Virus Induced Transformation in Cell Culture. New York, Springer-Verlag, 1971, p 30

11. Sutherland RM, McCredie JA, Inch WR: Growth of multicellular spheroids in tissue culture as a model of nodular carcinomas. J Natl Cancer Inst 46:113–120, 1971

12. Tischler AS, Dichter MA, Biales B, et al: Neuroendocrine neoplasms and their cell of origin. N Engl J Med 296:919–925, 1977

13. Pearse AGE: Neurocristopathy, neuroendocrine pathology and the APUD concept. Z Krebsforsch 84:1–18, 1975

14. Lauweryns JM, Cokelaere M, Dellersnyder M, et al: Intrapulmonary neuroepithelial bodies in newborn rabbits. Influence of hypoxia and hyperoxia, hypercapnia, nicotine, reserpine, L-DOPA and 5-HTP. Cell Tissue Res 182:425–440, 1977

15. Falck B, Owman C: A detailed methodological description of the fluorescence method for the cellular demonstration of biogenic amines. Acta Univ Lund, Sect II (7):1–23, 1965

16. El-Badawi A, Schenk EA: Histochemical methods for separate, consecutive and simultaneous demonstration of acetylcholinesterase and norepinephrine in cryostat sections. J Histochem Cytochem 15:580–588, 1967

17. Pascual JSF: A new method for easy demonstration of argyrophil cells. Stain Technol 51:231–235, 1976

18. Sorenson GD, Pettengill OS, Brinck-Johnsen T, et al: Hormone production by cultures of small cell carcinoma of the lung. Cancer 1980.

19. Brinck-Johnsen T, Pettengill OS, Brinck-Johnsen K, et al: Estrogen production by an established cell line from pulmonary small cell anaplastic carcinoma. J Steroid Biochem 10:339–340, 1979

20. Bertagna XY, Nicholson WE, Sorenson GD, et al: Corticotropin, lipotropin, and β-endorphin production by a human nonpituitary tumor in culture: Evidence for a common precursor. Proc Natl Acad Sci USA 75:5160–5164, 1978

21. Bertagna XY, Nicholson WE, Tanaka K, et al: Ectopic production of ACTH, lipotropin, and β-endorphin by human cancer cells. Structurally related tumor markers. Recent Results Cancer Res 67:16–25, 1979

22. Bertagna XY, Nicholson WE, Pettengill OS, et al: Ectopic production of high molecular weight calcitonin and corticotropin by human small cell carcinoma cells in tissue culture: Evidence for separate precursors. J Clin Endocrinol Metab 47:1390–1393, 1978

23. Szabo M, Berelowitz M, Pettengill OS, et al: Somatostatin (SRIF) secretion by cultured human small cell carcinoma of the lung. Abst 287. 61st Annual Meeting, Endocrine Society, Anaheim, 1979

24. Lauweryns JM, Cokelaere M, Lerut T, et al: Cross-circulation studies on the influence of hypoxia and hypoxaemia on neuro-epithelial bodies in young rabbits. Cell Tissue Res 193:373–386, 1978

25. Wharton J, Pollak JM, Bloom SR, et al: Bombesin-like immunoreactivity in the lung. Nature 273:769–770, 1978

26. Pettengill OS, Curphey TJ, Cate CC, et al: Animal model for small cell carcinoma of the lung. Effect of immunosuppression and sex of mouse on tumor growth in nude athymic mice. Exp Cell Biol 48:278–297, 1980

4

IN VITRO CLONING OF SMALL CELL CARCINOMA OF THE LUNG

Desmond N. Carney
Adi F. Gazdar
Paul A. Bunn, Jr.
John D. Minna

Cell culture and cloning techniques have long been applied to the study of the biology of normal and malignant mammalian cells. An extension of this demonstrated by Hamburger and Salmon is the ability of freshly isolated human tumor cells to form colonies in soft agar.[1] Colony-forming cells have now been quantitated from a number of human tumors including: multiple myeloma, ovarian carcinoma, transitional cell carcinoma of the bladder, neuroblastoma, melanoma, and breast and colon cancer.[2-9] This assay may be useful in predicting response to therapy. Salmon et al. found evidence of a correlation between in vitro drug sensitivity and clinical response for multiple myeloma and ovarian carcinoma.[10] Such information is potentially of great value in optimizing therapy for small cell lung cancer patients.

Although many tumor types may clone in the two-layer assay, the growth requirements for the individual tumor types have not been established. Colony formation for myeloma cells is dependent on the presence of conditioned medium from oil-primed mouse-spleen adherent cells.[1] Colony formation for other types of tumor cells has not demonstrated a

We are indebted to Virginia Bertness and Joan Wilson for their assistance in specimen collection and cytology preparation of specimens and colonies.

Table 4-1
Correlation of Histology with Agarose Clonogenicity

Specimen Source	No.	Pathologic Diagnosis of Specimen	
		SCC Positive*	SCC Negative*
Bone marrow	60	13/14	6/46
Pleural effusion	15	6/8	1/7
Lymph node	9	9/9	—
Liver	7	4/5	0/2
Total	91	32/36 (89%)	7/55

*Number of specimens with colony formation/number of specimens plated.

requirement for this conditioned medium.[5] Using the present system for different tumors, approximately one colony-forming cell is found per 10^3–10^4 nucleated cells plated. As culture conditions are improved and specific growth factors are identified for individual tumors, one would expect an increase in colony formation from the present minimum estimate.

Although small cell carcinoma of the lung (SCC) grows rapidly in patients, it is difficult to grow in tissue culture. The in vitro growth requirements of SCC have been so stringent, both in our work and in that of others,[11,12] that no systematic studies have been undertaken on the clonogenicity in a semisolid medium of SCC obtained directly from patients. We describe here the successful cloning of tumor cells from specimens of metastatic human SCC obtained directly from patients and compare the results with those obtained using established cultures of SCC treated under identical conditions.

Materials and Methods

Specimens from patients with histologically documented SCC were obtained simultaneously with those biopsies and aspirates that were routinely acquired for initial staging and restaging to assess response to therapy or relapse. Specimens were obtained from bone marrows, pleural effusions, lymph node aspirates and biopsies, and liver biopsies obtained under direct vision at peritoneoscopy. Part of each specimen was processed for cytological examination and histological examination (except for pleural effusions which were examined only cytologically) and for testing in the clonogenic assay. The detailed methods used for preparing the SCC specimens, their cloning in 0.3 percent agarose, and analysis by cytology and flow cytometry (FCM) are reported elsewhere,[13-15] as are the details of establishment and characterization of the continuous lines of small cell carcinoma.[11]

Results

Ninety-one specimens were obtained from 53 patients with SCC. Fifty-five specimens were from untreated patients and the remainder from patients undergoing staging procedures after receiving induction therapy or in relapse from primary cytotoxic therapy. Sixty specimens were obtained from bone marrow aspirates, 15 from pleural effusions, 9 from lymph node aspirations, and 7 from liver biopsies (Table 4-1). Pathological examination of the clinical biopsy specimens revealed evidence of SCC in 36 specimens. Colony formation was observed in 32 out of 36 specimens (89 percent) with histocytopathological evidence of SCC and in 7 out of 55 specimens histocytopathologically negative for SCC. In SCC positive specimens, colonies consisted of approximately 100–1000 tightly packed cells forming spherical aggregates (Fig. 4-1). No free layer of cells was observed at the periphery of these colonies, a feature typical of macrophage colonies. Cell doubling was observed 24–48 hr after plating, and colonies reached their peak size 7–10 days after plating, indicating an in vitro doubling time of less than 24 hr (1000 cells in 10 days). Although initial growth was brisk, cell death usually occurred 14–21 days after plating. No attempt was made to refeed these agarose plates. The number of colonies per plate ranged from 3 to 262, yielding a colony-forming efficiency (CFE) per plated nucleated cell of 0.003–0.26 percent (Table 4-2). The mean number of colonies per plate was 66.6, with a median of 22. Thus, the maximum CFE was 0.26 percent, but more often the CFE was considerably less. No difference in the generation of colonies between untreated and treated patients was observed. In addition, colony formation was observed equally in specimens obtained from the 4 metastatic sites of SCC tested.

The percentage of malignant cells in each positive specimen ranged from <1/1000 to up to 75 percent of the total specimen. The calculated CFE per plated SCC ranged from 0.05 to 1.5 percent, very similar to that observed for the established SCC lines (Table 4-3). In a small number of specimens, plating of cells over a concentration range of 10^2–10^6 cells provided evidence of linearity between the number of SCC cells plated and the number of colonies formed.

Cytological examination of multiple colonies from each positive specimen revealed only cells with the typical morphological appearance of SCC

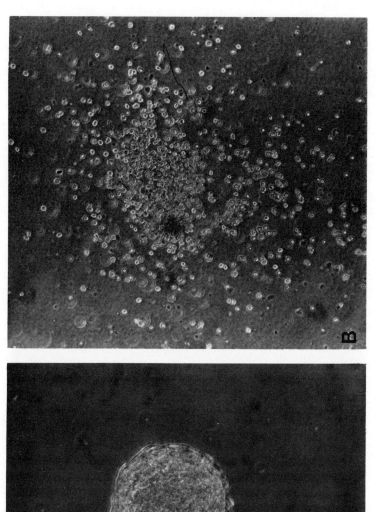

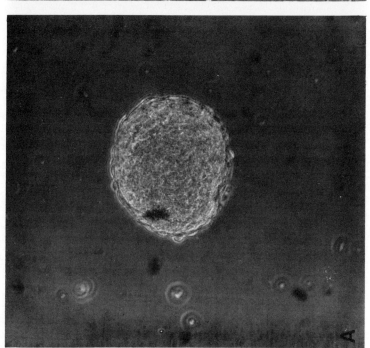

Figure 4-1. *Comparison of (A) a typical SCC colony with (B) a hemopoietic stem cell colony, both cultured from patients with SCC. The SCC cells are in tightly packed spherical aggregates, in contrast to the more loosely arranged bone marrow hemopoietic stem cell colony. Phase contrast × 32.*

82

Table 4-2
Colony-Forming Efficiency of SCC Stem Cells

Specimen Source	No. colonies per 10^5 cells plated	CFE per plated SCC*
Bone marrow	6–135	0.3 –1.0
Pleural effusion	3–250	0.4 –1.5
Lymph node	15–96	0.05–1.0
Liver	62–262	0.09–1.0
Range	3–262†	0.05–1.5

*Colony-forming efficiency (CFE) = $\dfrac{\text{number of colonies} \times 100}{\text{number of SCC cells plated}}$

†Mean, 66; median, 22.

(Fig. 4-2). Mitoses were evident in the majority of colonies examined. The cells had the same morphological characteristics as the tumor cells in the original biopsy specimen.

Examination (macroscopic and microscopic) of the colonies in the 7 specimens pathologically negative for SCC revealed colonies with the typical characteristics of SCC in 3 specimens. A review of the concentrated cytology specimen prepared from the cell suspension of these 3 specimens immediately prior to plating revealed typical SCC cells, suggesting that sampling problems had accounted for the initial discrepancy. In the 4 remaining specimens, colonies morphologically different from those observed in the positive SCC specimens were observed. These colonies ranged from 3 to 85 per plate and, unlike the typical SCC colonies, showed heterogeneity of clone size with varying proportions of compact and diffuse colonies, features typical of granulocytic, mixed, and macrophage bone marrow cell colonies (Figure 4-2). Cytological examination of these colonies revealed large mononuclear cells that appeared to be immature members of the granulocytic series.

The influence of conditioned medium from an established SCC cell line on the CFE of fresh tumor specimens is indicated in Table 4-4. The CFE was increased in the majority of specimens (10 out of 18), and, although the increase in number was modest (1.5–2.0), the size of individual colonies in these specimens was greatly increased (Fig. 4-3). Conditioned medium did not have any influence on the growth of hemopoetic stem cell colonies.

Flow cytometry of clinical specimens before culture demonstrated aneuploid tumor cells in the majority of specimens with pathologic evidence of SCC.[15] FCM analysis of cells pooled from agarose colonies revealed DNA histograms with a single aneuploid peak, proving that, as expected,

Table 4-3
Colony-Forming Efficiency, Subculture, and
Tumorigenicity of SCC Colonies

Specimen Source	Colony-Forming Efficiency*	Subculture in Liquid Medium	Tumorigenicity in Athymic Nude Mice
Cell Lines			
NCI H60	1.0	8/8	+
NCI H64	1.0	—	+
NCI H69	2.5	—	+
NCI H128	0.8	5/8	+
NCI H146	1.3	—	+
NCI H187	1.6	—	+
NCI N231	5.6	8/10	+
Total	0.8–5.6	21/26	7/7
Clinical Specimens			
Bone marrow	0.3–1.0	0/40	1/1
Pleural effusion	0.4–1.5	0/15	—
Lymph node	0.05–1.0	0/45	—
Liver	0.09–1.5	0/25	—
Total	0.05–1.5	0/125	1/1

*Per plated small cell.

the cells growing in agarose were the tumor cells and not normal cells (Fig. 4-4). The aneuploid peak observed in the colonies was identical to the aneuploid peak in the clinical specimen, showing that no change in DNA content occurred with growth in agarose.

A major question regarding the tumor cells growing in agarose is whether they are capable of continuous growth (self-renewal). We tested this by transferring individual colonies to microwell cultures. None of the subcloned colonies from fresh tumor specimens yielded continuous replicating cell lines. In contrast, colonies cultured from established SCC cell lines continued to replicate in 80 percent of cases (Table 4-3).

It is possible that some aspect of tissue culture was not optimal for the growth of the fresh SCC colonies. Therefore, we tried another approach. In prior studies with established SCC cell lines we had found that the brain of the nude mouse allowed growth of these cells with 100–1000-fold greater sensitivity than regular routes of inoculation. We pooled agarose colonies from a fresh tumor specimen and inoculated them intracranially into an athymic nude mouse. The animal developed signs of intracranial tumor after 12 wks and was sacrificed. Histologic examination of the brain

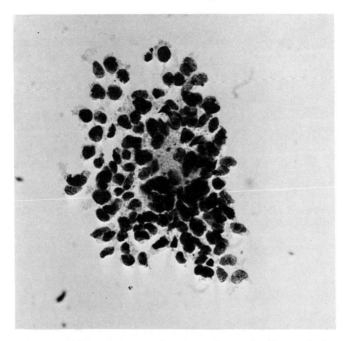

Figure 4-2. *Dispersed cells from a single SCC colony revealing typical cytological characteristics of SCC cells: scant cytoplasm nuclear molding, finely granular chromatin, and inconspicuous nucleoli. Hematoxylin and eosin. Original magnification × 400.*

revealed typical SCC cells with infiltration of the meninges and brain parenchyma. The DNA content of this tumor measured by FCM was identical to the original clinical specimen and to agarose colonies of the clinical specimen. Cells from this mouse tumor have remained proliferating in culture medium for over 3 mo.

Discussion

To date, many of the in vitro studies on the biology of SCC have been carried out on established tissue-culture cell lines. Whereas these studies have provided data on the growth and biochemical characteristics of SCC, the passage of these cells in culture or in an intermediate animal host may favor the selection of subpopulations of tumor cells during the many months of adaption and transplantation required to develop an autonomous cell line. Such selected cell lines may not be entirely representative of the tissue origin and are likely to have an expanded stem cell capacity.

Table 4-4
Influence of SCC-Conditioned Medium on the CFE of
SCC Positive Specimens

Specimen Source	Total No.	No. Demonstrating Increased CFE with CM	Range of Increased CFE*
Bone marrow	6	4	1.2–2.8
Pleural effusion	5	2	2.0[†]
Lymph node	4	2	1.1–2.0
Liver	3	2	1.6–1.8
Total	18	10	1.1–2.8

*No. colonies in CM/No. colonies in culture medium.
[†]In one specimen, colonies were observed only in the plates containing CM.

The direct culture of clonogenic cells from involved patient specimens in a semisolid medium would avoid such selection and subcloning. The cell-line approach has advantages over short-term colony assays, however, including the ability to perform repeated experiments, to prepare large quantities of cellular material, and to have absolute control over cellular growth conditions. Obviously both approaches are complementary.

Methods of culturing human tumors directly from biopsies of patients in a clonogenic assay in a semisolid medium should permit study of the biology of human cancers and identification of specific growth factor requirements of each tumor type, and may predict for chemotherapeutic responses.[10] If therapeutic and biologic studies are to be based on the clonogenic assay, however, one must provide evidence for the neoplastic origin of the colonies, correlate the generation of colonies with tumor involvement with the patient specimens, test for the "stem cell" (self-renewing) nature of the tumor cells in vitro, and correlate in vivo with in vitro responses. In this study we have demonstrated that specimens containing histologically identifiable metastatic tumor from patients with SCC form colonies in agarose with an efficiency of up to 1.5 percent per plated SCC and 0.003–0.26 percent of the nucleated cells plated. This compares favorably with the CFE for the established SCC culture cell lines and also with other fresh tumor specimens from a variety of tumor types.[2-9] Overall colony formation was observed in 89 percent of specimens with histocytopathological evidence of SCC. This excellent correlation between pathological examination of specimens and the development of colonies confirms the usefulness of this system in selectively favoring the growth of tumor cell colonies to the exclusion of non-neoplastic cells, including fibroblasts and other stromal cells. If approximately 1 percent of the cytolog-

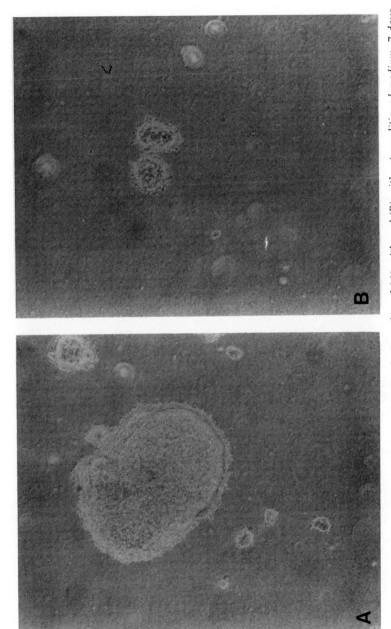

Figure 4-3. *Morphological appearance of SCC colonies cultured (A) with and (B) without conditioned medium, 7 days after plating a pleural effusion cytologically positive for SCC. Note increased size of colonies cultured with conditioned medium. Phase contrast × 100.*

87

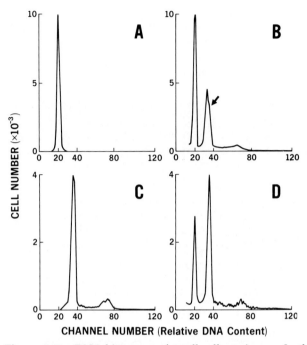

Figure 4-4. *DNA histogram of small cell carcinoma. In this study the electronics of the instrument were adjusted so that the G_0/G_1 peak of the diploid standard was in channel 20 (A). (B) FCM analysis of a pleural fluid specimen cytologically positive for SCC reveals two peaks: a large diploid peak in channel 20 and a smaller aneuploid peak in channel 37 (arrow). FCM analysis of agarose colonies cultured from this specimen reveals only a single aneuploid leak (C), which was confirmed by the addition of standard diploid lymphocytes to the specimen (D). Cytological examination of the colonies revealed only cells with typical SCC morphology.*

ically identifiable SCC cells in fresh tumor specimens can form colonies in vitro, then one can estimate that cytologically negative specimens without colony formation contain less than 0.1–0.01 percent of the nucleated cells plated as SCC cells. The formation of SCC cell colonies in specimens pathologically negative for SCC suggests that this assay may be more sensitive than standard pathological methods in detecting tumor cells in clinical specimens. This sensitivity would be greatly increased by conditions that would permit more of the SCC cells to replicate and form colonies.

The correlation between the development of SCC colonies and histo-

cytopathological evidence of SCC in the patient specimens is highly suggestive that these colonies are of neoplastic cell origin. However, the occasional growth of nontumorigenic colonies in bone marrow specimens
stresses the need for further studies to confirm the origin of colonies in
this assay. Cytological examination of multiple individually picked colonies from SCC positive specimens revealed only cells with the typical morphology of SCC, confirming that in these specimens colony growth was
caused by the proliferation of SCC in vitro. The demonstration of aneuploidy in colonies and the ability of colonies from a single specimen to
form a typical SCC tumor in athymic mice lends further confirmation to
the neoplastic origin of the colonies.

The development of bone marrow stem cell colonies in a small number of specimens without the use of specific growth factors is not altogether surprising, as one might expect to see a small number of such colonies when 1×10^5 cells are plated.[17] The appearance of these colonies in
patients with SCC might also suggest that the neoplastic cells may be producing hemopoietic humoral regulators capable of stimulating bone marrow stem cell colony formation. Morphologically these bone marrow stem
cell colonies were very different from the SCC stem cell colonies, and cytological examination of these colonies clearly distinguished them from typical SCC colonies.

The wide range in CFE from specimen to specimen, and the variation
in individual colony size in the same specimens suggests that heterogeneity of SCC may exist. Heterogeneity of SCC has been demonstrated in
vivo,[16] and it is possible that these variations in CFE and colony size
among colony-forming cells in vitro represent different subpopulations of
SCC cells in the tumor specimen. Studies using monoclonal antibodies or
cytogenetic analysis of cells in individual colonies may give us a clearer
indication of the homogeneity of the stem cells in the tumor specimen. We
have studied the behavior of SCC stem cells from metastatic sites only.
Clearly, studies of stem cells from the site of origin of the tumor and comparison to metastatic clones will be important and may be helpful in the
elucidation of the metastatic process.

The rapid growth of SCC stem cells, with a calculated in vitro doubling time of approximately 24 hr, is considerably more rapid than the
population doubling times found in patients and in established SCC cell
culture lines.[11,18] This significantly more rapid doubling time of stem cell
colonies compared with the clinical in vivo situation has also been reported for multiple myeloma stem cells (in vitro doubling time of 3 days
compared with an in vivo population doubling time of 2–6 mo for a
myeloma clone in the clinical phase) and for ovarian carcinoma stem

cells.[2,4] This phenomenon, coupled with the low CFE of fresh tumor specimens, suggests that a very small subpopulation of cells in a given tumor specimen has sufficient proliferative potential for colony formation in vitro and suggests that, in vivo, the tumor population and growth are maintained by activity of this subpopulation. Other factors, including cell death in vivo, differences in the in vivo environment, feedback regulation, or exit of cells from the proliferative cycle, may also be of importance. It appears, therefore, that the SCC tumor cell population is heterogenous in its growth potential, consisting of a majority of cells with little proliferative capacity which are maintained by the activity of a small subpopulation of cells with proliferative potential.

Although the source of the specimen did not influence the ability of SCC stems cells to proliferate, the number of colonies was lowest in the lymph node specimens. This result may be explained by the influence of the process of mechanical dissociation on the subsequent ability of the neoplastic cells to proliferate or on immunologic features. That techniques necessary to generate single-cell suspensions from solid tumor specimens thus often result in a suspension of nonviable cells may limit our ability to perform clonogenic experiments from solid tumors. Methods to improve the means of obtaining a viable single-cell suspension, including the use of a variety of enzymes, such as trypsin, collagenase, pronase, and mixtures of these, with and without mechanical dissociation may extend the use of the clonogenic assay to a large variety of solid tumors.[19] Some of these enzymes have been demonstrated to be of value in freeing tumor cells from surrounding stroma without decreasing the CFE of fresh specimens.[8,19]

Prior therapy did not influence either the development of colonies or the morphological appearance of these colonies in the stem cell assay. With only one exception there were no instances where, after therapy, a biopsy specimen was positive for SCC and the stem cell assay was negative, which might have suggested that sterilization of the stem cells of the tumor and visual persistence of nonclonogenic stem cells had occurred.

Attempts to subclone SCC stem cells and to test their ability to replicate continuously in a liquid medium demonstrated that a large number of colonies failed to replicate under conditions where identically handled clones from established SCC cell lines exhibited continuous replication. Studies in which stem cells colonies have been subcloned in agarose have demonstrated the self-renewal capability of multiple myeloma stem cells.[2] The failure of SCC colonies to replicate suggests that (1) the cells generating these colonies do not have an unlimited self-renewal capacity and (2) the cells require specific growth factors for continuous growth not supplied in our culture system. The latter possibility is more likely, as colonies inoculated intracranially into nude mice formed tumors, suggesting that at least some cells that grow in agarose are capable of self-renewal. The ability of these colonies to form tumors and the relative ease with which continuous cell lines may be established from these nude mouse heterotransplants indicates another function of the clonogenic assay.[11] The nude mouse brain assay may be a useful way of growing large quantities of tumor for drug testing.[20] The in vitro clonogenic assay of fresh tumor specimens has been specifically designed for detailed studies of the drug sensitivity of tumor stem cells. It has been estimated that, given the low CFE of these specimens, approximately $1-5 \times 10^6$ cells are required for the adequate evaluation of a single drug. Of greater significance, it appears that a minimum number of clones will be required for the control plates to properly evaluate drug responses in vitro and correlate these responses with clinical in vivo responses. The mean number of SCC stem cell colonies per plate was 66 (median, 22; range, 3–250). The identification of factors that would increase either the CFE of this tumor or the number of available cells would be of great importance.

All cloning procedures require careful consideration of factors affecting the survival and growth of isolated cells. In the development of cloning techniques it has been recognized that cells leak essential nutrients and secrete chemical messengers that are required for survival and growth. The medium containing these nutrients and chemical messengers—"conditioned medium"—has been shown to improve the cloning and growth of cells that are similar in origin to the cells "manufacturing" this medium.[10,21] We have previously demonstrated that the establishment of SCC cells in culture is greatly enhanced by using conditioned medium from an established, rapidly dividing SCC cell line.[11] The use of this medium in the growth of SCC stem cell colonies increased the number of colonies in the majority of specimens, in addition to greatly increasing the size of individual colonies. The use of this medium and the identification of specific chemical nutrients for SCC may allow us to develop selective cloning media for fresh SCC tumor specimens and thereby to increase the CFE of these specimens sufficiently to permit the in vitro testing of drug sensitivity.

Whereas the major focus of the stem cell assay has been on clinical drug testing and prediction of response, it is clear that the in vitro assay may have many other uses. In the vast majority of SCC stem cell colonies picked for cytological examination many mitoses were evident. Studies of ovarian and bladder stem cell colonies have demonstrated that colonies specifically prepared for cytogenetic analysis can be excellently maintained and that detailed karyotypic assessment is readily accomplished.[4] Thus, the culture conditions of this two-layer agarose system, which allows preferential and early rapid proliferation of tumor cells to the exclusion of normal stromal cells, may potentially expand the number and range of neoplasms, including SCC, available for cytogenetic studies.

Other potential uses of this assay include the identification of specific growth requirements for different tumor types, and, in addition to preclinical screening of cytotoxic, hormonal, and immunotherapeutic agents, may allow the study of promising new and innovative therapeutic modalities.

Conclusion

In conclusion, we have demonstrated that:

1. SCC cells from metastatic sites form colonies in agarose with a CFE of 0.003–0.26 percent of the nucleated cells plated and up to 1.5 percent of the SCC cells plated.
2. The CFE of SCC stem cells does not vary with metastatic site or between treated and untreated patients.
3. The colonies are of neoplastic origin, as shown by the excellent correlation between histocytopathological involvement of specimens with SCC and the generation of colonies, the cytological appearance of the colonies, the demonstration that colonies were aneuploid, and the ability of colonies to form tumors in nude mice.
4. Growth factors not supplied in our culture system are required for the long-term culture of these cells, as is suggested by the failure of colonies to demonstrate continuous replication when transferred to liquid medium. In future studies the use of this two-layer agarose assay system for growth of tumor stem cells should provide a means of identifying specific growth requirements; allow cytogenetic studies of many solid tumors that presently are not amenable to these studies; aid in the detection of malignant cells in clinical specimens; and provide a basis for testing therapeutic sensitivities of many tumor types, including SCC, in vitro.

References

1. Hamburger AW, Salmon SE: Primary bioassay of human tumor stem cells. Science 197:461–463, 1977
2. Hamburger AW, Salmon SE: Primary bioassay of human myeloma stem cells. J Clin Invest 60:846–854, 1977

3. Courtenay VD, Selby PJ, Smith IE, Mills J, Peckhan MJ: Growth of human tumor cell colonies from biopsies using two soft-agar techniques. Br J Cancer 38:77–82, 1978

4. Hamburger AW, Salmon SE, Kim MB, Trent JM, Soehnlen BJ, Alberts DS, Schmidt HJ: Direct cloning of human ovarian carcinoma cells in agar. Cancer Res 38:3438–3444, 1978

5. Buick RN, Stanisic TH, Fry SE, Salmon SE, Trent JM, Krasovich P: Development of an agar-methyl cellulose clonogenic assay for cells in transitional cell carcinoma of the bladder. Cancer Res 39:5051–5056, 1979

6. Kinball PM, Brattain MG, Pitts AM: A soft-agar procedure measuring growth of human colonic carcinoma. Br J Cancer 37:1015–1019, 1978

7. Buick RN, Fry SE, Salmon SE: Application of in vitro soft-agar techniques for growth of tumor cells to the study of colon cancer. Cancer 45:1238–1242, 1980

8. Rosenblum MD, Vasquez DA, Hoshine T, Wilson CB: Development of a clonogenic cell assay for human brain tumors. Cancer 41:2305–2314, 1978

9. Van Hoff DD, Johnson GE, Glaubiger DL: Secretion of tumor markers in the human tumor stem cell system. Proc Am Assoc Cancer Res 20:206, 1979

10. Salmon SE, Hamburger AW, Soehnlen B, Durie BGM, Alberts DS, Moon TE: Quantitation pf d fferential sensitivity of human tumor stem cells to anticancer drugs. N Engl J Med 298:1321–1327, 1978

11. Gazdar AF, Carney DN, Russell EK, et al: Small cell carcinoma of the lung; establishment of continuous clonable cell lines having APUD properties. Cancer Res 40:3502–3507, 1980

12. Pettingill OS, Sorenson GD, Wurster-Hill DH, et al: Isolation and growth characteristics of continuous cell lines from small-cell carcinoma of the lung. Cancer 45:906–918, 1980

13. Carney DN, Gazdar AF, Minna JD: Positive correlation between histologic tumor involvement and generation of tumor cell colonies in agarose in specimens taken directly from patients with small cell carcinoma of the lung. Cancer Res 40:1820–1823, 1980

14. Bunn PA Jr, Whangpeng J, Carney DN, et al: DNA content analysis by flow cytometry and cytogenetic analysis in mycosis fungoides and the Sezary syndrome. J Clin Invest, 1980, (in press)

15. Bunn PA Jr, Schlam M, Gazdar AF: Comparison of cytology and DNA content analysis by flow cytometry in specimens from lung cancer patients. Proc Am Assoc Cancer Res 21:160, 1980

16. Baylin SB, Abeloff MD, Goodwin G, Carney DN, Gazdar AF: Activities of L-dopa decarboxylase and diamina oxidase (histaminase) in

human lung cancers and decarboxylase as a marker for small (oat) cell cancer in tissue culture. Cancer Res 40:1990–1994, 1980

17. Pike BL, Robinson WA: Human bone marrow colony growth in agar-gel. Cell Physiol 76:77–94, 1970
18. Brigham BA, Bunn PA Jr, Minna JD, Cohen MH, Ihde DC, Shackney SE: Growth rates of small cell bronchogenic carcinoma. Cancer 42:2880–2886, 1978
19. Slocum HK, Rustum YM, Creaven PJ, et al: Mechanical disaggregation and enzymatic disaggregation of human melanoma, sarcoma and lung carcinoma. Proc Am Assoc Cancer Res 21:749, 1980
20. Rice JM, Houchens DP, Sanchez MS, Ovejera AA: Correlation of drug sensitivity on human tumor cells grown in soft agar and in nude mice. Proc Am Cancer Res 21:1099, 1980
21. Jones SE, Hamburger AW, Kim AB, Salmon SE: Development of a bioassay for putative human lymphoma stem cells. Blood 53:294–303, 1979

5

STUDIES ON XENOGRAFTS OF SMALL CELL CARCINOMA OF THE LUNG

George D. Sorenson
Olive S. Pettengill
Charles C. Cate

Origin of Nude Athymic Mouse

The mutant nude mouse was first described by Flanagan in 1966 and designated by the symbol Nu.[1] Only 2 years later, Pantelouris reported the most interesting characteristic of these mice when he indicated that they had, at most, a small rudimentary thymus.[2] Thus was provided a system for a wide variety of immunological studies and, in particular, a great spectrum of experimental manipulations which might be made in animals without a functioning thymus. The characteristics of these mice and many studies related to them have been summarized in recent reviews.[3-5] The early studies indicated that nude mice were quite susceptible to hepatitis and pneumonia and were short lived. It is now clear, however, that, if they are isolated from other mice and maintained in a reasonably sterile environment that limits exposure to pathogenic organisms, their survival will approximate that of conventional mice.

This work was supported in part by U.S. Public Health Service Grants CA17710 and CA25845 and National Cancer Institute Contract No. 1 CP65776.

Immunological Characteristics

Although nude mice have congenital thymic aplasia and are devoid of mature T cells, they do have T cell precursors, which are already committed to the pathway of T lymphocytes. The thymus-dependent areas of peripheral lymphoid tissues contain few lymphocytes,[6] and circulating lymphocytes are diminished.[7] However, an irradiated thymus grafted into a nude mouse is repopulated by precursors from the nude host.[8] They are incapable of rejecting allografts, responding to T cell–dependent antigens, or rejecting MSV-induced tumors.

In addition, there has been general agreement that, except for IgM, nude mice tend to have low immunoglobulin levels relative to nu/+ littermates or normal mice. These data were obtained from several strains of nude mice, not all of which were identified. IgA and IgG$_1$ levels are usually less than 10 percent of control, and IgG$_{2A}$ and IgG$_{2B}$ are depressed to 20 percent.[7] Nudes also seem to have a weak complement system.[9] More recent work suggests that caution must be used before such immunoglobulin values can be universally applied, in that wide variations (some overlapping normal levels) have been reported from BALB/c-derived nude mice, particularly among IgG$_1$ and IgG$_2$ subclasses.[10,11] In our own studies[12] baseline values of five immunoglobulin subclasses assayed at three time points in untreated nude mice derived from BALB/c stock clearly demonstrated significant age-related differences. In addition, serum IgG$_1$ concentrations in older mice frequently reached normal values (Table 5-1). Another unexpected finding was the appearance of relatively low levels of IgM in all age groups. This latter finding was consistent even in tumor-bearing mice injected with small cell carcinoma of the lung (SCC) cell lines and seemed to be uninfluenced by treatment with antilymphocyte sera (ALS). In contrast, serum IgG$_1$ and IgG$_2$ (the latter usually being significantly elevated in tumor-bearing mice relative to age-matched controls) were markedly reduced by ALS and antithymocyte serum (ATS) treatments.

Sensitivity to ALS, and particularly to ATS, was also seen in the antibody response of non–tumor-injected mice to sheep erythrocytes as measured by plaque assays. A noteworthy finding was that these data also indicated a sex-related difference in plaque-forming capability, suggesting that females were immunologically more responsive than males (Fig. 5-1).

Depressed T cell–dependent antibody synthesis, T cell–mediated cytolytic function, and immunoglobulin levels return to normal when nude mice are inoculated with thymocytes or T cell thymic replacing factors, or when they receive thymic grafts.

Table 5-1
Serial Serum Immunoglobulin Levels (mg/ml) in
Untreated BALB/c-Derived Nude Mice*

Age (wks)	Sex	Immunoglobulin Class				
		IgM	IgA	IgG_1	IgG_{2A}	IgG_{2B}
5	M	0.06–0.49[†] (0.15)	TLTM[‡]	0.02–3.44 (0.39)	TLTM	TLTM
	F	0.06–0.22 (0.13)	TLTM	0.00–0.24 (0.05)	TLTM	TLTM
11	M	0.16–0.61 (0.28)	TLTM	0.12–9.95 (4.15)	0.00–0.02 (TLTM)	0.00–0.32 (0.14)
	F	0.16–0.44 (0.29)	0.00–0.17 (0.02)	0.00–11.94 (2.51)	0.00–2.36 (0.43)	0.00–0.59 (0.20)
19	M	0.22–1.22 (0.28)	0.00–0.05 (0.01)	1.40–11.94 (7.53)	0.00–1.23 (0.22)	0.04–1.20 (0.40)
	F	0.29–0.61 (0.45)	0.00–0.25 (0.04)	0.38–9.74 (4.60)	0.00–1.31 (0.40)	0.16–1.07 (0.42)

*Mice bled orbitally at 5 and 11 wk and by cardiac puncture at 19 wk.
†Range and (mean) values from 10 male and 10 female mice.
‡Too low to measure (TLTM).

Natural killer cells (NK) are elevated in nude mice as compared with their levels in conventional littermates.[13] If the thymic function is reconstituted by grafting fetal thymuses in the young nude mice of BALB/c background, T cell function is restored and the NK activity is decreased to conventional levels.

Tissue Transplantation in Nude Mice

The important functional effect of the extensive impairment of T cell immunological function is that it allows nuce mice to tolerate a wide variety of transplanted tissues. It has been shown that these animals will accept xenografts from a wide variety of closely and distantly related mammals, and even skin grafts from nonmammalian vertebrates such as birds, reptiles, and amphibians.[14] This has made possible numerous studies of the xenotransplantation of a wide variety of tumors. Among these, the studies with human tumors—with which hundreds of mice have been now inoculated—are of particular interest.[15-17] Since the initial report by Rygaard and Poulsen,[18] the take rate has been described as variable and as depending somewhat on the tumor. In one series of 342 tumors trans-

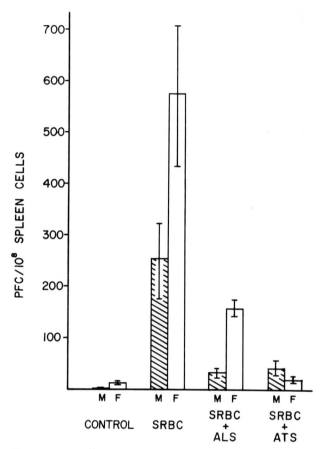

Figure 5-1. *Effect of ALS or ATS on immune response of nude mice immunized with sheep red blood cells (SRBC), as measured by localized hemolysis in gel assay. Plaque-forming cells assayed 5½ days after SRBC injection. ALS and ATS injected i.p. 1 day prior to and 1 and 3 days following SRBC injection.*

planted subcutaneously, it was 35.7 percent.[16] In general, it appears that tumors from lymphoreticular tissues and prostate grow less readily in nude mice.[15,16,19,20] The growth may be affected by the site of inoculation. Lymphoma cell lines,[21,22] as well as cultures of SCC,[23] grow better intracranially than subcutaneously. In most cases, the tumors resulting in the nude mice have been described as being quite comparable to the original neoplasm.[24] Occasionally, some increase in differentiation in the tumor in the nude mouse has been described.[25-27]

Transplantation of Pulmonary Tumors in Nude Mice

There are relatively few reports on transplantation of pulmonary tumors in nude mice. In the series of tumors and transplants reported by Reid et al.,[15] 5 out of 10 lung tumors were successfully transplanted, and, in this group, there was at least one adenocarcinoma, one epidermoid carcinoid, and one small cell (oat cell) carcinoma. In the largest study, by Sharkey et al.,[16] 35 of a series of 342 transplanted tumors were primary lung tumors. Growth occurred in 7 out of 13 (54 percent) of the hetero-transplanted epidermoid carcinomas, in none of the 7 attempts with well-differentiated adenocarcinoma, and in 10 out of 14 (71 percent) miscellaneous primary carcinomas including clear cell, mixed granular, epidermoid, large cell, and SCC. Tumors from metastatic sites were successfully transplanted. In general, the more poorly differentiated tumors were those that grew best in the nude mice. Hattler et al.[28] have reported the successful transplantation of 10 out of 14 squamous cell carcinomas. More recently, Mattern et al.[29] described the progressive growth of epidermoid and adenocarcinoma xenografts in 50 percent of 22 transplants attempted. The number of SCC transplanted to nude mice has been relatively small. This is probably because this tumor is not usually resected surgically. Besides those mentioned by Sharkey et al.,[16] several other small cell tumors have been transplanted by workers who were interested particularly in hormone production.[30,31]

Metastases in Nude Mice

Human tumors transplanted directly into nude mice usually do not metastasize. This is true even though the primary tumor will spread widely in the original host. In a recent study of a wide variety of human tumors, including those from the breast, lung, colon, endometrium, and other sites, the incidence of metastases seems to be influenced by the age of the recipient mice, the type of tumor, and the route of administration.[32] Where metastases have been described, this has frequently been when the tumor cells used were in culture prior to inoculation in nude mice[24,31,33,34]; thus, some modification or selection, or both, may have occurred during the in vitro period. When carcinoma is transplanted into neonatal mice, the incidence of metastases has been reported to be increased.[34] The route of administration may also affect metastatic potential, since intraperitoneal tumors spread more readily than those inoculated subcutaneously.[33] In most reports, control studies that would exclude changes in metastatic potential with the number of passages or time have not been included. The duration of the transplant may also affect metastatic potential, in that after tumors have been present for several months, metastases can be observed in a small percentage of animals. This involves, of course, not only the duration of the tumor, but also the fact that the mouse is aging. The metastases may be related to one of both of these factors. In one study, rat tumors that had lost their metastatic potential were metastatic when inoculated into nude mice and retained metastatic potential when subsequently inoculated into rats.[35]

The reason for this resistance to metastasis in nude mice is not clear. The occurrence of metastasis is a complicated phenomenon which depends upon the characteristics of the cell type as well as the host. The lack of metastases in nude mice has been correlated with increased numbers of NK cells, and this may be a partial explanation. It has been demonstrated that, if tumors are inoculated into very young mice, metastases occur; NK cell numbers are not increased at this time,[36] although they are increased in older mice.[13] In our studies with a number of SCC cell lines (see Chapter 3, this monograph), and with SCC directly transplanted from the patient into nude mice, the incidence of metastases has been very low. Metastases seemed to occur most often when the tumor had been in place in the mouse for many months (Fig. 5-2) and thus in relatively old mice.

Growth Characteristics of SCC in Nude Mice

Xenografts in This Laboratory

We have studied in detail the growth characteristics of tumors developing in nude mice after the inoculation of established cultures of SCC.[12] For these experiments, 10^7 cultured SCC were inoculated subcutaneously, and tumor growth was monitored over a 90-day period. The effect of ALS and ATS on tumor growth was also evaluated. In these groups ALS and ATS was inoculated i.p., 1 day prior to and at 1, 3, and 7 days following tumor cell inoculation, and then at weekly intervals during the 3-mo period. Tumors were measured weekly in three dimensions with calipers, and tumor volume data were fitted to previously described growth functions in order to estimate latent periods and doubling times, given in Table 5-2.[12] Since ALS was not found to have any significant effect on tumor growth, these data were not given. In a few instances, mice have been maintained with tumors for up to 20 mo. In these cases, the tumors became necrotic and the mice became wasted, but their survival was remarkably long. A latent period occurred prior to significant growth of the tumors, and this was variable with the different cell lines and even within a

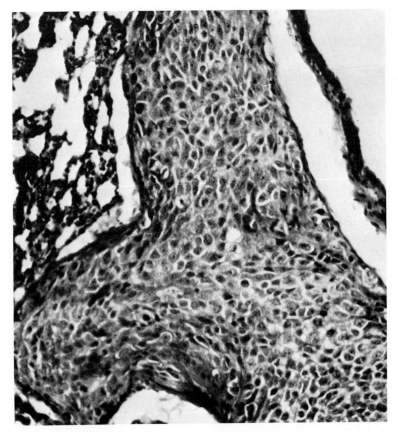

Figure 5-2. *Lung metastasis from male mouse inoculated with DMS 114 cells, subcutaneously. The tumor had infiltrated the peritoneal cavity and, when autopsied 90 days after inoculation, the tumor weighed 55.7 g. The mouse had been treated regularly with ATS. Hematoxylin and eosin stain. Original magnification × 500.*

group of animals inoculated with the same cell line. The latent period was defined as the time necessary for a tumor to reach a volume of 0.1 cm³; it varied from 3 to 6 wk among the 6 cell lines studied. A representative growth curve is illustrated in Figure 5-3. Late in the 3-month period, the rate of growth generally decreased. The change in growth rate with increasing tumor size appeared to be related to increased central necrosis in tumors of other SCC cell lines.

When fewer than 10⁷ DMS 79 cells were inoculated, tumors did not usually occur unless the mice were immunosuppressed with ATS (Table 5-3).[23]

The appearance of the tumor cells under the electron microscope re-

Table 5-2
Effect of Antithymocyte Serum on Tumor Incidence and
Growth in Mice Inoculated with 10^7 SCC-Cultured Cells

Cell Line Inoculated	Tumor Incidence		Mean Latent Period (days)		Mean Doubling Period (days)	
	M	F	M	F	M	F
DMS 79						
Control	9/10	6/9	33	43	6.5	15.4
ATS	10/10	10/10	35	30	7.4	15.7
DMS 92						
Control	9/10	5/9	44	60	10.8	11.7
ATS	5/5	4/4	43	45	13	9.7
DMS 114						
Control	9/10	4/10	20	36	7.8	2.9
ATS	5/5	5/5	17	21	5.4	16.4
DMS 153						
Control	5/5	8/9	24	43	6.1	6.0
ATS	5/5	4/4	25	62	10.0	7.9
DMS 187						
Control	5/5	1/5	56.2	45.2	13.1	13.9
ATS	5/5	5/5	51.2	62.9	7.7	12.7
DMS 235						
Control	5/5	3/5	40.7	43.6	13.1	11.4
ATS	5/5	4/5	46.3	50.4	8.6	13.5
DMS 55						
Control	0/5	0/5	—	—	—	—
ATS	0/5	0/5	—	—	—	—

Table 5-3
Effect of ATS on Tumor Incidence and Growth at Low
Cell Dose of DMS 79 Cells in Nude Mice

Group	Number Cells Inoculated	Tumor Incidence	Mean Latent Period (days)	Mean Doubling Time (days)
Untreated mice	10^6	1/5	20.9	6.5
Mice inoculated weekly with ATS	10^6	4/5	40.7	7.5
Mice inoculated weekly with ATS	10^5	0/5	—	—

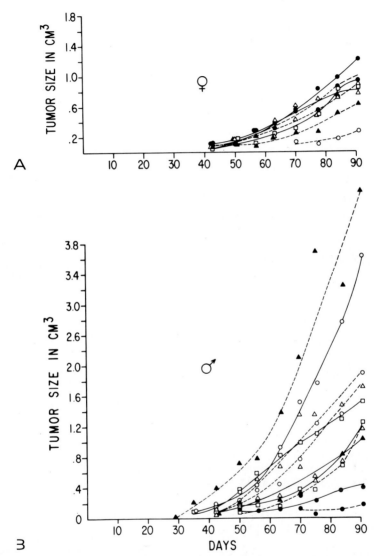

Figure 5-3. *Growth curves of DMS 235-cultured cells (10⁷/mouse) inoculated subcutaneously in nude athymic mouse. (A) Growth of individual tumors in female mice. (B) Growth of individual tumors in male mice. Solid lines indicate mice inoculated only with tumor cells; dotted lines indicate mice inoculated regularly i.p. with ATS in addition to tumor cells.*

mained constant when the original biopsy from the patient, the cell line from the biopsy, and the xenograft from the culture were compared (Fig. 5-4).

Influence of Sex on the Transplantation of SCC

The influence of the sex of the recipient mouse on the success of transplantation and the subsequent growth or other characteristics of the transplanted tumor in nude mice has not been systematically studied by others, and, in many reports, the sex of the mouse is not indicated. In others, either male or female mice have been used without apparent concern. However, hormone treatment does facilitate the growth of certain tumors derived from hormonally dependent tissue, and prostatic carcinoma grows better in male than in female mice.[15]

When cultures of SCC were inoculated into male mice, the incidence of tumors was greater in most instances than with comparable inoculations in female mice (Tables 5-2 and 5-4). This was true for 6 cell lines studied in detail, where the incidence of tumors in untreated males was 42 tumors in 45 mice (93 percent), as compared with 27 tumors in 47 female mice (57 percent).

Influence of Immune Status of Host on Transplantability of SCC

Our evidence indicates a role for immunity in this difference in susceptibility between the sexes, as the difference can be eliminated by ATS. This suggests that the hormonal differences are but indirectly involved via their effect on host immune function and thus the greater immune resistance to tumor transplantation observed in female mice can be abrogated by the effects of ATS. It is of interest that ALS did not affect tumor incidence, and this may be attributable to its lesser effect on T cell function, at least as measured by its effect on reactivity to sheep red blood cells (SRBC) (Fig. 5-1).[12]

SCC cell line DMS 55 produced no tumors in nude mice when 10^7 cells were inoculated into both male and female mice, untreated or given either ATS or ALS, according to the standard protocol (Table 5-2).[12] There is suggestive evidence, however, that the tumorigenicity of this line increased during the next 2 yr in culture. At that time, this cell line was again tested in male nude mice which were immunosuppressed by either irradiation with 450 rads (cobalt-60 source) or treatment with ATS under the same conditions as previously. Tumor growth was monitored for 90 days and, at

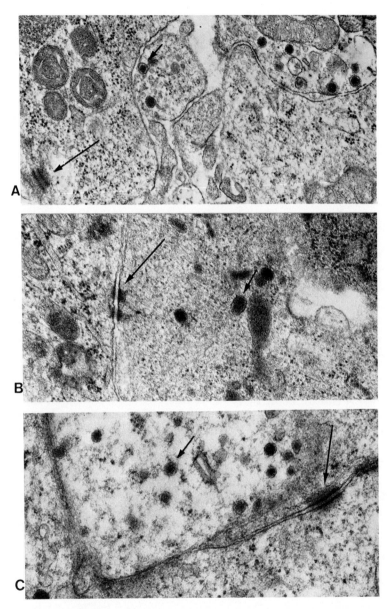

Figure 5-4. *Comparison of ultrastructural features of cells from (A) bone marrow aspirate, (B) cell line DMS 235 derived from aspirate, and (C) tumor resulting in nude mice after inoculation of cultured cells. All three specimens contain dense-core vesicles (short arrow), an identifying structure for SCC, as well as desmosomes (long arrow). Original magnification × 35,000.*

Table 5-4
Comparison of Growth of DMS 273 Cell Line with Nu
273, Transplanted Tumor

No. of Cells Inoculated	Males			Females		
	Tumor Incidence	Latent Period (days)	Doubling Time (days)	Tumor Incidence	Latent Period (days)	Doubling Time (days)
Nu 273						
5×10^6 + ALS	5/5	16.8		5/5	23.7	4.33
10^6 + ALS	3/5	20.6	8.65	1/5	51.1	5.17
10^6	0/5	—	—	0/5	—	—
DMS 273						
5×10^6 + ALS	5/5	19.59	1.9	5/5	19.06	2.8
10^6 + ALS	2/5	26.31	4.0	5/5	31.58	3.8
10^6	2/5	37.18	4.0	1/5	44.6	1.3

autopsy, tumors were dissected and weighed. By this time, tumors had occurred not only in the irradiated mice; now one was also observed in an ATS-treated mouse. This tumor was small and it did not reach a volume of 0.1 cm³. (See Table 5-5.) One of the tumors from an irradiated mouse was transplanted to a normal nude mouse in which it grew. When returned to cell culture, a cell population similar to the parent DMS 55 was obtained, which grew continuously in vitro. However, the transplanted tumor did not grow when inoculated into mice for a second passage.

Comparison of Growth of SCC Cells In Vitro and In Vivo

In vivo and in vitro growth rates were compared using DMS 79 cells in culture and tumors derived from their inoculation in nude mice. Autoradiographic analysis of ³H-thymidine uptake was made to determine the cell-cycle time by the method of percent-labeled metaphases.[37] For these experiments, 10^7 cells were inoculated subcutaneously in male nude mice, which received regular i.p. inoculations with ALS as previously described. (This was subsequently shown to have no significant effect on tumor growth.) Both labeling indices and percent-labeled metaphase data were obtained by autoradiographic analysis. (See Table 5-6.)

The labeling indices obtained here are in close agreement for DMS 79 cells growing either in vitro or in vivo. They are also in close agreement

Table 5-5
Influence of Immunosuppression on Tumogenicity of
DMS 55 after Extended Culture in Vitro

Inoculum*	Tumor Incidence	Final Tumor Weight[t] (g)
Irradiated mice	9/10	0.31
ATS-treated mice	1/5	0.032

*10^7 cells/mouse.
[t]Mean given.

with similar data obtained from SCC cells in patients. The more direct
method of estimating actual primary tumor doubling time in patients with
SCC has been carried out by measuring tumor area on x-ray films.[40] The
doubling times estimated from a series of 12 patients from this type of
measurement averaged 81–83 days. These data are influenced by cell
growth as well as cell loss, and therefore doubling times are much greater
than from estimates based on ^{3}H-thymidine incorporation. The latter reflects the growth potential of tumor cells, as only viable cells can be evaluated by this technique.

Comparison of Growth of Transplanted Tumors versus Tumors from Cultured Cells

One of the prominent observations in examining tumor growth data of
SCC cells inoculated in nude mice was the wide variation within each
treatment group. One explanation was thought to be the lack of genetic
homogeneity inherent in nude mice currently available. However, the cell
lines used for inoculation had not been cloned, although they were be-

Table 5-6
Comparison of Growth Rates of Cells by
Autoradiographic Analysis

Tumor and Cultured Cells	Labeling Index	Cycle Time (hr)
DMS 79 cells in vitro	16.2	28 (approx.)
DMS 79 cells in vivo	15.0	28 (approx.)
SCC in patients (ref. 38)	13.2 2.5–12.6	—
(ref. 39)	7.2–23.8 (median 16.7)	18.8

lieved to be homogeneous. Because of the variable results from the tumors derived from cultured cells, the growth of serially transplantable tumors was investigated. Two lines of transplantable SCC tumors were used. DMS 79 cultured cells were inoculated, resulting in a tumor which was then serially transplanted (Fig. 5-5). The effect of inoculum size was measured for transplanted tumor cells (Nu 79; Table 5-7) for comparison with data for cultured DMS 79 cells (Table 5-2).

In another instance, a continuous cell line as well as a transplantable tumor were initiated simultaneously from a single pleural fluid specimen (Fig. 5-6). Growth of tumor in the first tumor transplant passage was compared with that derived from cells cultured 8 or more months in vitro, when a homogeneous, continuously growing cell line had been established. These data are shown in Table 5-4. No statistically significant differences in tumor incidence or growth rate were observed between cultured and transplanted tumor cells, suggesting that a system was available for both in vitro and in vivo evaluation of treatment effects on the same tumor cell.

Morphological Characteristics of SCC in Nude Mice

The human tumors that have been transplanted to nude mice have been reported to retain their original morphological characteristics in most cases, although an exception to this was observed in melanomas.[41] This persistence of morphological features gives support to the hope that the tumor in the nude mouse retains important features of the original neoplasm and thus represents a model of the human tumors from which results of experimental study will have application to cancer in man.

A priori, it would not be surprising if the tumor did change with transplantation, because human tumors in their host often become less well differentiated and proliferate more rapidly with time. Therefore, this would not be an unexpected observation in transplanted tumors in nude mice, and increased rates of proliferation have been described with serial transplantation.[42]

Tumors in nude mice derived from cultures or primary transplants of SCC, or both, have maintained a close morphological similarity with the tumor obtained directly from the patient. Because some cellular selection has certainly occurred during the establishment of the cell cultures, it would not be unexpected if the tumors derived from these cultures differed somewhat from the original specimens. However, the morphologic features at the light- and electron-microscopic level are maintained (Figs.

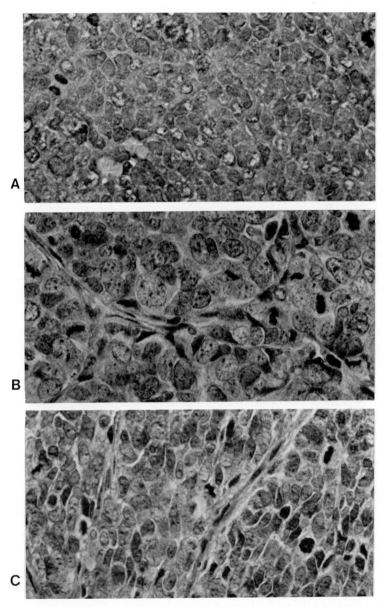

Figure 5-5. *Comparison of cultured DMS 79 cells, with tumor produced from them and with serially transplanted tumor. All paraffin sections of formalin-fixed tissue. (A) Section of pellet of cultured cells prepared by centrifugation. (B) Section of tumor produced from cultured cells. (C) Transplanted Nu 79 tumor. Hematoxylin and eosin stain. Original magnification × 500.*

Table 5-7
Tumor Incidence and Growth Rate of Nu 79 Tumor
Transplanted in Nude Mice

No. of Cells Inoculated	Males			Females		
	Tumor Incidence	Mean Latent Period (days)	Mean Doubling Time (days)	Tumor Incidence	Mean Latent Period (days)	Mean Doubling Time (days)
10^7	5/5	11.11	3.6	5/5	14.8	3.9
5×10^6	5/5	31.04	12.59	5/5	19.2	6.1
10^6	4/5	66.46	11.50	0/3	—	—

5-7 through 5-10). This would seem to indicate that the morphologic features which produce the general light and electron microscopic appearance of these tumors are quite stable, even under presumably significant, although undefined, selective pressure both in culture and in the nude mice.

Hormonal Characteristics of SCC in Nude Mice

The cell lines that we have inoculated into nude mice are producing a wide variety of peptide and glycoprotein hormones, as well as estrogens.[43,44] Thus, one might expect to find some morphological or physiological effect of hormone production by the tumors in the recipient mice. In one study, an adrenal trophic effect has been described from a SCC tumor transplanted in nude mice.[45] Although several of the DMS cell lines studied were producing ACTH in vitro, and one (DMS 79) was producing large amounts, we have not been able to demonstrate convincingly that adrenocortical hypertrophy occurred in mice with tumors derived from these cell lines. The explanation for this is not clear, as we have evidence that the tumors in mice contain and secrete large amounts of ACTH (*vide infra*). However, much of the ACTH produced by these tumors is in the form of precursors to the usual circulating $ACTH_{1-39}$, and because these precursor forms have much less biological activity, the lack of adrenal hypertrophy may be explained in this way.

We also sought evidence for the biologic effects of a tumor derived from a cell line that produced relatively large amounts of growth hormone releasing factor (GHRF).[43] In these studies, the growth of relatively mature animals with these tumors was compared over 3 mo with that of control

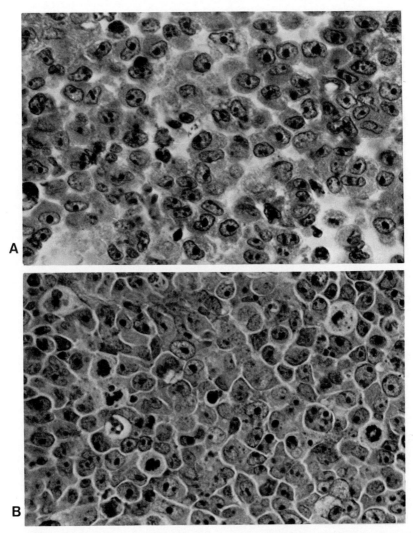

Figure 5-6. *Comparison of cell line DMS 273 and transplantable tumor Nu 273, both initiated from the same pleural fluid specimen. Paraffin sections. (A) Cell pellet prepared by centrifugation of cultured cells. (B) Sections of subcutaneously transplanted tumor. Hematoxylin and eosin stain. Original magnification × 500.*

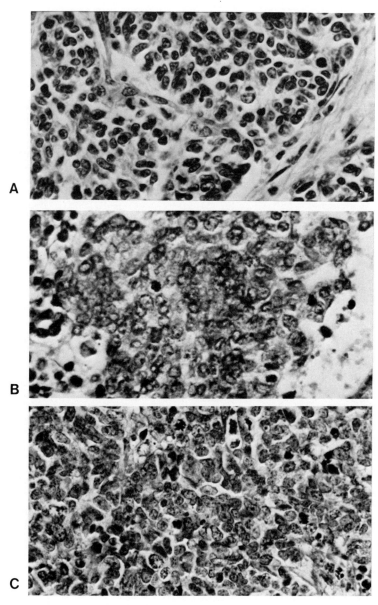

Figure 5-7. *DMS 153. Comparison of tumor from which cell line originated and tumor produced in nude mouse from inoculated cultured cells. Paraffin sections. (A) Section of liver metastasis obtained at autopsy. (B) Pellet of cultured cells obtained by centrifugation. (C) Nude tumor section. Hematoxylin and eosin stain. Original magnification ×500.*

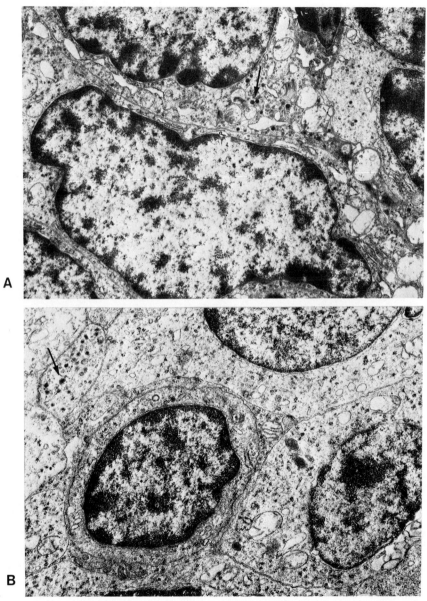

Figure 5-8. *Ultrastructural comparison of tissues of Figure 5-7. (A) Liver metastasis, obtained at autopsy. Note dense-core vesicles (arrow), characteristic of SCC. (B) Section of nude mouse tumor resulting from subcutaneous inoculation of cultured tumor cells, DMS 153. Dense-core vesicles (arrow) present. Original magnification × 8000.*

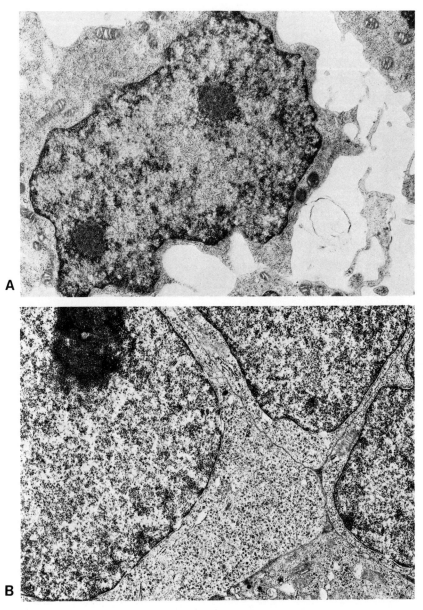

Figure 5-9. *Electron micrograph of pleural fluid specimen from which both a transplantable tumor (Nu 273) in nude mice and a continuous cell line (DMS 273) were initiated. (A) Pleural fluid, showing tumor cell with higher nuclear–cytoplasmic ratio and condensed chromatin. (B) Nu 273, tumor in which cells have similar ultrastructural features as seen in pleural fluid. Dense-core vesicles are also present. Original magnification × 8000.*

114

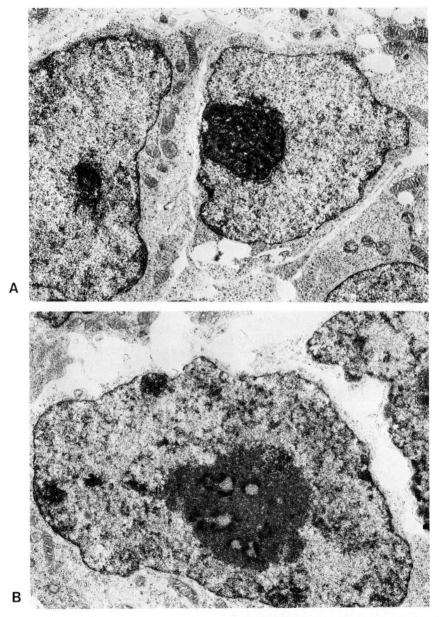

Figure 5-10. *Ultrastructural comparison of cell line DMS 273 obtained from pleural fluid (Fig. 5-9, panel A) and tumor resulting from inoculation of cultured cell for comparison with tumor (Fig. 5-9, panel B). (A) Cell line. Original magnification × 14,500. (B) Tumor. Original magnification × 8000.*

115

animals. No significant differences were observed in body weight, either whole or corrected for tumor weight at autopsy. An effect would have been dependent on the stimulation of the mouse pituitary, and apparently this did not occur. The material from the cells does stimulate the release of GH by rat pituitary cells in vitro, but the effect on mouse pituitary has not been tested. It is also possible that younger animals would have been more responsive.

The studies above, in which biological effects of hormones produced by the cells in culture have not been demonstrable in nude mice with the tumors, would suggest that perhaps the tumors did not synthesize the same hormones or at least the same amounts as the cell lines. However, available evidence is to the contrary. In fact, it appears that there is a remarkable persistence of the hormone-producing capability of these cells when they form tumors in nude mice.

Studies that focused particularly on ACTH show the pattern of intracellular ACTH to be quite consistent between cell lines and their nude mouse tumors. In addition, serial transplantation in nude mice does not appear to alter peptide synthesis significantly. In these evaluations, DMS 79, a high producer of ACTH, was used to compare production in other cell lines (Table 5-8).

In additional studies the immunoreactive ACTH isolated from SCC culture supernatants, cells, and xenograft tumors, was characterized by separation on Sephadex G-50 fine columns. Essentially all protein and immunoreactive material eluted with the void volume, suggesting that the peptide existed as large precursor molecule(s) in all preparations, which possibly accounts for its low biological activity.[46]

Conclusions

The tumors that develop in nude mice following the inoculation of SCC cells provide the first useful experimental model for this important human neoplasm. Even though this does not represent a primary tumor in these animals, which would be another type of model with desirable attributes, the xenografts permit one to study tumors derived from man under experimental conditions. A priori this would seem to be a great advantage if one hopes to extrapolate results more or less directly to patients with this disease. The apparent stability of certain morphological and endocrinological features of these tumors within the xenografts is both desirable and encouraging. The extensive computer-assisted mathematical evaluation of multiple growth parameters of tumors derived from different

Table 5-8
Comparison of Percent Yields of Immunoreactive ACTH
Produced by SCC Cell Lines

Cell Line	Source of ACTH		
	4-Day Culture Medium	Cultured Cell Extract	First Passage Xenograft Tumor Extract
DMS 79	100.0	100.0	100.0
DMS 153	4.0	6.8	26.5
DMS 92	0.5	3.1	8.7
DMS 114	0.4	1.6	6.6
Nu 79*	n.d.	n.d.	92.9

*Nu 79 was a DMS 79-induced tumor in its sixth continuous serial passage in nude mice.

cell cultures indicates that the pattern of tumor growth was distinctive in each instance studied.[12] Thus, although all were similar, each behaved in a somewhat individualistic manner. This feature also can be considered as simulating the natural situation, because this tumor is somewhat variable among individual patients. Thus, for many reasons, the use of xenografts of SCC in nude mice should be a valuable approach for future investigations.

References

1. Flanagan SP: "Nude," a new hairless gene with pleiotropic effects in the mouse. Genet Res Camb 8:295–309, 1966
2. Pantelouris EM: Absence of thymus in the mouse mutant. Nature 217:370–371, 1968
3. Nomura T, Ohsawa N, Tamachi N, et al (eds): Proceedings of the Second International Workshop on Nude Mice. Stuttgart, Fischer Verlag, 1977
4. Houchens DP, Ovejera AA (eds): Proceedings of the Symposium on the Use of Athymic (Nude) Mice in Cancer Research. New York, Fischer, 1978
5. Fogh J, Giovanella BC: The Nude Mouse in Experimental and Clinical Research. New York, Academic Press, 1978
6. de Sousa MA, Parrott DVM, Pantelouris EM: The lymphoid tissues of mice with congenital aplasia of the thymus. Clin Exp Immunol 4:637–644, 1969
7. Wortis HH: Immunological studies of nude mice, in: Cooper MD,

Warren NL (eds): Contemporary Topics in Immunobiology vol 3. New York, Plenum Press, 1974, p 243

8. Pritchard H, Micklem HS: Haematopoietic stem cells and progenitors of functional T-lymphocytes in the bone marrow of "nude" mice. Clin Exp Immunol 14:597–607, 1973

9. Koene R, Cerlay R, Jansen J, et al: Rejection of skin grafts in the nude mouse. Nature 251:69–70, 1974

10. Brogen CH, Warren HS, Mielsen E, et al: Quantitative immunoelectrophoretic analysis of serum proteins and immunoglobulins in the serum and produced by spleen cell cultures of individual nude mice, in Nomura T, Ohsawa N, Tamachi N, et al (eds): Proceedings of the Second Workshop on Nude Mice. Stuttgart, Fischer Verlag, 1977, p 157

11. Okudaira H, Komagata Y, Ghoda A, et al: Thymus-independent and -dependent aspects of immunoglobulin synthesis and specific antibody formation in nude mice, in Nomura T, Ohsawa N, Tamachi N, et al (eds): Proceedings of the Second Workshop on Nude Mice, Stuttgart, Fischer Verlag, 1977, p 167

12. Pettengill OS, Curphey TJ, Cate CC, et al: Animal model for small cell carcinoma of the lung. Effect on Immunosuppression and sex of mouse on tumor growth in nude athymic mice. Exp Cell Biol 48:278–297, 1980

13. Herberman RB, Nunn ME, Lavrin DH: Natural cytotoxic reactivity of mouse lymphoid cells against syngeneic allogeneic tumors. 1. Distribution of reactivity and specificity. Int J Cancer 16:216–229, 1975

14. Reed ND, Manning DD: Present status of xenotransplantation of non malignant tissue to the nude mouse, in: Fogh J, Giovanella BC (eds): The Nude Mouse in Experimental and Clinical Research. New York, Academic Press, 1978, p 167

15. Reid LM, Holland J, Jones C, et al: Some of the variables affecting the success of transplantation of human tumors into the athymic nude mouse, in Houchens DP, Ovejera AA (eds): The Use of Athymic (Nude) Mice in Cancer Research. New York, Fischer, 1978, p 107

16. Sharkey FF, Fogh JM, Hajdu SI, et al: Experience in surgical pathology with humor tumor growth in the nude mouse, in Fogh J, Giovanella BC (eds): The Nude Mouse in Experimental and Clinical Research. New York, Academic Press, 1978, p 187

17. Giovanella BC, Stehlin JS Jr, Williams LJ Jr, et al: Heterotransplantation of human cancers into nude mice. A model system for human cancer chemotherapy. Cancer 42:2269–2291, 1978

18. Rygaard J, Poulsen CO: Heterotransplantation of a human malignant tumor to nude mice. Acta Pathol Microbiol Scand 77:758–760, 1969
19. Poulsen CO, Rygaard J: Growth of human tumors in nude mice, in Bloom BB, David JR (eds): In Vitro Methods in Cell Mediated and Tumor Immunity. New York, Academic Press, 1976, pp 701–711
20. Sordat B, Fritsche R, Mach J-P, et al: Morphological and functional evaluation of human solid tumours serially transplanted in nude mice, in Rygaard J, Poulsen CO: Proceedings of the First International Workshop on Nude Mice. Stuttgart, Fischer Verlag, 1973, p 269
21. Arnstein P, Taylor DON, Nelson-Rees WA, et al: Propagation of human tumors in anti-thymocyte treated mice. J Natl Cancer Inst 52:71–81, 1974
22. Epstein AL, Kaplan HS: Biology of the human malignant lymphomas. I. Establishment in continuous cell culture and heterotransplantation of diffuse histiocytic lymphomas. Cancer 34:1851–1872, 1974
23. Chambers WF, Pettengill OS, Sorenson GD: Subcranial growth of pulmonary small cell carcinoma cells in nude athymic mice. Exp Cell Biol (in press)
24. Giovanella BC, Yim SO, Morgan AC, et al: Metastases of human melanomas transplanted in "nude" mice. J Natl Cancer Inst 50:823–833, 1973
25. Helson L, Das SK, Haydju SI: Human neuroblastoma in nude mice. Cancer Res 35:2594–2599, 1975
26. Giovanella BC, Stehlin JS, Williams LJ: Heterotransplantation of human malignant tumors in "nude" thymusless mice. II. Malignant tumors induced by injection of cell cultures derived from human solid tumors. J Natl Cancer Inst 52:921–930, 1974
27. Takahashi S, Konishi Y, Nakatani K, et al: Conversion of a poorly differentiated adenocarcinoma to ascites form with invasion and metastasis in nude mice. J Natl Cancer Inst 60:925–929, 1978
28. Hattler BG, Soehnlen B, Seaver NA, et al: Heterotransplantation of human malignant neoplasms to the mouse mutant nude. Surg Forum 25:127–129, 1974
29. Mattern J: Different growth rates of lung tumors in man and their xenografts in nude mice. Eur J Cancer 16:289–291, 1980
30. Shin S, Kadish AS, Bancroft FC: Host response to heterologous tumor transplants in nude mice, in Houchens DP, Ovejera AA (eds): Proceedings of the Symposium on the Use of Athymic (Nude) Mice. New York, Fischer, 1978, p 133

31. Kameya T, Shimasoto Y, Hayashi H, et al: Growth and differentiation of hormone-producing tumors in nude mice, in Nomura T, Ohsawa N, Tamachi N, et al (eds): Proceedings of the Second International Workshop on Nude Mice. Stuttgart, Fischer Verlag, 1977, p 405

32. Sharkey FE, Fogh J: Metastases of human tumors in athymic nude mice. Int J Cancer 24:733–738, 1979

33. Kyriazis AP, Persio LD, Michael GJ, et al: Growth patterns and metastatic behavior of human tumors growing in athymic mice. Cancer Res 38:3186–3190, 1978

34. Sordat BC, Merenda C, Carrel S: Invasive growth and dissemination of human solid tumors and malignant cell lines grafted subcutaneously into newborn nude mice, in Nomura T, Ohsawa N, Tamachi N, et al (eds): Proceedings of the Second International Workshop on Nude Mice. Stuttgart, Fischer Verlag, 1977, p 313

35. Kim U, Shin SI, Freedman VH: Restoration of hematogeneously metastasizing capacity of rat mammary tumors (MT) by athymic nude mice: immunological manifestation of tumor–host interaction. Proc Am Assoc Cancer Res 20:122, 1979

36. Nabil H: Natural killer cells in nudes. Frederick Cancer Research Center's Workshop on Design of Models for Screening of Therapeutic Agents, Warrendon, Virginia, 1980

37. Pettengill OS, Sorenson GD, Wurster-Hill DH, et al: Isolation and growth characteristics of continuous cell lines from small cell carcinoma of the lung. Cancer 45:906–918, 1980

38. Muggia FM, Krezoski SD, Hause HH: Cell kinetic studies in patients with small cell carcinoma of the lung. Cancer 34:1683–1690, 1974

39. Straus MJ, Moran RE: Cell cycle parameters in human solid tumors. Cancer 40:1453–1461, 1977

40. Brigham BA, Bunn PA Jr, Minna JD, et al: Growth rates of small cell bronchogenic carcinomas. Cancer 42:2880–2886, 1978

41. Aubert C, Chirieceanu E, Foa C, et al: Ultrastructural and biochemical changes in cultured human malignant melanoma cells after heterotransplantation into nude mice. Cancer Res 36:3106–3112, 1976

42. Nakatani K, Takahashi S, Shiratori T, et al: Heterotransplantation of human gastric carcinomas into nude mice. World J Surg 3:641–650, 1979

43. Sorenson GD, Brinck-Johnsen T: Hormone production by cultures of small cell carcinoma from lung. Am Assoc Cancer Res 18:248, 1977

44. Sorenson GD, Pettengill OS, Brinck-Johnsen T, et al: Hormone pro-

duction by cultures of small cell carcinoma of the lung. Cancer (in press)

45. Reid LCM, Shin S: Transplantation by heterologous endocrine tumor cells in nude mice, in: Fogh J, Giovanella BC (eds): The Nude Mouse in Experimental and Clinical Research. New York, Academic Press, 1978, pp 348–352

46. Cate CC, Pettengill OS, Sorenson GD. Manuscript in preparation.

6

ENDOCRINE BIOCHEMISTRY IN THE SPECTRUM OF HUMAN LUNG CANCER: IMPLICATIONS FOR THE CELLULAR ORIGIN OF SMALL CELL CARCINOMA

Stephen B. Baylin
Adi F. Gazdar

The number of contributions to this text testifies to the intense interest that has arisen in small (oat) cell lung carcinoma (SCC) in recent years. Indeed, many properties of this neoplasm have led clinicians and investigators to focus upon it as an entity quite separate from the other major histopathologic types of human lung cancer. This focus has certainly been reasonable considering the major differences that SCC manifests in a number of parameters relative to the other types of lung cancer. In its growth pattern, SCC exhibits a relatively high growth fraction and extremely early potential for metastatic dissemination.[1-4] These growth characteristics have, of course, correlated with a high degree of sensitivity to

Portions of the work included were funded by Grant RO1-CA-18404 from the National Institutes of Health and by Grant PDT-108 from the American Cancer Society. Dr. Baylin has been supported by Research Career Development Award 1-KO4-CA-000-27. The authors deeply appreciate the collaboration of Dr. Martin Abeloff, Dr. Joseph Eggleston, Dr. Geoffrey Mendelsohn, Dr. David Ettinger, Dr. Charles Berger, and Dr. Desmond Carney in some of the studies cited. We also acknowledge the expert technical assistance of Kathleen Wieman, Sara Lyles, RoxAnna Thompson, and Gregory Goodwin, as well as the secretarial assistance of Sandra Lund and Alverta Fields.

radiation therapy and/or chemotherapy for this cancer as opposed to most other types of lung neoplasms.[2,4] Finally, the endocrine behavior of SCC has been emphasized; the propensity for the tumor to cause clinical syndromes due to excess production of small polypeptide hormones is now well known[5,6] (see Chapter 8, this monograph).

Each of the above features of SCC, in addition to generating intense interest in this tumor, led to the evolution of a theory that SCC might have a separate cell of origin in the bronchial epithelium from the other major types of human lung cancer. The endocrine properties of SCC were instrumental in the development of such theories. The documentation of a propensity for SCC to produce biologically active small polypeptide hormones such as adenocorticotropin (ACTH) and antidiuretic hormone (ADH), plus the findings of neurosecretory granules in electronmicroscopy studies of the tumor, led many investigators to include SCC as a neoplasm of amine precursor uptake and decarboxylation (APUD) endocrine cells.[7] In turn, in the early evolution of Pearse's thinking about endocrine cells, SCC was postulated to be among the APUD cells that have a probable embryologic origin in the neural crest.[7,8] This view was strengthened by the finding that certain functions present in neural cells, such as the ability to generate short-duration electrical action potentials, could be demonstrated in a number of normal and neoplastic APUD cells including cultured SCC.[9] More recent studies also have described the presence of certain neural antigens in SCC as opposed to other types of human lung cancer.[10] Thus, the proposal that SCC might be of neural origin would implicate an entirely separate cell lineage for this cancer in comparison to the other major lung tumors, which evolve in the endodermally derived epithelium of the bronchial mucosa. This degree of separation would carry important clinical and biological ramifications for SCC.

Over the past five years, an emerging body of data has raised serious questions about a separate cell of origin for SCC. First, the concept of a neural origin for all APUD endocrine cells is no longer maintained.[11-14] Elegant studies involving chimera formation between neural crest derivatives of chick and quail have apparently proven the neural crest origin of such endocrine cells as the thyroid C cells and adrenal medullary cells[15,16]; however, the same techniques have not confirmed a neural origin for APUD cells in the pancreatic islets and in the intestinal tract.[11-13] Proposals that a single endodermal progenitor cell may give rise to all of the specialized cell types in the intestinal mucosal epithelium, including the small numbers of APUD endocrine cells, have important ramifications for our thinking about the development of the endodermally derived bronchial mucosa. Second, an increasing number of biochemical studies have indicated that various forms of multiple small polypeptide hormones are indeed found in each of the histopathologic types of human lung cancer and are not restricted to SCC.[17-19] Third, there has been a renewed interest in findings known to pathologists for many years; namely, that the same patient may harbor lesions that demonstrate SCC histology in combination with the morphologic characteristics of other human lung cancers.[20-22] This phenomenon has been dramatically emphasized in recent studies showing that a percentage of patients with well-confirmed initial diagnoses of SCC may die after eventual failure of chemotherapy protocols and have only non-SCC lung cancer found at the time of postmortem examination[21,22] (see Chapter 10, this monograph).

All of the above data, then, raise questions about the relationship of SCC to the other human lung cancers. Among the issues involved are: (1) What is the precise cellular origin of SCC, and is it truly separate from that for the other human lung cancers? (2) If, indeed, all human lung cancers, including SCC, have a common cellular origin, what are the possible clinical and biological relationships which they may share? (3) What directions should clinical and basic investigation take in order to clarify further these important questions concerning human lung cancer? It is the purpose of this chapter to describe a subset of biochemical information which appears to shed some further light on the relationships of SCC to other human lung cancers and on the possible cell of origin for this important tumor. Chapters 4 and 7 also contain information from morphologic and tissue culture studies that bear on this question. The biologic and clinical ramifications of the data presented below are discussed and speculated upon, and some suggestions for lines of future research are put forth.

Biochemical Markers Selected for Study

The concept of the APUD endocrine cell system involves the possession of certain biochemical properties by the cells so classified. Theoretically, then, all normal and neoplastic cells from diverse regions belonging to the system share these characteristics. Our approach to studying relationships between SCC and the other major types of lung cancer has involved tissue measurements of a subset of biochemical indices which have established relationships to APUD cells outside the lung. A detailed discussion of each of these parameters is important for an understanding of the implications of the data obtained.

L-Aromatic Amino Acid Decarboxylase or L-dopa Decarboxylase (DDC) Activity

The activity of this enzyme constitutes an important element of the APUD cell concept.[7] The theory states that many types of small polypeptide-secreting endocrine cells also contain the biochemical machinery for biogenic amine synthesis. DDC catalyzes the conversion of precursor amino acids (tryptophan, 5-hydroxytryptophan, L-dopa) to their corresponding amines (tryptamine, 5-hydroxytryptamine or serotonin, and dopamine); this decarboxylation step for the conversion of L-dopa to dopamine is depicted in Figure 6-1. The enzyme DDC, then, is represented by the "D" in the acronym "APUD."[7] Theoretically, if SCC is a typical APUD tumor, high levels of DDC ought to be present in this tumor. Also, if SCC has a neural cell origin which distinguishes it from the other, endodermally derived, lung cancers, DDC might, theoretically, be absent in the other tumors. It is important to note, however, that high levels of DDC activity are present in some tissues, such as kidney and liver,[23] that are clearly not of neural origin. The precise cellular origin of the DDC in these tissues has not been defined.

Calcitonin (CT)

Production of this small polypeptide hormone is, of course, the hallmark feature of the APUD endocrine tumor, medullary thyroid carcinoma.[24] The parent cell for this tumor, the C cell of the thyroid, is the tissue normally responsible for producing significant quantities of CT in many species, including man.[25,26] The relationship between CT and the first marker described, DDC, is a well-defined one; DDC levels correlate closely with the numbers of CT-producing C cells in the thyroid gland of many species,[27] and DDC is present in varying levels in medullary thyroid carcinoma.[28,29] Increased circulating levels of CT[19,30] and presence of the hormone in tumor tissues[31] have now been described in patients with all histologic types of lung cancer.

Diamine Oxidase or Histaminase Activity (DAO)

This enzyme activity does not bear a specific relationship to APUD cells,[32] but is consistently found in high amounts in human medullary thyroid carcinoma tissue[29,33] and in some other human neoplasms.[34-36] This established relationship between DDC, CT, and DAO, although of a

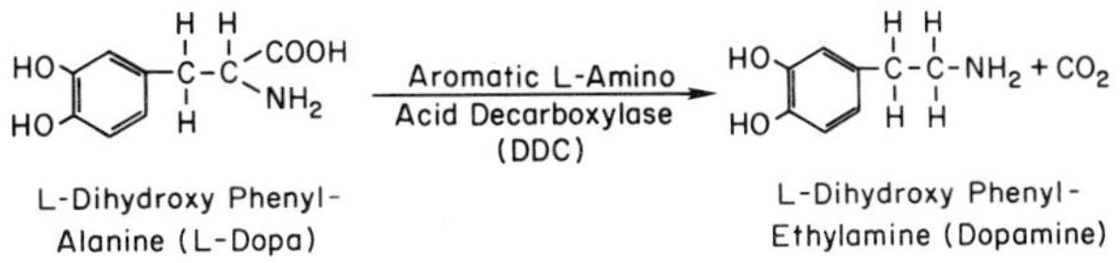

Figure 6-1. *The role of L-dopa decarboxylase (DDC) in the conversion of amine precursor amino acids to their corresponding amines. The reaction is shown here for the conversion of L-dopa to dopamine.*

still undefined nature in medullary carcinoma,[29] led us to include DAO in our studies of lung cancer.

β-Endorphin

In some studies, measurements of the polypeptide hormone, β-endorphin, have been included. This peptide is important because it is synthesized as a portion of the precursor molecule that contains ACTH and β-lipotropin; β-endorphin comprises the last 30 amino acids in β-lipotropin, which, in turn, is contained in the carboxy-terminal portion of the precursor protein.[37,38] The studies of several investigative groups have documented the frequency with which lung cancer tissues contain ACTH[17,39]; synthesis of the precursor protein containing both ACTH and β-lipotropin has also been identified in lung cancer cells.[40] For these reasons, β-endorphin is a potentially useful biochemical parameter for investigation in an endocrine-oriented biochemical study of lung cancer tissues.

Biochemical Patterns in SCC Tissues

The initial phases of our studies were restricted to SCC among the different lung cancers.[41,42] The findings emphasized the heterogeneous nature of the cell populations that constitute this neoplasm; these populations differ between SCC tissues from different patients, between primary and metastatic lesions within the same patient, and even within individual SCC lesions.[41,42] This heterogeneity is well exemplified in studies of DAO alone. Activity of this enzyme was almost always high in primary SCC lesions as compared with values for surrounding lung and bronchial mucosa.[41,42] As shown in Figure 6-2, however, the level of activity varied drastically among tumors from different patients and among lesions from

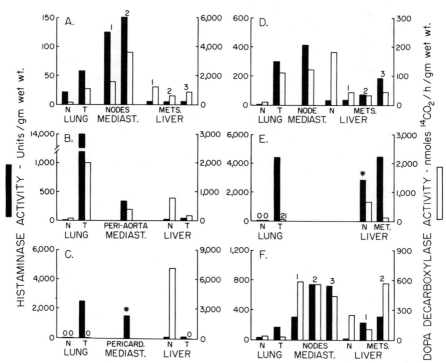

Figure 6-2. *Levels of DAO and L-decarboxylase activities in homogenates of SCC tumor tissues from 6 different patients. The numbers 0 and 21 in (C, E) indicate the actual activity above the assay blank. The other numbers above the bars designate separate metastatic lesions studied. N, normal tissue; T, tumor;*, L-dopa decarboxylase was not measured in the mediastinal tumor (C) and liver tissue could not be separated from the extensive metastatic tumor (E). Also note that normal human liver is known to have considerable L-dopa decarboxylase activity. (Reprinted, by permission of the N Engl J Med, from Baylin et al.[42])*

individual patients.[41,42] In most patients, metastatic lesions contained lower activity than primary lesions (Fig. 6-2); however, in a lesser number of individuals, high values were found in all lesions sampled.[41,42]

The varied distribution of DAO among SCC lesions appears to result from the heterogeneity of cell populations that contain significant quantities of the protein. This heterogeneity can be appreciated, through immunohistochemistry studies, even within single primary SCC lesions (Fig. 6-3).

The variable distribution found for DAO was also characteristic of the

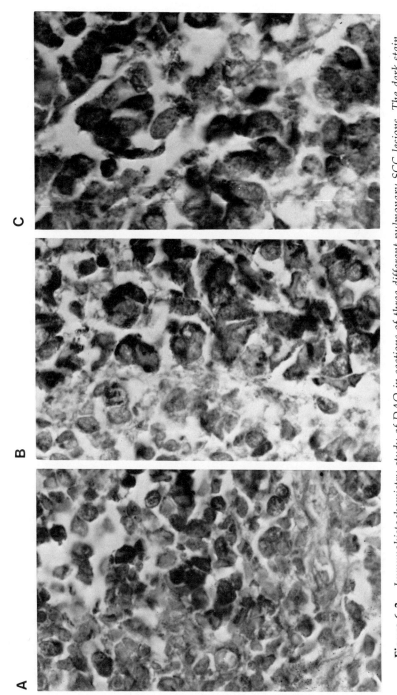

Figure 6-3. *Immunohistochemistry study of DAO in sections of three different pulmonary SCC lesions. The dark stain indicates presence of DAO in the cell cytoplasm; note the heterogeneous pattern of staining in each tumor with many cells showing a positive reaction, but no reaction in other adjacent cells. (Sections kindly provided by Dr. Geoffrey Men-delsohn.[42])*

129

other biochemical parameters studied in SCC. Consistent with the proposed APUD nature of SCC, values of DDC were almost always higher in tumor tissue than in adjacent non–tumor-involved lung. Again, however, tumor tissue values differed drastically between patients and between individual lesions[42]; as for DAO, values were often lower in distant metastases than in primary tumor (Fig. 6-2). Similar findings have been found for CT,[42] which is often present in SCC tissue but usually in small amounts.

Portions of the above data are compatible with the assigning of APUD characteristics to SCC. Certainly, the relatively high levels of DDC in many SCC lesions is consistent with this; to a lesser extent, the presence of CT would also fit this hypothesis. However, the biochemistry data emphasize the heterogeneous nature of SCC; one must conclude, therefore, that a variety of cell types, with unknown relationships between them, constitute SCC lesions at any given point in time. The admixture of morphologic cell types which characterizes SCC, including, to a variable degree, the histologic features of other lung cancers,[20-22] suggests that these different cell types could play a role in the biochemical heterogeneity found. This possibility raises the important question of how the subset of biochemistry under investigation relates to the entire spectrum of human lung cancer as well as to SCC alone. Our subsequent studies have sought to address this issue and are described below.

Biochemical Patterns in the Spectrum of Human Lung Cancer

We have now simultaneously studied the concentrations of four biochemical parameters in a large number of SCC and non-SCC lesions.[43,44] The findings might be summarized as demonstrating that the APUD and other characteristics studied, to a degree, quantitatively, but *not* qualitatively, separate SCC from non-SCC lung cancers. Individual non-SCC tumors, even quantitatively, may fully resemble SCC for the entire set of biochemical parameters studied. The extensive overlap between SCC and non-SCC tumors is well demonstrated for DDC and DAO activity levels in Figure 6-4. The SCC lesions, as a population, clearly have higher values of DDC and DAO activities than do the other types (note that the graph is plotted on a log scale). Even for DDC, however, extensive overlap exists particularly between lung adenocarcinomas and SCC. Note that two adenocarcinoma lesions have DDC activity values far above those for the

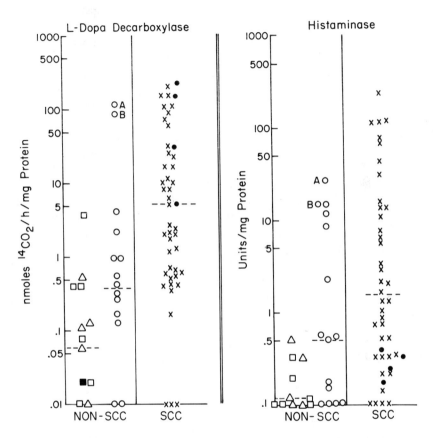

Figure 6-4. *L-dopa decarboxylase and histaminase (diamine oxidase) activities in surgical and autopsy specimens from patients with the major types of lung cancer (note log scale).* Δ, *squamous cell carcinoma, surgical;* ○, *adenocarcinoma, surgical;* □, *large cell carcinoma, surgical;* ■, *large cell carcinoma, autopsy;* X, *small cell carcinoma, autopsy;* ●, *small cell carcinoma, surgical. Two adenocarcinomas are designated (A) and (B) so that they may be followed in the text.* ---, *Median. (Data are updated from Baylin et al.[43])*

131

other tumors in their group, and as high as the top values for SCC. These two tumors also had the highest DAO values among the adenocarcinomas, findings which emphasize the degree to which SCC and non-SCC tumors can share even theoretically APUD-specific features such as high DDC activity.

Our biochemical studies of the spectrum of human lung cancer tissues have also included measurements of the two polypeptide hormones, calcitonin and β-endorphin. Concentrations of these peptides showed even greater overlap among the major histopathologic types than did the enzyme activities discussed above. Significant quantities of calcitonin were found consistently in each of the tumors except for squamous cell cancers; similar findings have been obtained in other studies.[30,45] It is particularly important to note that the two adenocarcinoma lesions discussed above as having very high DDC and DAO activity levels (and designated by A and B in Fig. 6-4) also had the highest concentrations of calcitonin in the current study. The incidence of significant concentrations of β-endorphin was highest in SCC tumors; among these lesions, the highest value was found in a patient with SCC and ectopic ACTH syndrome. In summary, the data for the peptide hormones showed great overlap among the major types of human lung cancer, and neither of the hormones qualitatively separated SCC from the other types.

After having analyzed all the data on tumor lesions, in which all four biochemical markers were simultaneously determined, we sought to derive a quantitative value which would indicate the incidence of a high value for more than one marker occurring in any given tumor type. We derived a simple value which was the product of each of the four markers in each tumor lesion and defined this as an endocrine index.[44] The distribution of these values clearly shows the tendency for endocrine activity to group with SCC as opposed to the other tumor types. Little or no overlap exists between the index values for SCC and the values for the other lung cancers. However, the two adenocarcinomas that had high values for three out of the four markers also had index values higher than the top figures obtained for SCC. As for each of the lesions which comprise the study, the histology of these tumors was reviewed carefully by three or more pathologists; no morphologic features of SCC could be observed on routine studies. One of the two tumors did have a mildly positive Grimelius stain, indicating the presence of some neurosecretory type granules. The index values for these two adenocarcinomas further emphasize that high values for the entire set of biochemical parameters studied can occur in occasional non-SCC tumors.

Biological and Clinical Implications of the
Biochemical Data

We have presented data showing that biochemical properties once thought to be exclusive for SCC are indeed shared among the major histopathologic types of lung cancer. Quantitatively, the index values for the set of markers examined are higher in SCC; however, we have presented firm evidence that some tumors with no morphologic characteristics of SCC may contain high values for multiple markers.

We feel that the data presented are most consistent with the postulation that the major forms of lung cancer share a common cell lineage. Certainly, we have demonstrated that the presence in SCC of a major APUD property, such as DDC, cannot be interpreted as evidence for a separate neural cell origin for this tumor. Moreover, the sharing of the biochemical parameters investigated among the different tumors suggests that all bronchial epithelial neoplasms may indeed arise from a single cell system. This situation might be best visualized by considering briefly, as we have done in detail previously,[32] the known differentiation pathways in the hematopoietic cell system and the mucosa of the gastrointestinal tract.

The evolution of differentiation characteristics is much better understood and characterized in the hematopoietic cell system than in most epithelial systems. In the production of blood cell elements, it is now accepted that a single multipotential stem cell may give rise to the different types of mature cell elements.[46-49] In this concept, the multipotential cell of origin gives rise to a series of cells which retain proliferative capacity but have an increasing degree of commitment along separate differentiation lines. Thus, separate stem cells emerge from the parent cell and give rise to the erythroid, lymphoid, and granulocyte series. Shared differentiation characteristics between the groups appear to be more evident in the early stages of stem cell development than in the stages of more terminal and committed differentiation. The evidence for a single hematopoietic stem cell is also apparent in neoplasms arising within this cell system: in patients with chronic myelogenous leukemia, both the frankly neoplastic cells and most of the more normal-appearing elements of the bone marrow may all apparently arise in a single clone of transformed cells.[50]

The concept of multiple types of differentiated cells arising from a common cell of origin has also been discussed for epithelial cell systems. As mentioned at the outset of this chapter, some investigators have postulated that a multipotential progenitor cell in the crypt region of the gastrointestinal mucosa may give rise to each of the differentiated cells found in this epithelium.[11] Most importantly, for our considerations of the cell of origin of SCC, is the postulation of Cheng and LeBlond that the occasional endocrine or APUD cells scattered throughout the gastrointestinal mucosa are among the cells formed from the common progenitor cell.[11]

The relationships among the major types of human lung cancer could well be appreciated if these neoplasms are viewed in the context of the above proposals for cellular differentiation. It is probable that a common basal progenitor cell in the bronchial epithelium gives rise, through progressive differentiation, to several cell types.[51] Neoplastic transformation would then be superimposed on this complex pathway for cell renewal and differentiation in the normal epithelium. The tumor type that emerges as predominant may be determined by the level of differentiation of the cell(s) in which the final malignant transformation takes place. Alternatively, the level of differentiation achieved in epithelium injured by chronic smoking might determine the level of differentiation of the subsequent neoplasm. In this setting, the frequencies for the types of neoplasms would somewhat parallel the frequencies for the various cell types populating the normal mucosa. Thus, a particular developmental stage of a multipotential columnar mucous cell might be principally involved in the squamous metaplastic changes which take place in the bronchial epithelium of many smokers. This involvement, in turn, might be reflected in the fact that squamous cell carcinoma is the most common type of lung cancer in man. Similarly, some workers have predicted that a multipotential mucous cell with the capacity for mucin production may also be involved in the formation of lung adenocarcinoma.[51]

The position of SCC in the spectrum of human lung cancer and bronchial differentiation is somewhat harder to explain. If the tendency for this tumor to express APUD properties is interpreted as evidence that the tumor originates from endocrine or K cells which are scattered in sparse numbers throughout the bronchial epithelium,[52,53] the incidence of SCC might be predicted to be much lower. If, however, SCC arises in a mucosal cell with multipotential differentiation capabilities, including those of an endocrine cell, the incidence of this neoplasm might be much better explained. The cell of origin for the tumor would not have to be a fully committed endocrine cell at the time of neoplastic transformation; rather, the endocrine characteristics may emerge during a differentiation process which subsequently occurs in the neoplastic tissue itself. Such differentiation might evolve from the commitment level that had been reached by the cell in which the tumor originated. Alternatively, as we have previously discussed, certain APUD cell properties may be more characteristic of all primitive cells in the bronchial mucosa.[32] Occasional endocrine cells may maintain this differentiation as they mature, while most of the other mucosal cell types might lose most of these biochemical characteristics. If, as has been proposed by Yesner, SCC most closely resembles the basal cell component of the bronchial epithelium,[20] then its endocrine biochemical patterns might be expected on this basis.

Whichever sequence of events ultimately proves to explain the relationships among the major types of human lung cancer, there is an increasing body of biochemical evidence that differentiation features are shared among the major types. There is thus a great need for several lines of research. First, the biochemical profile we have investigated and markers studied by other investigators must be placed into perspective in terms of normal bronchial mucosa differentiation. Factors involved in APUD activity, such as DDC, must be related to each of the cell types that constitute the normally renewing epithelium. Through such studies, we might learn whether DDC activity is indeed a generalized property of multipotential basal progenitor cells in the epithelium, as well as of the occasional terminally differentiated endocrine cell. Second, the biochemical events must be related to stages of neoplastic development in the epithelium. The ways in which individual biochemical markers relate to progressive stages of atypia and to the different histologic types of atypia may provide valuable information regarding the distribution of these markers in fully formed lung cancers. Third, studies of this type in other epithelial cell systems will also prove rewarding. For example, we have studied the distribution of two of the markers investigated in the current study in the GI mucosa of the rat.[54] DDC activity is present at very high levels in the intestinal mucosa; the levels found would be poorly explained by the presence of enzyme activity solely in occasional endocrine cells. Rather, it is probable that this enzyme activity is present to some degree in most cells of the mucosa. Studies relating the level of enzyme activity to stage of cell maturation in the renewing mucosa indicate that the specific activity of DDC is some twofold higher in cells from the proliferative crypt region than in cells from the nonproliferative, terminally differentiated villus tip area.[54] Conversely, DAO activity in GI mucosal cells is some sixfold higher in mature villus tip cells than in proliferative cells from the crypt region.[54] Similar relationships between cell kinetic and differentiation features and the biochemical parameters studied may be important in defining the heterogeneous cell populations that constitute SCC and other lung cancers.

Finally, the biochemical data presented also stress the need for the development of in vitro model systems that will permit more detailed studies of the relationships between kinetic and differentiation parameters and biochemical markers. The establishment of cell culture systems for SCC and other types of human lung cancer has been the emphasis of several investigative groups, and studies with these systems are outlined in Chapters 3, 4 and 7 of this monograph. Some of the biochemical parameters discussed in this chapter, bear important relationships to lung cancer cells in culture, however, and it is appropriate to discuss these data here briefly. DDC activity appears to be a constant marker of SCC cells in cell culture.[43] As shown in Figure 6-5, there is much less overlap between SCC and non-SCC cancers in DDC activity in cell culture than we have found in analyses of autopsy and surgical tissues (Fig. 6-4). The reasons for this difference have not yet been defined, but may relate in part to the selection of cell populations that can be established in culture from each tumor type. Also, differences in the direction and degree of differentiation of the cultured tumor cells versus the cells in vivo may be involved. One certain implication of the data is that the constantly high DDC activity found in SCC culture lines appears to make the activity level of this enzyme an important marker for identifying SCC cells in culture.

Interestingly, the activity of DAO bears an opposite relationship for SCC in cell culture as compared to SCC in surgical and autopsy specimens.[43] DAO activity is low in the majority of SCC culture lines thus far investigated and does not separate SCC from other types of lung cancer cells in culture. Again, the explanation for this difference between in vivo and in vitro findings may involve (1) the particular clones of cells which are able to be established in culture; (2) the preferential selection of proliferative cells by culture techniques; or (3) the direction and degree of cellular differentiation achieved by the cultured cells. It is of interest in this regard that, when the cultured cells are grown in the athymic or nude mouse, the distribution of the activity values for both DDC and DAO more resemble those for the in vivo specimens shown in Figure 6-4.[43] More detailed investigation of the relationships between the cell types present in culture and their expression of the biochemical markers we have studied follows in Chapter 7 of this monograph.

The precise implications of the discussed biochemistry for the clinical arena are not yet defined. However, there are some important possibilities that merit discussion. First, the ramifications of the shared biochemical parameters for defining the types of cells that populate each form of lung cancer must be considered. We previously discussed the findings, outlined in Chapter 10, regarding the presence of mixed histologies within single lesions of lung cancer. One must raise the possibility that more subtle mixtures of cell types, which might not be grossly apparent in routine histologic studies, might be reflected in the variable biochemical patterns we have obtained. For example, SCC lesions with a relatively low endocrine index might contain cells with biologic features of the other

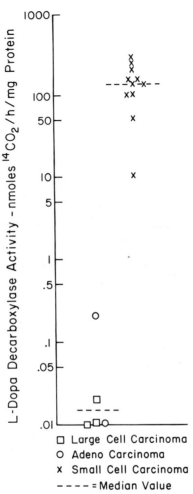

Figure 6-5. *L-dopa carboxylase activity in sonicates of cultured cells of SCC and non-SCC tumors. (Data are updated from Baylin et al.[43])*

types of human lung cancer; the relationships between SCC and large cell carcinoma which are outlined in Chapter 7 may be illustrative of this possibility. Conversely, adenocarcinoma lesions with a high endocrine index might contain cell types with biologic features of SCC. Given the high susceptibility of SCC cells to radiation and/or chemotherapy and the relatively lower sensitivity of the other types of human lung cancer, these postulations merit serious consideration. The emergence of drug resistance in patients on long-term chemotherapy for SCC could involve the selection of cell types or the transition of SCC cells to resistant types that might be marked by changes in the types of biochemical parameters we have considered. These possibilities have been discussed in some detail in Chapters 7 and 10 of this monograph. Alternatively, it is known that a small percentage of adenocarcinomas may initially be quite responsive to combination chemotherapy treatment. Could those lesions be represented by the occasional adenocarcinomas with a high endocrine index as we have illustrated in the present studies? As in vitro techniques capable of testing for the presence of cell populations in single tumors with differing drug sensitivities become more sophisticated, the relationships between biochemical expression of various cells and their response to therapeutic modalities might become further clarified.

Finally, the biochemical data we have obtained and studies from other investigators have ramifications for the use of endocrine biomarkers in monitoring the course of lung cancer. The heterogeneous nature of SCC for the modalities studied suggests that it is unlikely that any single peptide hormone yet investigated may serve as a universal biomarker for this tumor. In light of the data presented, it is not difficult to see why only a certain percentage of patients with SCC and other lung cancers will have an elevated value in the circulation of any given marker[17,18,30,32,39,45] and also why, on many occasions, the sequential measurements of the circulating marker may not behave concordantly with the changes in tumor mass.[41,55] Furthermore, the data clearly indicate that no one marker will serve to suggest the underlying histology of the lung neoplasm involved. By contrast, the use of multiple markers might be much more valuable for these purposes. The data presented on the derived endocrine index suggest the degree to which multiple endocrine parameters may group towards SCC cancers; therefore, the finding of a combination of elevated values for multiple endocrine parameters in the circulation of a patient with lung cancer might correlate more closely with SCC.[44] Also, such a combination of markers would be more likely to define one or more parameters that are indeed elevated in the circulation. The combination would also possibly obviate the false information derived from discordant behavior of a single marker during changes in tumor burden.

Summary

In this chapter, we have discussed data concerning the distribution of a small subset of endocrine-related biochemistry among the spectrum of human lung cancers. We have presented evidence that the biochemical parameters investigated have a heterogeneous distribution in SCC lesions both between patients and among SCC tumor lesions within the same patient. The underlying dynamics for this heterogeneity appears to involve different cell populations in the tumor which variably express the biochemical parameters being investigated. We have shown that the endocrine properties are not qualitatively restricted to SCC among the human lung cancers and are shared to a variable degree among all the histologic types. Quantitatively, the endocrine parameters tend to group more with SCC than with the other tumors, although occasional lung cancers, such as adenocarcinoma, may fully express the biochemical activity. We suggest, from these data and from analyses of studies by other investigators, that evidence is emerging against a separate neural cell origin for SCC in the bronchial mucosa, and that it appears much more likely that the spectrum of human lung cancers represents neoplastic changes within a common cell lineage. The potential biologic implications of the current findings must be realized through detailed studies of biochemical relationships between differentiating cells in the normal bronchial mucosa and of the manner(s) in which these relationships are either retained or distorted, or both, in various stages of neoplastic transformation. The potential clinical importance depends on the degree to which biochemical classifications of lung tumors may or may not serve as a valuable adjunct to histologic classifications in predicting the course and/or treatment sensitivity of individual lesions.

References

1. Muggia FM, Krezoski SK, Hansen HH: Cell kinetics in patients with small cell carcinoma of the lung. Cancer 34:1683–1690, 1974
2. Straus MJ: The growth characteristics of lung cancer and its application to treatment design. Sem Oncol 1:167–174, 1974
3. Matthews MJ: Problems in morphology and behavior of bronchopulmonary malignant disease, in Israel L, Chahinian AP (eds): Lung Cancer: Natural History Prognosis and Therapy. New York, Academic Press, 1976, p 23
4. Greco FA, Oldham RK: Small-cell lung cancer. New Engl J Med 301:355–358, 1979
5. Meador CK, Liddle GW, Island DP, et al: Cause of Cushing's syndrome in patients with tumors arising from "non-endocrine" tissue. J Clin Endocrinol Metab 22:693–703, 1962
6. Amatruda TT Jr, Mulrow PJ, Gallagher JC, et al: Carcinoma of the lung with inappropriate antidiuresis: Demonstration of antidiuretic-

hormone-like activity in tumor extract. N Engl J Med 269:544–548, 1963

7. Pearse AGE: The cytochemistry and ultrastructure of polypeptide hormone producing cells of the APUD series and the embryologic, physiologic and pathologic implications of the concept. J Histochem Cytochem 17:303–313, 1969

8. Tischler AS: Small cell carcinoma of the lung: Cellular origin and relationship to other neoplasms. Sem Oncol 5:244–252, 1978

9. Tischler AS, Dichter MA, Biales B, et al: Neuroendocrine neoplasms and their cells of origin. N Engl J Med 296:919–925, 1977

10. Bell EC, Seetharam S: Expression of endodermally derived and neural crest-derived differentiation antigens by human lung and colon tumors. Cancer 44:13–18, 1979

11. Cheng H, LeBlond CP: Origin, differentiation and renewal of the four main epithelial cell types in the mouse small intestine. V. Unitarian theory of the origin of the four epithelial cell types. Am J Anat 141:537–562, 1974

12. Andrew A: Further evidence that enterochromaffin cells are not derived from the neural crest. J Embryol Exp Morphol 31:589–598, 1974

13. Fontaine J, LeDouarin NM: Analysis of endoderm formation in the avian blastoderm by the use of quail-chick chimeras: Problem of the neuro-ectodermal origin of the cells of the APUD series. J Embryol Exp Morphol 41:209–222, 1977

14. Pearse AGE, Takor Takor T: Embryology of the diffuse neuroendocrine system and its relationship to the common peptides. Fed Proc 38:2288–2294, 1979

15. LeDouarin NM, LeLièvre C: Sur l'origine des cellules à calcitonine du corps ultimobranchial de l'embryon d'oiseau. C R Assoc Anat 152:558–568, 1971

16. Teillet MA, LeDouarin NM: Determination par la méthode des graffes hétérospécifiques d'ébauches neurales de caille sur l'embryon de poulet, du niveau du néuraxe dont derivent les cellules médullo-surrenaliennes. Arch Anat Micr Morph Exp 63:51–62, 1974

17. Gewirtz G, Yalow RS: Ectopic ACTH production in carcinoma of the lung. J Clin Invest 53:1022–1032, 1974

18. Odell WD, Wolfsen AR, Bachelot I, et al: Ectopic production of lipotropin by cancer. Am J Med 66:631–638, 1979

19. Silva OL, Becker KL, Primack A, et al: Increased serum calcitonin levels in bronchogenic cancer. Chest 69:495–499, 1976

20. Yesner R: Spectrum of lung cancer and ectopic hormones. Pathol Ann 13:217–240, 1978

21. Brereton HD, Matthews MM, Costa J, et al: Mixed anaplastic small-cell and squamous-cell carcinoma of the lung. Ann Int Med 88:805–806, 1978

22. Abeloff MD, Eggleston JC, Mendelsohn G, et al: Changes in morphologic and biochemical characteristics of small cell carcinoma of the lung—A clinico-pathologic study. Am J Med 66:757–764, 1979

23. Christenson JG, Dairman W, Udenfriend S: On the identify of DOPA decarboxylase and 5-hydroxy tryptophan decarboxylase. Proc Natl Acad Sci USA 69:343–347, 1972

24. Tashjian AH Jr, Howland BG, Melvin KEW, et al: Immunoassay of calcitonin, clinical measurement, relation to serum calcium, and studies in patients with medullary carcinoma. N Engl J Med 283:890–895, 1970

25. Foster GV, MacIntyre I, Pearse AGE: Calcitonin production and the mitochondrion-rich cells of the dog thyroid. Nature 203:1029–1030, 1964

26. Williams ED: Histogenesis of medullary carcinoma of the thyroid. J Clin Pathol 19:114–118, 1966

27. Hakanson R, Owman C, Sundler F: Aromatic-L-amino acid decarboxylase in calcitonin-producing cells. Biochem Pharmacol 20:2187–2190, 1971

28. Atkins FL, Beaven MA, Keiser HR: Dopa-decarboxylase in medullary carcinoma of the thyroid. N Engl J Med 289:545–548, 1973

29. Baylin SB, Mendelsohn G, Weisburger WR, et al: Levels of histaminase and L-dopa decarboxylase activity in the transition from C-cell hyperplasia to familial medullary thyroid carcinoma. Cancer 44:143–149, 1979

30. Schwartz KE, Wolfsen AR, Forster B, et al: Calcitonin in nonthyroidal cancer. J Clin Endocrinol Metab 49:438–444, 1979

31. Becker KL, Snider RH, Silva OL, et al: Calcitonin heterogeneity in lung cancer and medullary thyroid cancer. Acta Endocrinol 89:89–99, 1978

32. Baylin SB, Mendelsohn G: Ectopic (inappropriate) hormone production by tumors: Mechanisms involved and the biological and clinical implications. Endocrinol Rev 1:45–77, 1980

33. Baylin SB, Beaven MA, Engelman K, et al: Elevated histaminase activity in medullary carcinoma of the thyroid gland. N Engl J Med 283:1239–1244, 1970

34. Lin C-W, Orcutt ML, Stolbach LL: Elevation of histaminase and its concurrence with Regan isoenzyme in ovarian cancer. Cancer Res 35:2762–2765, 1975

35. Lin C-W, Inglis NR, Rule AH, et al: Histaminase and other tumor markers in malignant effusion fluids. Cancer Res 39:4894–4899, 1979

36. Ettinger DS, Rosenshein NB, Parmley TH, et al: Tumor cell origin of histaminase activity in ascites fluid from patients with ovarian carcinoma. Cancer 45:2568–2572, 1980

37. Mains RE, Eipper BA, Ling N: Common precursor to corticotropins and endorphins. Proc Natl Acad Sci USA 74:3014–3018, 1977

38. Eipper BA, Mains RE: Structure and biosynthesis of pro-adrenocorticotropin/endorphin and related peptides. Endocrinol Rev 1:1–27, 1980

39. Wolfsen AR, Odell WD: Pro-ACTH: Use for early detection of lung cancer. Am J Med 66:765–772, 1979

40. Bertagna XY, Nicholson WE, Sorenson GD, et al: Corticotropin, lipotropin, and β-endorphin production by a human nonpituitary tumor in culture: Evidence for a common precursor. Proc Natl Acad Sci USA 75:5160–5164, 1978

41. Baylin SB, Abeloff MD, Wieman KC, et al: Elevated histaminase (diamine oxidase) activity in small-cell carcinoma of the lung. N Engl J Med 293:1286–1290, 1975

42. Baylin SB, Weisburger WR, Eggleston JC, et al: Variable content of histaminase, L-dopa decarboxylase and calcitonin in small-cell carcinoma of the lung—Biologic and clinical implications. N Engl J Med 299:105–110, 1978

43. Baylin SB, Abeloff MD, Goodwin G, et al: Activities of L-dopa decarboxylase and diamine oxidase (histaminase) in human lung cancers and decarboxylase as a marker for small (oat) cell cancer in cell culture. Cancer Res 40:1990–1994, 1980

44. Berger CL, Goodwin G, Mendelsohn G, et al: Endocrine biochemistry in the spectrum of human lung carcinoma. J Clin Endocrinol Metab (in press)

45. Roos BA, Lindall AW, Baylin SB, et al: Plasma immunoreactive calcitonin in lung cancer. J Clin Endocrinol Metab 50:659–666, 1980

46. Cline MJ, Golde DW: Controlling the production of blood cells. Blood 53:157–165, 1979

47. Quesenberry P, Levitt L: Hematopoietic stem cells (part 1). N Engl J Med 301:755–760, 1979

48. Quesenberry P, Levitt L: Hematopoietic stem cells (part 2). N Engl J Med 301:819–823, 1979

49. Quesenberry P, Levitt L: Hematopoietic stem cells (part 3). N Engl J Med 301:868–872, 1979

50. Fialkow PJ, Jacobsen RJ, Papayannopoulou T, et al: Chronic myelocytic leukemia: Clonal origin in a stem cell common to the granulocyte, erythrocyte, platelet and monocyte/macrophage. Am J Med 63:125–130, 1977

51. McDowell EM, Barrett LA, Glavin F, et al: The respiratory epithelium. I. Human bronchus. J Natl Cancer Inst 61:539–549, 1978

52. Bensch KG, Corrin B, Parienta R, et al: Oat cell carcinoma of the lung. Its origin and relationship to bronchial carcinoid. Cancer 22:1163–1170, 1968

53. Bonikos DS, Bensch KG: Endocrine cells of bronchial and bronchiolar epithelium. Am J Med 63:765–771, 1977

54. Baylin SB, Stevens SA, Shakir KMM: Association of diamine oxidase and ornithine decarboxylase with maturing cells in rapidly proliferating epithelium. Biochem Biophys Acta 541:415–419, 1978

55. Hansen M, Hommer L: Ectopic hormone production in small cell carcinoma, in Muggia TM, Rozencweig M (eds): Lung Cancer: Progress in Therapeutic Research. New York, Raven Press, 1979, p 207

7

SMALL CELL CARCINOMA OF THE LUNG: CELLULAR ORIGIN AND RELATIONSHIP TO OTHER PULMONARY TUMORS

Adi F. Gazdar
Desmond N. Carney
John G. Guccion
Stephen B. Baylin

For some years small cell carcinoma of the lung (SCC) has been recognized as a distinct clinical, pathological, and biological entity.[1] These features, in addition to the unique responsiveness of SCC to cytotoxic therapy, divide the major forms of lung cancer into two broad groups: SCC and non-SCC tumors. The realization, over a decade ago, that SCC and their presumptive precursor cells were part of a diffuse network of cells having amine-handling properties[2] led to a new theory of histogenesis. Whereas the rest of the bronchial mucosa, and the tumors derived from it, were of endodermal origin, Pearse suggested that amine precursor uptake and decarboxylation (APUD) cells were derived from the neural crest.[2] However, gradual accumulation of new data, together with a re-evaluation of previously known facts, has led some investigators to revive the older, unitarian theory of histogenesis.

This chapter discusses the cells of the normal bronchial mucosa and their possible histogenesis, the tumors arising from them, and the complex interrelationships among these tumors. We review the important lessons that can be learned from the endocrine cells of the gastrointestinal tract. In addition, we describe experimental models that we have developed for examining the histogenesis and biology of SSC and its relationships to other tumors. Finally, we outline theories explaining the relationships among the various forms of lung cancer.

Whereas the histogenesis of a tumor is primarily of interest to the embryologist, anatomist, and biologist, it may also be of importance to the clinician. An understanding of the etiology of a tumor may lead to the development of new methods of prevention and treatment. This chapter contains a mixture of both fact and speculation about the etiology of SCC. Whenever possible, we have tried to clearly delineate one from the other.

The Respiratory Mucosa

The respiratory mucosa and the alveolar lining cells are of endodermal origin. The lungs begin as a ventral diverticulum of the foregut, which elongates caudally and branches laterally to form the lung buds. The buds branch repeatedly to form the bronchopulmonary buds. These are surrounded by mesoderm, from which arise the vascular, cartilaginous, muscular, and fibroelastic components. The pleura is also of mesodermal origin.

The tracheobronchial mucosa is pseudostratified and consists of several cell types.[3] The small dark basal cells form a nearly continuous layer covering the basement membrane. They do not reach the luminal surface. Basal cells proliferate in response to many stimuli and probably represent the progenitor cells of many, if not all, of the other cell types. Another form of basal cell has a lighter cytoplasm and contains dense-core neurosecretory granules. It is described in greater detail in a following section. The luminal cells consist mainly of goblet cells, distended to varying degrees with mucin, and tall columnar ciliated cells. Other, relatively undifferentiated cell types have also been described.[3] They probably represent the immediate precursors of the fully differentiated luminal cells. Occasionally, ciliated cells will contain mucin granules, indicating that they and the goblet cells originate from a common precursor.[3] Ciliated and goblet cells are fully differentiated end-stage cells; they do not incorporate thymidine. Because of their scarcity in the adult lung, relatively little is known about the replicative capacities of the neurosecretory granule-containing cells. Bronchioles are lined by a single layer of cuboidal ciliated cells and cuboidal or columnar glycogen-containing Clara cells. Alveoli are lined by a single layer of flattened type I pneumocytes and plump type II pneumocytes, the latter containing osmiophilic lamellar bodies—the apparent source of surfactant. Alveolar cells apparently arise by replication and migration of bronchiolar cells.

In response to injury, infection, or exposure to carcinogens, a proliferation of basal and undifferentiated columnar cells occurs—basal cell hyperplasia. Frequently, goblet cell hyperplasia is also noted, and the mucosa is distended by multiple layers of mucin-distended cells. Further or continued injury results in a shedding of the superficial mucosa and its replacement by metaplastic squamous cells.[4] The metaplastic cells may arise directly from undifferentiated cells or from mucous granule-containing cells.[4] With time, progressive anaplasia of the metaplastic cells occurs, with eventual development of squamous cell carcinoma in situ.[5] These changes frequently require exposure to carcinogens over several years.[5] All of the changes, except carcinoma in situ, are believed to be reversible.

The Pathology of Lung Cancer

A detailed description of the pathology of lung cancer is beyond the scope of this chapter. However, an outline is required for an understanding of the origin of and complex interrelationships among the various forms of lung cancer. More than 90 percent of pulmonary malignancies are of four major types. By light microscopy, two of these are regarded as "differentiated" and two as "undifferentiated" carcinomas. For more detailed accounts of lung cancer pathology than that presented below, see Matthews and Gordon,[6] Mackay et al,[7] and Chapter 2 of this monograph.

The commonest form of lung cancer is squamous cell or epidermoid. This type of cancer usually presents as bulky, central tumors. The tumor cells frequently stratify and are connected by "intercellular bridges." Better-differentiated tumors elaborate keratin, which is visible intra- or extracellularly. Ultrastructurally the most prominent feature is the presence of numerous, prominent desmosomes (the "intracellular bridges"), which are associated with bundles of tonofilaments. Keratin may be deposited on the latter. Squamous carcinomas are often associated with, and presumed to arise from, foci of atypical squamous metaplasia. Carcinoma in situ may be present, and almost certainly precedes the onset of invasive carcinoma.[8]

Most adenocarcinomas arise peripherally, and are unconnected to the major bronchi. Many of the peripheral tumors are the classic bronchiolar–alveolar carcinomas, which consist of cuboidal or columnar cells forming papillary structures and tending to line air spaces. They may be associated with, and presumably arise from, hyperplastic atypical columnar alveolar cells; however, their original cell of origin is probably bronchiolar. A minority of adenocarcinomas arise centrally, from the surface epithelium or from bronchial glands. Whatever their origin, adenocarcinomas have a basic tendency to form acinar structures. Luminal cell borders frequently have microvilli. Complex interdigitations exist between adjacent cells, and tight junctions are often present adjacent to the lumen. Intra- and extracellular mucin may be noted by light or electron microscopy. Ciliated cells are rarely present.

Large cell carcinoma is a designation for epithelial neoplasms that do not show evidence of maturation by light microscopy and that lack the characteristic nuclear cytology of SCC. They are composed of polygonal, spindle, or oval cells containing abundant cytoplasm and pleomorphic nuclei. Nucleoli frequently are prominent. By electron microscopy, some tumors show feeble attempts at differentiation towards adenocarcinomas (small microvilli, mucin formation) or squamous cell carcinomas (well-formed desmosomes, tonofilaments).[7,9] Some tumors lack all evidence of differentiation. It has been reported that some large cell carcinomas contain neurosecretory granules,[10,11] and thus may be related to SCC. Whether such tumors actually exist, or whether they represent polygonal cell variants of SCC mistakenly called large cell carcinomas, is debatable. Because many large cell carcinomas are distinguished from poorly differentiated carcinomas only by their relatively greater percentage of undifferentiated cells, the very concept of large cell carcinoma as a separate entity has been questioned. The concept incorporates a heterogeneous collection of tumors composed of undifferentiated or poorly differentiated cells, so that the term "large cell carcinoma" serves as a convenient wastebin for carcinomas that do not readily fit into other pigeon holes. As our methods of diagnosis become more sophisticated and are routinely applied to surgical specimens, we may restrict the term to a relatively small group of tumors that appear to be truly undifferentiated (and thus possibly represent a stem cell carcinoma).

The pathology of SCC and its subtypes is described in Chapter 2 of this monograph. Some of its features require emphasis and are restated here. The cells are relatively small and have high nuclear–cytoplasmic ratios. Their distinguishing feature is not size, but nuclear characteristics. Nucleoli are small and inconspicuous. The chromatin is finely granular and dispersed in a "salt and pepper" fashion. Ultrastructurally, the distinguishing feature is the presence of neurosecretory granules (see below). The cytoplasm appears relatively lucent, because of the lack of organelles. As discussed in Chapter 2, subtyping appears to have little or no clinical or biological importance.

Carcinoid tumors, very similar to those appearing in the foregut, usually occur centrally and may be associated with the carcinoid syndrome.[12] The cells have vesicular nuclei, and mitoses are rare. They metastasize late and have a relatively good prognosis. Whereas most of them arise from the large bronchi, some of the peripheral ones may histologically resemble SCC and are more highly malignant.[13,14]

A discussion of other, rarer, forms of lung cancer and mesotheliomas is beyond the scope of this chapter.

Endocrine Cells of the Respiratory Tract and the APUD Cell Concept

In a series of papers spread over many years, the Austrian pathologist Feyrter described a system of epithelial cells with characteristic morphological and histological characteristics.[15] Most of these cells were found in the gut, but later some were identified in a variety of organs, including the lung. He named them Helle-Zellen cells because of their clear cytoplasm, and they frequently stained with argentophil or argyrophil silver techniques. Feyrter considered them endodermal in origin and ascribed to them a hormonal function with either distant (endocrine) or local (paracrine) effects. He considered them the precursors of carcinoid tumors.

Pearse, during the 1960s, identified a similar group of cells present in many endocrine and nonendocrine organs. The cells either stored amines or could take up precursor substances and decarboxylate them to amines. The decarboxylase, aromatic amino acid decarboxylase, acted on a number of substrates, and is also referred to as L-dopa decarboxylase (DDC; see Chapter 6, this monograph.) Pearse named the cells amine precursor uptake and decarboxylation (APUD) cells, after their principal properties.[2] Ultrastructurally, their most consistent feature was the presence of cytoplasmic dense-core granules that resembled those found in certain nerve endings and hence were called neurosecretory granules.

Pearse contended that APUD cells possessed common metabolic functions and that their major function was the formation of polypeptide and amine hormones, which were stored in the neurosecretory granules. He postulated that there were at least two mechanisms by which these cells of multiple organ systems could have developed similar properties: (1) they were of diverse origin but had evolved similar biochemical and functional properties; or (2) they shared a common embryological origin, and had retained, usefully or not, a distinct set of ancestral functions. Because certain APUD cells (melanoblasts, pheochromoblasts, thyroid C cells) were of known neural crest origin, if all APUD cells had a common ancestry, they had to evolve from the neural crest. Pearse subsequently became a strong proponent of the theory that all APUD cells arose from the neural crest,[16,17] although he has modified his views recently.[18]

While Feyrter and others had long ago suggested that endocrine cells were present in the lung, ultrastructural confirmation was slow in arriving.[19,20] Much of the difficulty may have been attributable to the scarcity of the cells in the adult respiratory tract; however, they are relatively abundant in the fetal lung.[21] Whereas only one morphological cell type has been described in the adult lung, the fetal lung has at least three morphologically distinguishable cell types.[21] The characteristic feature of these endocrine cells is the presence of neurosecretory granules; the number, size, and appearance of the granules are variable, however. The cells are often flask shaped, and their apices may reach the luminal surface.[22] They have been identified in segmental bronchi, bronchioles, and bronchial glands. Usually the cells are single, but they may occur in small groups. Neurosecretory granules have been found in a small percentage of mucin-containing cells,[23] suggesting that cellular interconversions may occur.

In addition to their ultrastructural resemblance to APUD cells, the respiratory endocrine cells fluoresce after exposure to formaldehyde vapor, provided that they are first exposed to an amine precursor.[24] This indicates precursor uptake and decarboxylation, with either a failure to store amines or the storage of an unknown, nonfluorogenic amine. A major function of APUD cells is the secretion of polypeptide hormones, and several biologically active peptides have been identified in normal lung, including substance P, bombesin, and a distinct "spasmogenic peptide."[25,26] A variety of other hormones, including bombesin, ACTH and a hypothetical "pneumokinin," have been suggested as possible products.[17] Until the recent finding of intracytoplasmic calcitonin,[27] however, no polypeptide hormone had been identified directly in the pulmonary endocrine cells. Masson[28] described the intimate relationship between nerve endings and intestinal endocrine cells, coining the term "neurocrine cells." Intramucosal nerves have been described in rat airways and are often associated with basal cells.[29] In addition, intramucosal collections of cells with APUD properties, "neuroepithelial bodies," have been described in various species, including man, and are associated with nerve endings.[30] Under conditions of experimental hypoxia, the cells of these bodies discharged their granules, suggesting that they were hypoxia-sensitive neuroreceptors.

Despite the above-mentioned findings, our knowledge of the endocrine cells of the lung remains at a relatively primitive level.[31] This is attributable partly to the failure to isolate pure or enriched populations of the cells and partly to the lack of knowledge of their secretory products. Whether functionally different endocrine cells exist in the lung, or whether one cell type can secrete multiple products is also unknown. The recent finding that carcinogens may induce experimental proliferation of pulmonary APUD cells[32,33] may aid these studies.

The endocrine cells of the lung are known by several terms, including: K, Kultschitzky (or Kulchitsky); neurosecretory; neurocrine (or neuroendocrine); argyrophilic; argyrophilic-fluorescent-granulated (AFG), or APUD cells.

APUD Cell Properties of SCC and Bronchial Carcinoids

The finding of neurosecretory granules in SCC and bronchial carcinoids[34,35] provided the major impetus for investigating their possible origin. The granules are present in only some SCC cells and in such cells tend to be small, relatively scarce, and localized mainly near the cell border and in cytoplasmic processes. In contrast, neurosecretory granules in carcinoid cells are larger, more abundant, variable in size and shape, and present in most, if not all, cells. They are distributed throughout the cytoplasm.[7,20,22,36] The larger size and greater numbers of granules present in carcinoids accounts for the greater frequency with which the granules stain positive with silver stains.[37] Argyrophil granules may also be demonstrated in SCC, especially when the Grimelius stain is used.[38] Pulmonary tumorlets, minute lesions occurring in the peripheral bronchi and bronchioles, also contain argyrophil-staining neurosecretory granules.[39] The tumorlets may be related to or may represent early or in situ forms of peripheral carcinoids.

Biochemical evidence links these tumors to APUD tumors as well, and, in particular, to the carcinoid tumors of the gut and to their precursor cells. Whereas the carcinoid syndrome may occasionally occur with bronchial carcinoids and SCC,[12,40,41] the detection of catechols, indoles, their amines, and other substances implicated in the carcinoid syndrome occur more frequently.[34,36,42] The demonstration of the key APUD enzyme, DDC, in SCC tumors and cultures[43-45] confirmed Pearse's inclusion of SCC in his list of APUD cell tumors.[2]

Occasional reports of syndromes of hormonal excess in patients with SCC have been described for many years. However, the development of sensitive radioimmunoassays for serum hormone levels demonstrated a much greater frequency of "ectopic" hormone secretion. Because the secreted peptide hormones are frequently in the form of relatively inactive precursor molecules, the incidence of clinical symptoms is relatively low. Whereas many, and often multiple, forms of peptides may be secreted,[46] the ones most commonly detected are ACTH, calcitonin, and arginine vasopressin[47-51] (see also Chapter 8, this monograph). Elevated levels of hormones in serum or tumors may be caused by many mechanisms, but hormonal secretion by continuous cultures of SCC and their clones confirms their endocrine properties.[52,53]

SCC, bronchial carcinoids, and other APUD tumors generate all-or-nothing short-duration action potentials similar to those in neurons.[54,55] Whereas these findings were thought to indicate a neuroectodermal origin for APUD tumors, action potentials are also present in muscle and pancreatic islet cells.[56]

The Morphological and Biochemical Spectrum of Lung Cancer

The findings reported above indicate that SCC is a distinct biological entity and that the cells have APUD properties. At first most investigators, including ourselves, accepted Pearse's hypothesis that all APUD cells were derived from the neural crest. However, several new, and some previous, data indicate a relationship among the major forms of lung cancer, including SCC, and suggest a common embryological origin.

The classic histological descriptions of SCC by Barnard[57] and Azzopardi[58] identified tubular formation, rosettes, squamous nests, giant cells, and even mucin secretion. The presence of foci of squamous carcinoma or adenocarcinoma in SCC tumors is recognized by the World Health Organization classification as a separate category, whereas the more common composite tumor, consisting of small and large cell carcinoma components, is not.[59] Our experience with 360 patients over the last 7 yr indicates that 6 percent of untreated SCC cases present with mixed histology. After therapy, 39 percent of SCC cases have mixed histology at autopsy, and in a few cases the residual tumor is of a completely different histological type.[60] Similar observations have been made by others[61,62] (see also Chapter 10, this monograph). Changes in morphology may be accompanied by loss of DDC activity and other tumor markers.[62] In addition to tumors having mixed histology, multiple lung cancers may arise simultaneously or metachronously. The premalignant changes preceding the onset of squamous cell carcinoma and SCC are similar,[5] and there is a high incidence of in situ or invasive squamous cell carcinoma occurring metachronously with SCC.[63] Although there are many explanations for these findings (see Chapter 10, this monograph), ultrastructural evidence indicates that SCC cells may undergo squamous metaplasia.[7,64] Nitrosamine-induced pulmonary neoplasia in the hamster is preceded by bronchial endocrine-cell hyperplasia. These cells subsequently undergo squamous metaplasia.[32]

Biochemical evidence also links all forms of lung cancer[44] (see also Chapter 6, this monograph). Therefore, although levels of DDC and hormone secretion or content are highest and most frequent in SCC, they can be found in any morphological type of lung cancer, especially adenocarcinoma. These findings suggest that lung cancers cannot be rigidly compartmentalized. Rather, they present a continuous and changing histological and biological spectrum of interrelated tumor types.

Development of Model Systems

In an effort to study the biology and interrelationship of lung cancers, we have developed models of human lung cancer by serially transplanting tumors in athymic nude mice and establishing continuous cell cultures.[45] Tumor specimens, both primary and metastatic, are obtained from untreated and relapsed patients and are injected subcutaneously into nude mice and cultured. The basic scheme is outlined in Figure 7-1. We have found that serially transplanted tumors are excellent sources of cultures, and use them as a secondary source when attempts to culture the parent tumor directly fail. In addition, cultured cells are injected into nude mice to confirm their tumorigenicity as well as determine their histological cell type.

Heterotransplanted tumors arise at the site of injection and grow progressively as crcumscribed or locally invasive tumors. Distant metastases do not occur. The heterotransplanted tumors, at least initially, closely resemble the histological type of the original human tumor. The tumors are serially transplanted at 4- to 10-wk intervals.

SCC cultures initially replicate very slowly and display considerable dependence on growth factors released by other growing SCC cells or accompanying stromal cells[45] (see also Chapters 3 and 4, this monograph). Once established as independent continuous cultures, free of stromal cells, they replicate relatively slowly as aggregates of floating cells, and clone in semisolid medium at low efficiencies. All cultures are aneuploid, with a wide range of chromosome number, ranging from hypodiploid to

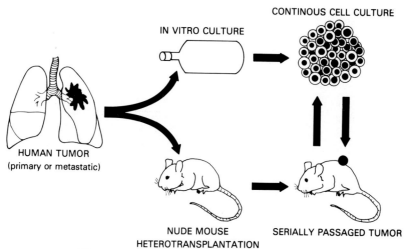

Figure 7-1. *Development of experimental models.*

near-tetraploid. Cultured cells resemble SCC cytologically (Fig. 7-2), although careful examination of the cultured cells usually reveals small numbers of cells with larger nuclei, moderate amounts of cytoplasm, and eosinophilic nucleoli. In contrast, non-SCC cultures (Table 7-1) are readily established as rapidly growing cultures without the need for additional growth factors, and they replicate faster and frequently adhere to the substrate. They clone relatively efficiently and retain their characteristic morphology and cytology.

Using these techniques, we have established 16 continuous SCC cultures, 6 non-SCC cultures, and 7 serially transplanted SCC tumors. Of these, 12 SCC cultures and 5 tumors have been studied serially for periods of 6–50 mo. Initial characterization of the SCC models revealed remarkable uniformity in expression of APUD cell markers. All cultures had exceedingly high levels of the key APUD cell enzyme, DDC, whereas non-SCC cultures had low or absent levels (Fig. 7-3). In addition, SCC cultures had neurosecretory granules in the cytoplasm of at least some of their cells (Fig. 7-4). As in SCC tumors, the granules occurred in the peripheral cytoplasm or in cellular processes. Exposure of cultured SCC cells to formaldehyde-induced vapor resulted in weak fluorescence, but the fluorescence was bright and uniform after incubation with amine precursors. Many, but not all, of the cultures secrete one or more of the polypeptide hormones ACTH, arginine vasopressin, or calcitonin.[53,65] Calcitonin was secreted initially by 75 percent of the SCC cultures[65] and was selected for

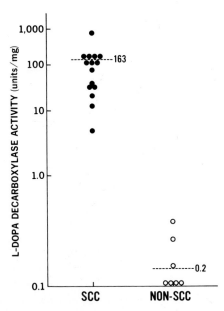

Figure 7-2. *Comparison of L-dopa decarboxylase activities of SCC and non-SCC lung cancer cultures.*

Table 7-1
Properties of Lung Cancer Cultures

Property	SCC	Non-SCC	SCC → Non-SCC
Morphology	SCC	Non-SCC	Non-SCC
Growth characteristics	Floating clusters	Usually adherent	Adherent or floating
Doubling time	Long	Relatively short	Variable
Cloning efficiency	Low	Relatively high	Relatively high
Ploidy	Aneuploid	Aneuploid	Aneuploid
Tumorigenicity	Yes	Yes	Yes
DDC levels	High	Low or absent	Low or absent
FIF	Present	Absent	Absent
Neurosecretory granules	Present	Absent	Rare or absent
Polypeptide hormone secretion	Frequent	Occasional	Occasional

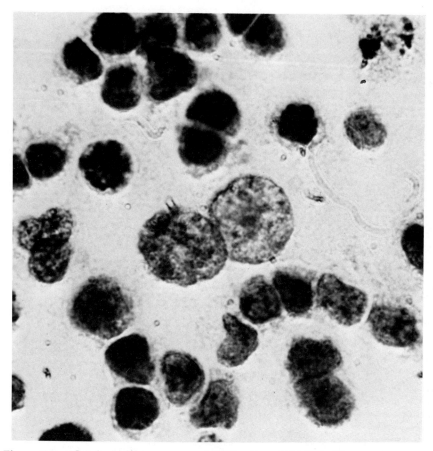

Figure 7-3. *Cytological appearances of SCC culture NCI H69. The vast majority of cells resemble the intermediate subtype of SCC. However, in the center of the field are two larger cells having more vesicular nuclei. A nucleolus is present in one of these cells. Hematoxylin and eosin stain. Original magnification × 400.*

serial studies. In contrast, the 6 non-SCC cultures (3 adenocarcinomas, 2 large cell carcinomas, and 1 mesothelioma) lacked APUD cell properties (Table 7-1).

The uniform expression of APUD properties by SCC cultures and their absence in non-SCC cultures contrasts with the findings in human tumors[44] (see also Chapter 6). In general, the human tumors show a much higher incidence of expression of APUD characteristics by SCC tumors, but there is considerable overlap with non-SCC tumors. In fact, the entire APUD machinery can be expressed by tumors having non-SCC morphol-

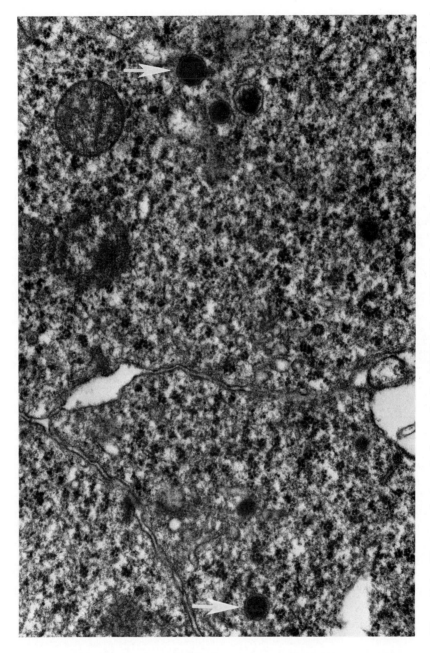

Figure 7-4. Electron micrograph of several cells of SCC culture NCI H60 demonstrating neurosecretory granules (arrows) in cytoplasm of two contiguous cells. Uranyl acetate and lead citrate stain. Original magnification × 16,000.

Table 7-2
Transition Time for Morphological Conversion of Small
Cell Carcinoma to Large Cell Carcinoma

	Months	
	Less than 24	24–60
Heterotransplanted tumors	0/7	4/6
Cell cultures	0/12	5/6

ogy. Some of the differences between the tumor and culture data may be explained by problems of sampling, varying number of stromal cells, tumor necrosis, and so forth, but the presence of APUD features in non-SCC tumors cannot be explained except by the concept that lung cancers present a continuing spectrum.

Long-Term Changes in SCC Models

The stability of the SCC models was monitored by sequentially studying their morphology and biological and biochemical features. Morphology was the most easily and frequently studied parameter. Cytological examination of the cultures was performed every few passages, and histological examination of transplanted tumors was done at every passage. Morphological change was not noted in 12 cultures or in 7 heterotransplants maintained for periods of 6–24 mo (Table 7-2). In models studied for periods of 24–60 mo, however, morphological change was noted in the majority. The major change was an increase in the number of large cells containing prominent nucleoli. Whereas initially only a few of these cells could be identified in almost all cultures, they now constituted a significant percentage of the total cell number. The change did not occur suddenly, but gradually, frequently over lengthy periods of time, and with the presence of transitional cells first being noted. Transitional cells retained the salt-and-pepper chromatin distribution characteristic of SCC, but had prominent eosinophilic nucleoli. With continued passage, transitional cells were partially or completely replaced by cells morphologically indistinguishable from large cell carcinoma (Fig. 7-5). Similar changes were noted in serially passaged heterotransplants (Fig. 7-6). Although the gross appearances and other characteristics of the transplanted tumors did not alter during this morphological change, the characteristics of the cultured cells altered visibly. The tightly packed aggregates characteristic of SCC cultures became looser and either remained as floating cells, but in

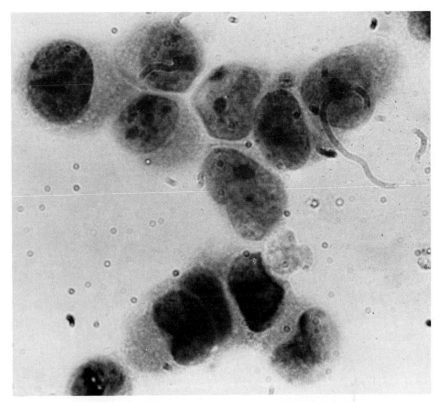

Figure 7-5. *Cytological appearances of cell culture NCI H60, subline 177. The cells have large nuclei with prominent nucleoli and moderate amounts of cytoplasm. The appearances are similar to large cell anaplastic carcinoma. Hematoxylin and eosin stain. Original magnification × 400.*

cord-like or single-cell arrangements, or adhered to the substrate and became a monolayer culture. Preliminary studies indicate an increased population doubling time and higher cloning efficiency accompany morphological change.

Biochemical and ultrastructural studies were performed at irregular intervals before, during, and after morphological change. Complete transition to large cell morphology was accompanied by loss of DDC, neurosecretory granules, and formaldehyde-induced fluorescence, but these were present during transitional stages. Formaldehyde-induced fluorescence studies indicated that the small clustered floating cells retained DDC activity, whereas the larger single or adherent cells had lost amine-handling properties. Calcitonin secretion, present initially in most SCC cultures,

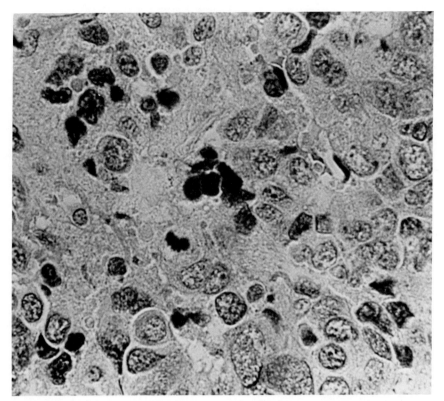

Figure 7-6. *Histological appearances of tumor induced in a nude mouse by injection of NCI H60, subline N177, cells. The appearances are those of a large cell carcinoma. Hematoxylin and eosin stain. Original magnification × 250.*

was sometimes absent during transitional stages and was always absent after complete morphological conversion. Sublines established from the same human tumor occasionally gave divergent results, with nude mouse tumors and their cultures contrasting with cultures established directly from the human tumor. In addition, cultures and heterotransplants were established from 2 patients whose tumors had mixed small cell–large cell carcinoma histology. The models established from these patients also had mixed histology at initial passages. In time, however, they completely converted to large cell morphology, with loss of APUD cell markers.

The properties of SCC cultures that have converted morphologically to large cell carcinomas are compared and contrasted to those retaining SCC morphology and to non-SCC cultures in Table 7-1. It is apparent that the characteristics of morphologically converted cultures are similar to those of non-SCC cultures.

Ultrastructural studies of culture N230 were of great interest. This tumor, originally established as a heterotransplant by Y. Shimosato, was sent to our laboratory and established as a culture after the ninth transplant generation. It remained as a floating culture with SCC morphology and APUD cell characteristics for an additional 2 yr (total in vitro time more than 4 yr). Subsequently, a large adherent cell subpopulation was noted. The mixed cell culture retained APUD cell properties, including calcitonin secretion. However, ultrastructural studies demonstrated that some of the cells of the mixed culture had prominent bundles of tonofilaments, sometimes in cells that retained neurosecretory granules (Figs. 7-7 and 7-8). Tonofilaments were not present in the cells that had a pure SCC morphology.

These studies, and the patient observations cited earlier, indicate that SCC tumors may alter their morphology, especially to large cell carcinoma, but to other histological cell types as well. The appearance and extent of the changes are time related, sometimes present at diagnosis, but much more commonly seen after therapy (in the patient) or after prolonged culture. Complete loss of SCC morphology is accompanied by loss of APUD markers. These changes could be explained by several possibilities:

1. Multiple oncogenic events may simultaneously or almost simultaneously transform cells in close proximity to each other. The transformed cells, of more than one histological type, then grow together to form a composite tumor.
2. A single transforming event may give rise to morphologically different cell types.
3. Tumors of one morphology may convert to tumors having a different morphology.

Because most of the cultures and lung cancers we have examined have had a single aneuploid peak, we believe that the first explanation cannot account for all the observations, but that a combination of the last two can do so (see sections below on Gut Lessons and The Interrelationship of Lung Cancers). The absolute proof that SCC tumors can undergo morphological changes resides in observing similar changes in clonal cultures. We have initiated such studies, but only lengthy observation periods will determine the correctness of our postulates. Our observations with culture N230 and the observations with nitrosamine induced tumors,[32] however, indicate that squamous differentiation may occur in APUD cells.

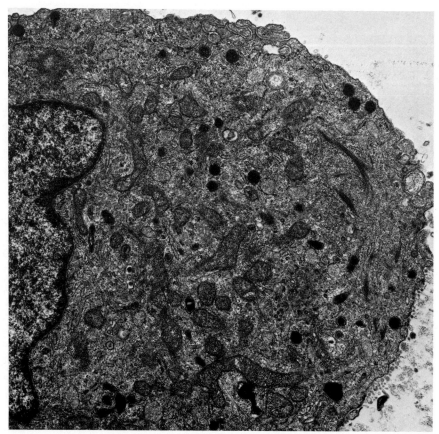

Figure 7-7. *Electron micrograph of SCC cell culture NCI N230, late passage, showing abundant cytoplasm rich in organelles, including mitochondria, lysosomes, peripherally distributed neurosecretory granules, and scattered bundles of tonofilaments. Uranyl acetate and lead citrate stain. Original magnification × 6300.*

Gut Lessons

A study of the normal endocrine cells of the gastroenteropancreatic (GEP) tract, their origin, and relationship to other mucosal cells, and the tumors that originate from them offers many useful lessons in understanding their counterparts in the respiratory tree. This subject is also discussed in Chapter 6 of this monograph. The GEP tract has been called the largest endocrine organ in the body, and only the brain secretes as many diverse

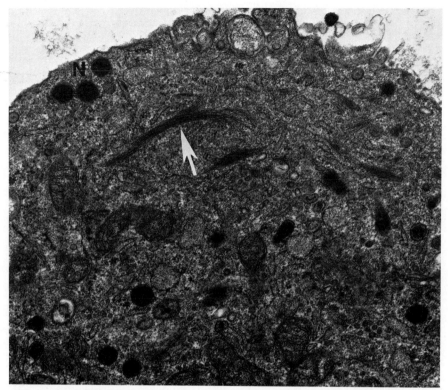

Figure 7-8. *Higher magnification of cell from NCI N230 culture illustrated in Figure 7-7. Neurosecretory granules (N) and bundles of tonofilaments (arrow) are more clearly illustrated in the cytoplasm. Uranyl acetate and lead citrate. Original magnification ×10,000.*

polypeptides with endocrine and paracrine functions. At least 15 morphologically or functionally different endocrine cells have been described, extending from the stomach to the anus,[66] with the expectation that many more remain to be discovered.

The mucosa of the GEP tract is endodermal in origin, as is that of the respiratory tract. Pearse originally suggested that the endocrine (APUD) cells in both these locations were of neural crest origin,[2] and later demonstrated migration of neural crest cells into the GEP tract.[16] The finding of many identical or similar peptides in the brain and GEP tract was regarded as further evidence of a common origin.[67] However, overwhelming evidence from several investigators using diverse techniques has demonstrated unequivocally that the endocrine cells of the GEP tract are not of neural crest origin,[68-70] and that the neural crest cells migrating into the GEP tract give rise to intramural autonomic ganglia.

Autoradiographic and mucosal graft studies demonstrate that all of the mucosal cells of the stomach, small intestine, and colon arise from common progenitor cells.[71-73] Rare cells contain both mucin globules and secretory granules, indicating the ability of stem cells to simultaneously differentiate along more than one pathway.[73] Numerous reports have documented the presence of multiple cell types, including endocrine, in GEP tumors (for review, see Sidhu[64]). Some of these reports document endocrine and other pathways of differentiation occurring simultaneously in individual tumor cells.

The APUD Concept Revisited

Pearse's ideas of a widely distributed system of endocrine cells sharing common amine-handling properties of probable neural crest origin were eagerly embraced by many investigators, including the authors. However, the overwhelming evidence against a neural crest origin of the endocrine cells of the GEP tract must lead us to a reevaluation of the entire concept. Currently only 6 of the approximately 36 identified APUD cells are of definite neural crest origin.[66] Pearse has recently modified his original views and now suggests that the APUD cells of the gut are derived from cells of the embryonic epiblast that invade the secondary hypoblast (the definitive endoderm of the gut)[18] and that all APUD cells are deemed to be "neuroendocrine programmed." Our interpretation of this theory is that it still implies that the endocrine cells of the GEP system have a different origin from that of the other mucosal cells. As such, it would be incompatible with many of the observations described in the preceding section.

We have investigated the APUD cell concept by measuring the levels of the key APUD cell enzyme, DDC, in a variety of fresh, transplanted, and cultured tumors of human and animal origin. We have concentrated on tumors with specific products or pathways of differentiation. Studies with continuous cultures having defined properties indicate that they fall into two categories: (1) those with very high levels of the enzyme, and (2) those with low or absent levels. Exceedingly few cultures have intermediate levels. Studies with tumors indicate greater heterogeneity. All of the histological types of tumors with consistently high levels are believed to be derived from progenitor cells whose normal differentiated function is peptide or amine production. Details of these studies will be published elsewhere, but some generalizations can be made:

1. All APUD cells are not of neural crest origin, with at least two and possibly all three germ cell layers involved.
2. Only those neural crest derivatives that have the ability to produce biologically active, fully packaged hormones possess APUD cell properties.
3. Some random tumors that lack APUD properties may secrete hormones, usually at low levels.
4. Cells and their tumors that secrete certain peptide hormones (e.g., parathyroid hormone) lack APUD properties.

In summary, we believe that the APUD cell concept has many merits, and that there undoubtedly is an easily identifiable population of cells, widely dispersed throughout the body, having amine-handling properties. Only the postulation of a common embryological origin of all APUD cells is unacceptable. Rather, APUD differentiation is one pathway of differentiation available to progenitor cells from diverse sources. We presume that APUD properties are required or desirable in cells secreting certain peptides, and absolutely essential in cells producing serotonin or catecholamines. In both neural crest and non-neural crest derived cells, microenvironmental factors probably determine the final pathways of differentiation and the acquisition of APUD cell properties.

The Interrelationship of Lung Cancers

We believe that the data presented in the preceding sections provide overwhelming evidence for a common origin of all the bronchial mucosal cells and the tumors derived from them. We propose, as have others,[50] that all the mucosal cells of the bronchial epithelium, and the tumors that arise from them, have a common stem cell origin (Figs. 7-9 and 7-10). The stem cell undergoes progressive differentiation, through morphologically undifferentiated intermediate stages that are committed to certain pathways of differentiation (differentiation-committed cells) to fully differentiated cells. The latter are end-stage cells, probably incapable of further division. The differentiation-committed cells may simultaneously differentiate along more than one pathway, or, when exposed to new environmental conditions (e.g., virus infections, carcinogens) switch from one pathway

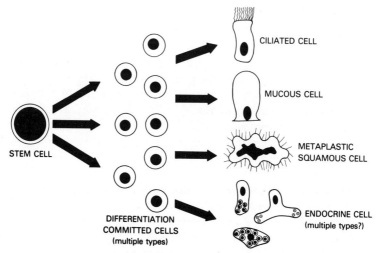

Figure 7-9. *Unitarian theory of the origin of the cells of the respiratory mucosa.*

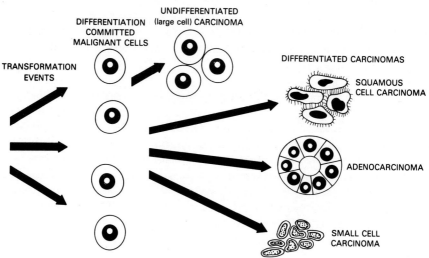

Figure 7-10. *Unitarian theory of the origin of lung cancers.*

to another. One set of stimuli may lead to the development of metaplastic squamous cells.

In our unitarian concept, the bronchial endocrine cells with APUD properties are one type of differentiated cell. Whether APUD properties develop with the onset of endocrine differentiation, or, as has been suggested by one of the authors,[74] develop in most if not all intermediate cells and are selectively retained in endocrine cells, is not currently known. We also postulate that more than one type of endocrine cell will eventually be identified in the respiratory mucosa.

Because most fully differentiated cells are end cells not capable of replication, it is unlikely that transforming events occur in them. Rather, transforming events must affect undifferentiated or partially differentiated cells. Depending on the level of differentiation at which transformation occurs, the resultant tumor will be differentiated or undifferentiated. In our concept, endocrine cell tumors, and thus SCC, are regarded as differentiated or partially differentiated tumors. We postulate that a stem cell or true undifferentiated tumor will morphologically resemble large cell carcinoma. The stem cell concept explains the presence of tumors having more than one morphological component and also the presence of APUD cell markers in occasional non-SCC cancers.

Morphological conversion from one cell type to another is more difficult to explain. The groundwork for the theory that follows is not as well founded as the above-mentioned concepts, and may have to be modified as more data become available. We believe, as do others,[75] that fully differentiated cells, whether normal or neoplastic, are capable of little or no division. Tumors are propagated by a core of undifferentiated or partially differentiated "stem" cells. Tumor stem cells are capable of infinite division; some of the progeny differentiate further, while others remain relatively undifferentiated and maintain the stem cell pool. The size of the stem cell pool may vary from tumor to tumor, and, with time, within a single tumor.

These concepts may be used to explain the conversion of SCC to other forms of lung cancer, especially to large cell carcinoma. If SCC cells are relatively differentiated, they are capable of only limited division. The tumor is maintained by a core of stem cells, which may appear morphologically different. Our observations that most SCC cultures contain a very small percentage of large cells have been described earlier. These cells may be the tumor stem cells of SCC. Changing tumor morphology cannot be explained on the basis of loss of differentiated functions and appearances by individual cells. Rather, loss of differentiation must be explained by progressive failure of stem cells to undergo differentiation. This concept is

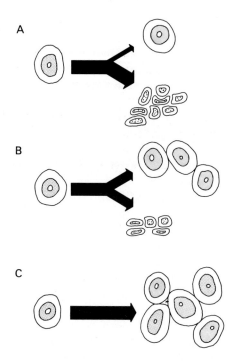

Figure 7-11. *Hypothetical method whereby a SCC tumor (A) may convert to large cell undifferentiated carcinoma (C). (B) shows a mixed small cell–large cell carcinoma.*

illustrated in Figure 7-11. Panel A depicts a "pure" SCC tumor. However, this tumor is in fact maintained by a core or more primitive stem cells (large cells). As the proportion of stem cells failing to mature increases, a mixed small cell–large cell carcinoma develops (panel B). Finally (panel C), all the stem cells fail to mature, and a large cell carcinoma evolves from a SCC. Two other pieces of data support the stem cell concept of SCC. Clonogenic assays indicate that only a very small percentage of SCC cells (about 1 percent) are capable of giving rise to progressively growing tumorigenic colonies, but that many cells are capable of limited replication[76] (see also Chapter 4). In addition, in mixed small cell–large cell tumors, autoradiography studies indicate greater thymidine uptake by the large cell component (B. Brigham and P. A. Bunn, personal communication), suggesting greater replicative ability of the latter. Our findings that conversion of small cell carcinomas to large cell carcinomas are accompanied by an increase in population doubling time and clonogenic efficiency sup-

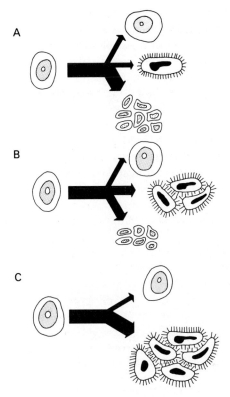

Figure 7-12. *Hypothetical method whereby a SCC tumor (A) may convert to a squamous cell carcinoma (C). (B) shows a mixed SCC–squamous cell carcinoma.*

port the concept that the stem cell is a relatively larger, morphologically different cell than the typical small cell of SCC. The stem cell concept almost certainly applies to teratomas, myeloproliferative malignancies, and the GEP tract. Its application to the respiratory tract, despite the paucity of suitable morphologically identifiable prospective candidates in the normal respiratory mucosa, explains the spectrum of lung cancers.

If all lung cancers arise from a single stem cell, conversion from one differentiated cell type to another can also be explained, as shown in Figure 7-12. Panel A of this figure depicts stem cells that are differentiating predominantly into SCC, with a few that are differentiating into squamous cells. Such a tumor might be interpreted as SCC with a minor squamous cell carcinoma component. With time, more stem cells may mature along the squamous pathway, resulting in a mixed SCC–squamous cell carcinoma (panel B). Finally, all the cells differentiate into squamous cells (panel C). In all instances, the stem cell pool replenishes itself. Thus a SCC tumor has converted into a squamous cell carcinoma. Likewise, a SCC tumor may convert into an adenocarcinoma.

A final relationship remains to be discussed—that between SCC and bronchial carcinoids. SCC are relatively primitive cells at the ultrastructural level, whereas carcinoids appear to more differentiated. It has long been proposed that SCC tumors are a primitive form of carcinoid and that both are developed from a common precursor K cell. The morphological spectrum between the two is regarded as additional evidence in support of this concept. Although this concept has certain merits and may not be entirely false, we regard both tumors as arising from endocrine cell precursors. If there are, indeed, multiple types of endocrine cells in the lung, they may arise from related but different precursor cells. Of course, ultimately they would have to arise from a common precursor stem cell. However, they would arise from immediate precursor cells more closely related to each other than to the immediate precursor cells of the other forms of differentiated lung cancers.

Very few ideas in science or in other disciplines are entirely new. Thus we have come full circle and have returned to Feyrter's ideas of the endodermal origin of the Helle-Zellen system. The unitarian theory has been revived and is replacing the concept of a separate histogenesis for SCC. Despite its common lineage to other lung cancers, SCC remains as a distinct biological entity.

References

1. Cohen MH, Matthews MJ: Small cell bronchogenic carcinoma: A distinct clinicopathologic entity. Sem Oncol 5:234–243, 1978
2. Pearse AG: The cytochemistry and ultrastructure of polypeptide hormone-producing cells of the APUD series and the embryologic, physiologic and pathologic implications of the concept. J Histochem Cytochem 17:303–313, 1969
3. McDowell EM, Barett LA, Glavin F, Harris CC, Trump BF: The respiratory epithelium. I. Human Bronchus. J Natl Cancer Inst 61:539–549, 1978
4. Trump BF, McDowell EM, Glavin F, Barrett LA, Becci PJ, Schurch W, Kaiser HE, Harris CC: Respiratory epithelium. III. Histogenesis of epidermoid metaplasia and carcinoma in situ in the human. J Natl Cancer Inst 61:563–573, 1978

5. Saccomanno G, Archer VE, Auerbach O, et al: Development of carcinoma of the lung as reflected in exfoliated cells. Cancer 33:256–270, 1974

6. Matthews MJ, Gordon PR: Morphology of pulmonary and pleural malignancies, in Strauss MJ (ed): Lung Cancer—Clinical Diagnosis and Treatment. New York, Grune & Stratton, 1977, pp 49–69

7. Mackay B, Osborne BM, Wilson RA: Ultrastructure of lung neoplasms, in Strauss MJ (ed): Lung Cancer—Clinical Diagnosis and Treatment. New York, Grune & Stratton, 1977, pp 71–84

8. Carter D, Marsh BR, Baker RR, et al: Relationship of morphology to clinical presentation in ten cases of early squamous cell carcinoma of the lung. Cancer 37:1389–1396, 1976

9. Churg A: The fine structure of large cell undifferentiated carcinoma of the lung. Hum Pathol 9:143–156, 1978

10. Gould VE, Chejfec G: Ultrastructural and biochemical analysis of 'undifferentiated' pulmonary carcinomas. Hum Pathol 9:377–384, 1978

11. Fisher ER, Paulson JD: A new in vitro cell line established from human large cell variant of oat cell cancer. Cancer Res 38:3830–3835, 1978

12. Warner RR, Southren AL: Carcinoid syndrome produced by metastasizing bronchial adenoma. Am J Med 24:903–914, 1958

13. Turnbull AD, Huvos AG, Goodner JT, et al: The malignant potential of bronchial adenoma. Ann Thorac Surg 14:453–463, 1972

14. Arrigoni MG, Woolner LB, Bernatz PE: Atypical carcinoid tumors of the lung. J Thorac Cardiovasc Surg 64:413–421, 1972

15. Feyrter F: Uber die peripheren endokrinen (parakrinen) Drusen des Menschen. Vienna, Wilhelm Mandrich, 1953

16. Pearse AG, Polak JM: Neural crest origin of the endocrine polypeptide (APUD) cells of the gastrointestinal tract and pancreas. Gut 12:783–788, 1971

17. Pearse AG: The APUD cell concept and its implications in pathology. Pathol Ann 9:27–41, 1974

18. Pearse AG, Takor-Takor T: Embryology of the diffuse neuroendocrine system and its relationship to the common peptides. Fed Proc 38:2288–2294, 1979

19. Bensch KG, Gordon GB, Miller LR: Studies on the bronchial counterpart of the Kultschitzky (argentaffin) cell and innervation of bronchial glands. J Ultrastruct Res 12:668–686, 1965

20. Gmelich JT, Bensch KG, Liebow AA: Cells of Kultschitzky type in bronchioles and their relationship to the origin of peripheral carcinoid tumors. Lab Invest 17:88–98, 1967

21. Capella C, Hage E, Solcia E, et al: Ultrastructural similarity of endocrine-like cells of the human lung and some related cells of the gut. Cell Tissue Res 186:25–37, 1978

22. McDowell EM, Barrett LA, Trump BF: Observations on small granule cells in adult human bronchial epithelium and in carcinoid and oat cell tumors. Lab Invest 37:202–206, 1976

23. Terzakis J, Sommers S, Andersson B: Neurosecretory appearing cells of human segmental bronchi. Lab Invest 26:127–132, 1972

24. Cutz E. Chan W, Wong V, et al: Ultrastructure and fluorescence histochemistry of endocrine (APUD-type) cells in tracheal mucosa of human and various animal species. Cell Tissue Res 158:425–437, 1975

25. Wharton J, Polak JM, Bloom SR, et al: Bombesin-like immunoreactivity in the lung. Nature 273:769–770, 1978

26. Said SI, Mutt V: Relationship of spasmogenic and smooth muscle relaxant peptides from normal lung to other vasoactive compounds. Nature 265:84–86, 1977

27. Becker KL, Monghan KG, Silva OL: Immunocytochemical localization of calcitonin in Kultschitzky cells of human lung. Arch Pathol Lab Med 104:196–198, 1980

28. Masson P: Carcinoids (argentaffin-cell tumors) and nerve hyperplasia of the appendicular mucosa. Am J Pathol 4:181–211, 1928

29. Jeffrey P, Reid L: Intra-epithelial nerves in normal rat airways: A quantitative electron microscopic study. J Anat 114:35–45, 1973

30. Lauweryns JM, Cokelaere M: Hypoxic-sensitive neuro-epithelial bodies: Intrapulmonary secretory neuroreceptors modulated by the CNS. Z Zellforsch 145:521–540, 1973

31. Bonikos DS, Bensch KG: Endocrine cells of bronchial and bronchiolar epithelium. Am J Med 63:765–771, 1977

32. Reznik-Schuller H: Ultrastructural alterations of APUD cells during nitrosamine-induced lung carcinogenesis. J Pathol 121:79–82, 1976

33. Blair WH, Heinen J, Tremback K: An in vitro cell line established from "oat-cell like" lung carcinoma experimentally induced in rodents. Proc Am Assoc Cancer Res 21:82, 1980

34. Hattori S, Matsuda M, Tateishi R, et al: Oat-cell carcinoma of the lung containing serotonin granules. Gann 59:123–129, 1968

35. Bensch KG, Corrin B, Pariente R, et al: Oat cell carcinoma of the lung: Its origin and relationship to bronchial carcinoids. Cancer 22:1163–1177, 1968

36. Hattori S, Matsuda M, Tateishi R, et al: Oat cell carcinoma of the lung: Clinical and morphological studies in relation to its histogenesis. Cancer 30:1014–1024, 1972

37. Salyer DC, Salyer WR, Eggleston JC: Bronchial carcinoid tumors. Cancer 36:1522–1537, 1975

38. Tateishi R, Horai T, Hattori S: Demonstration of argyrophilic granules in small cell carcinoma of the lung. Virchows Arch Path Anat Histol 377:203–210, 1978

39. Churg A, Warnock ML: Pulmonary tumorlet: A form of peripheral carcinoid. Cancer 37:1469–1477, 1976

40. Williams ED, Azzopardi JG: Tumors of the lung and the carcinoid syndrome. Thorax 15:30–36, 1960

41. Salyer DC, Eggleston JC: Oat cell carcinoma of the bronchus and the carcinoid syndrome. Arch Pathol 99:513–515, 1975

42. Warner RR, Kirchner PA, Warner GM: Serotonin production by bronchial adenomas without the carcinoid syndrome. J Am Med Assoc 178:1175–1179, 1961

43. Baylin SB, Weisburger WR, Eggleston JC, et al: Variable content of histaminase, L-dopa decarboxylase and calcitonin in small cell carcinoma of the lung—Biologic and clinical implications. N Engl J Med 299:105–110, 1978

44. Baylin SB, Abeloff MD, Goodwin G, et al: Activities of L-dopa decarboxylase and diamine oxidase (histaminase) in human lung cancers and decarboxylase as a marker for small (oat) cell cancer in culture. Cancer Res 40:1990–1994, 1980

45. Gazdar AF, Carney DN, Russell EK, et al: Establishment of continuous, clonable cultures of small cell carcinoma of the lung which have amine precursor uptake and decarboxylation properties. Cancer Res 40:3502–3507, 1980

46. O'Neal LW, Lipnis DM, Luse SA, et al: Secretion of various endocrine substances by ACTH-secreting tumors—Gastrin, melanotropin, norepinephrine, serotonin, parathormone, vasopressin, glucagon. Cancer 21:1219–1232, 1968

47. Gerwitz G, Yalow RS: Ectopic ACTH production in carcinoma of the lung. J Clin Invest 53:1022–1032, 1974

48. Rees LH: The biosynthesis of hormones by non-endocrine tumors—A review. J Endocrinol 67:143–175, 1975

49. Silva OL, Becker KL, Primack A, et al: Increased serum calcitonin levels in bronchogenic cancer. Chest 69:495–499, 1976

50. Yesner R: Spectrum of lung cancer and ectopic hormones, in Sommers SC, Rosen PP (eds): Pathology Annual, part I. New York, Appleton-Century-Crofts, 1978, pp 217–240

51. Yalow RS, Eastridge CE, Higgins G, et al: Plasma and tumor ACTH in carcinoma of the lung. Cancer 44: 1789–1792, 1979

52. Pettengill OS, Faulkner CS, Wurster-Hill DH, et al: Isolation and characterization of a hormone-producing cell line from human small cell anaplastic carcinoma of the lung. J Natl Cancer Inst 58:511–518, 1977

53. Radice PA, Dermody WC: Clonal heterogeneity of hormone production by continuous cultures of small cell carcinoma of the lung (SCCL). Proc Am Assoc Cancer Res 21:41, 1980

54. Tischler AS, Dichter MA, Biales B: Neural properties of cultured human endocrine tumor cells of proposed neural crest origin. Science 192:904–906, 1976

55. Tischler AS, Dichter MA, Biales B: Electrical excitability of oat cell carcinoma. J Pathol 122:153–156, 1977

56. Matthews EK, Sakamoto Y: Electrical characteristics of pancreatic islet cells. J Physiol 246:421–437, 1975

57. Barnard WG: The nature of the "oat-celled sarcoma" of the mediastinum. J Pathol Bacteriol 29:241–244, 1926

58. Azzopardi JG: Oat cell carcinoma of the bronchus. J Pathol Bacteriol 78:513–519, 1959

59. Yesner R, Sobel L: Histological typing of lung tumors. International Histological Classification of Tumors. Geneva, World Health Organization, 1977 (in press)

60. Matthews MJ, Gazdar AF: Pathology of small cell carcinoma of the lung and its subtypes: A clinicopathologic correlation, in Livingston RB (ed): Lung Cancers: Advances in Research and Treatment. The Hague, Martnus Nijhoff, (in press)

61. Brereton HD, Matthews MJ, Costa J, et al: Mixed anaplastic small-cell and squamous-cell carcinoma of the lung. Ann Int Med 88:805–806, 1978

62. Abeloff MD, Eggleston JC, Mendelsohn G, et al: Changes in morphological and biochemical characteristics of small cell carcinoma of the lung. Am J Med 66:757–764, 1979

63. Gazdar AF, Cohen MH, Ihde DC, et al: Bronchial epithelial changes in association with small cell carcinoma of the lung. In Muggia F, Rozencweig M (eds): Lung Cancer: Progress in Therapeutic Research. New York, Raven Press, 1979, pp 167–173

64. Sidhu GS: The endodermal origin of digestive and respiratory tract APUD cells. Am J Pathol 96:5–20, 1979

65. Becker KL, Gazdar AF, Carney DN, et al: Calcitonin secretion by small cell carcinoma of the lung cultures: Incidence and heterogeneity studies. (Submitted for publication.)

66. Pearse AG, Polak JM, Bloom SR: The new gut hormones; cellular

sources, physiology, pathology and clinical aspects. Gastroenterology 72:746–761, 1977

67. Pearse AG: Peptides in the brain and intestine. Nature 262:92–94, 1976

68. Pictet RL, Rall LB, Phelps P, et al: The neural crest and the origin of the insulin-producing and other gastrointestinal hormone-producing cells. Science 191:191–192, 1976

69. Andrew A: APUD cells, Apudomas and the neural crest. SA Med J 50:890–898, 1976

70. Fontaine J, LeDouarin NM: Analysis of endoderm formation in the avian blastoderm by the use of quail-chick chimaeras. J Embry Exp Morphol 41:209–222, 1977

71. Matsuyama M, Suzuki H: Differentiation of immature mucous cells into parietal, argyrophilic and chief cells in stomach grafts. Science 169:385–387, 1970

72. Chang WW, LeBlond CP: Renewal of the epithelium in the descending colon of the mouse. II Renewal of argentaffin cells. Am J Anat 131:101–109, 1971

73. Cheng H, LeBlond CP: Origin, differentiation of the four main epithelial cell types in the mouse small intestine. V. Unitarian theory of the origin of the four epithelial cell types. Am J Anat 141:537–562, 1974

74. Baylin SB, Mendelsohn G: Ectopic (inappropriate) hormone production by tumors: Mechanisms involved and the biological and clinical implications. Endocrinol Rev 1:45–77, 1980

75. Pierce GB, Shikes R, Fink LM: Cancer: A problem of developmental biology. Englewood Cliffs, New Jersey, Prentice-Hall, 1978

76. Carney DN, Gazdar AF, Minna JD: Positive correlation between histologic tumor involvement and generation of tumor cell colonies in agarose in specimens taken directly from patients with small cell carcinoma of the lung. Cancer Res 40:1820–1822, 1980

8

HORMONE PRODUCTION AND PARANEOPLASTIC SYNDROMES

F. Anthony Greco
John Hainsworth
Anna Sismani
Ronald L. Richardson
Kenneth R. Hande
Robert K. Oldham

Paraneoplastic syndromes often accompany neoplastic disease. They are disorders of organ function distant from the tumor that are caused neither by the direct space-occupying nature of the primary tumor nor by its metastases. Many tumors have been characterized by their ability to increase or decrease the metabolic function of distant organs. In some neoplasms "mediators" of particular syndromes have been isolated and identified.

Paraneoplastic syndromes as a group occur frequently. It has been estimated that, at any given time, nearly 20 percent of cancer patients in all stages of their disease will be suffering from a paraneoplastic syndrome.[1] The percentage is even higher over the entire course of their disease. Mortality and morbidity as a direct result of these syndromes is not uncommon. Management of the syndromes at times may be more effective than treatment of the cancer, although ideally the therapy should be directed at the underlying neoplastic disease.

This work was supported in part by Grants 1R01 CA27333-01, CA19429, and CA23909-01 from the National Cancer Institute and Grants JFCF 394A and JFCF 508 from the American Cancer Society.

Many neoplasms are associated with paraneoplastic syndromes but none are seen more often or have more diverse manifestations than those associated with small cell lung cancer (SCC). For the clinician these tumors are fascinating because they sometimes present in a dramatic fashion. They may be diagnostic enigmas, and they often pose complex problems in patient management. For the biochemist and physiologist they offer insights into differences between normal and neoplastic cells and may provide clues to the process involved in the transformation from a benign to a neoplastic state. For the histologist and embryologist these tumors are intriguing because of their peculiar staining characteristics and histogenesis.

The reason SCC is frequently associated with paraneoplastic syndromes is not clearly understood. It is tempting to speculate that most of the syndromes associated with SCC result from biologically active tumor-associated products. At least two hormones, antidiuretic hormone (ADH) and adenocorticotropin (ACTH), have been shown to mediate clinical syndromes. The capacity to produce these hormones might be directly related to the possible "neuroendocrine" origin of SCC from the amine precursor uptake and decarboxylation (APUD) cells.[2] The fact that many of the syndromes are related to the endocrine and neurologic systems may support this theory.

This chapter reviews the endocrinologic and neurologic syndromes associated with SCC. The discussion focuses on the tumor-associated peptide products and the clinical syndromes.

Hormone Production and SCC

After the first formal description and characterization of tumors that produce hormonelike substances by Liddle and his colleagues,[3,4] several other investigators have shown that several tumors may produce a variety of hormonelike products.[4-7] Several clinical effects are not explained by the mere physical presence of a tumor but rather must be attributed to a biologically active hormonelike material the tumor produces. It became obvious that other patients without recognizable clinical syndromes related to hormone production also had circulating products, which were either quantitatively insufficient to produce symptoms or qualitatively lacked biologic activity.

A general review of the "ectopic hormones" produced by all histologic types of lung cancer is illustrated in Table 8-1. There are problems in interpreting these data precisely, because the criteria for determining the

Table 8-1

Patients with Ectopic Hormone Production in Lung
Carcinoma by Cell Type

Hormone	Histologic Cell Type					
	Epidermoid	Small Cell	Adeno- carcinoma	Large cell Anaplastic	"Undiffer- entiated'	Not Specified
ACTH	8	120	3	—	3	56
MSH	—	15	—	—	—	—
ADH	1	95	—	1	2	10
Calcitonin	1	50	3	—	—	—
Serotonin	—	14	—	—	—	—
HCG	3	1	2	5	—	4
HGH	—	2	5	4	—	—
PTH	9	1	—	—	—	29
Prolactin	—	—	—	—	1	—
Insulin	—	—	—	—	1	—
Glucagon	—	6	—	—	1	—
Placental lactogen	1	1	—	2	1	—
Estradiol	1	—	—	—	—	—
Renin	—	1	—	—	—	—
Erythropoietin	—	—	—	—	1	—
Gastrin	—	2	—	—	1	4

From Primack,[8] Hansen,[9] and Richardson.[10]

"ectopic" nature of hormone production and the methods of measuring the products has varied. This survey demonstrates the strong association of SCC with several hormones, particularly ACTH, ADH, and calcitonin. It is likely that many of the "undifferentiated" and "not specified" tumors in Table 8-1 were also SCC, particularly those exhibiting ectopic ACTH and ADH. Table 8-2 lists the most common clinical syndromes in SCC that are caused by hormone production, and Table 8-3 shows those hormones or amines that are often elevated but do not necessarily produce a recognized clinical effect.

The term "ectopic" was first used by Liddle to describe hormonelike products arising from cells or tumors that do not normally produce the hormone in question.[3] The detailed study of tumor peptide production has provided insights into the normal biosynthetic mechanisms by which peptides are produced. In addition, ectopic hormone production is a useful model for investigating the general aspects of tumor synthesis of proteins and the relationship of these proteins to malignant transformation. For the purpose of discussion, it is useful to classify produc-

Table 8-2
Clinical Syndromes in Small Cell Lung Cancer Related to
Hormone Production

Syndrome	Hormone
Cushing's	ACTH
Inappropriate secretion of antidiuretic hormone (SIADH)	ADH
Hyperpigmentation	ACTH
Carcinoid	Serotonin and metabolites

tion of a particular peptide product by a specific tumor type as ectopic.
However, this designation should be considered only provisional because
it presumes that all normal sites of synthesis of every peptide are known.
Clearly this is not the case, as can be demonstrated by several examples.
Somatostatin is found in the D cells of the pancreatic islets and in the
gastrointestinal tract, even though it was originally isolated from the hy-
pothalmus. ACTH was originally thought to be synthesized only by
the pars distalis of the pituitary, but it now appears to be one of several
products cleaved from a single large glycopeptide precursor molecule[11]
that is also produced in the pars intermedia of the pituitary, in normal brain
and placenta, and in APUD cells located in several other areas.

Hormones are now beginning to appear to be much more widely distributed than was originally thought, and even "placental" hormones, or
very closely related peptides, are being found in normal adult male and
female tissues.[12] Thus, various genes responsible for peptide production
may not be completely repressed in nonendocrine cells. Furthermore, cells
such as the Kulchitsky cell—which may be the precursor of bronchial carcinoid tumors, thymomas (thymic carcinoid tumors), and SCC may normally secrete peptide hormones, and hormone secretion by tumors derived from these cells may not be ectopic—only exaggerated.

Table 8-3
Hormones or Amines Detected in
Plasma or Tumors Not Necessarily
Producing Recognized Clinical
Syndromes

Histaminase	ACTH
Dopa decarboxylase	ADH
Oxytocin	Growth hormone
Gastrin	Glucagon
	Calcitonin

Table 8-4
Criteria for Establishing Diagnosis of Ectopic Hormone
Secretion

---

1. Association of the neoplasm with a clinical syndrome.
2. Association with inappropriately elevated plasma or urine hormone levels, or both.
3. Failure of plasma or urine hormone levels, or both, to respond to normal suppression.
4. Exclusion of other possible causes.
5. Fall in hormone levels after tumor therapy.
6. Arteriovenous stepup gradient across the tumor.
7. Demonstration of hormone in tumor.
8. In vitro (tissue culture) or in vivo (xenograft in animal model) hormone synthesis and release from tumor tissue.
9. *In vitro* cell-free translation of tumor hormone-specific messenger RNA.

The subject of polypeptide formation and secretion by malignant tumors is extremely broad and complex. The criteria used to confirm ectopic hormone secretion are listed in Table 8-4. Only rarely have these criteria been met. In selected patients with SCC, several of these criteria have been fulfilled. The association of SCC with clinical ectopic hormone syndromes and increased circulating ectopic hormones without recognizable clinical abnormalities has been well established. In selected patients, these tumor-associated products have declined after tumor-specific therapy, and hormones have been demonstrated directly in tumor tissue or in vitro (tissue culture).[13-15] However, detailed analysis and serial investigation of polypeptide hormones in more than a few patients with SCC has not been done.

Various amines and peptide products have been observed in patients with SCC.[10] A number of these same products have also been reported to occur in poorly differentiated adenocarcinomas or large cell undifferentiated lung carcinomas. In view of the difficulty in classifying poorly differentiated tumors by light microscopy, however, it is likely that at least some of these tumors may have been the intermediate subtype of SCC, an entity not widely recognized in the past.[16] Ectopic hormone syndromes also occur in squamous lung cancer and adenocarcinoma; however, they are usually different from those seen in SCC.[17]

The true incidence of ectopic peptide production in SCC is not known, but a reasonable estimate of the clinical syndromes related to ectopic ACTH and ADH is in the range of 5–10 percent of all SCC patients.[10] However, the detection of one or more hormones or amines in plasma or tumor tissue in the absence of a clinical syndrome has frequently occurred. It is possible that all SCC synthesize one or more peptide products or amines that do not produce clinical manifestations. Further investigation into the relationship of polypeptide hormone production and synthesis by SCC may provide (1) important biologic information regarding the regulatory mechanisms of hormone production in this neoplasm and in normal cells, (2) biochemical characterization which may aid in classification and diagnosis, and (3) biologic products and markers useful in following the effects of therapy. A review of ADH, ACTH, and calcitonin in SCC is now presented.

Antidiuretic Hormone

In 1938, Winkler and Crankshaw[18] described a patient with bronchogenic carcinoma who had marked hypochloremia and urinary chloride wasting, without evidence of vascular collapse. The authors remarked that this syndrome was not due to adrenal insufficiency but did not speculate about its etiology. The syndrome was not described again until 1957 when Schwartz et al.[19] published detailed metabolic studies on 2 patients with bronchogenic carcinoma. These patients manifested persistent severe hyponatremia, hypoosmolality of the serum, and continued urinary sodium excretion with less than maximally dilute urine. Both patients had normal renal and adrenal function and showed no evidence of fluid volume depletion. The authors postulated that all of these abnormalities were caused by a sustained inappropriate secretion of ADH. This hypothesis has been subsequently confirmed, and very little has been added to their description of the syndrome.

The pathogenesis of the metabolic abnormalities in the syndrome of inappropriate secretion of antidiuretic hormone (SIADH) is illustrated in Figure 8-1. Increased serum levels of ADH cause water retention by increasing the permeability of the renal collecting tubules to water. The extracellular fluid volume expands, with subsequent increase in glomerular filtration rate (GFR) and inhibition of aldosterone secretion. Failure of renal conservation of sodium results both from an increase in the filtered sodium load (GFR × serum sodium) and from decreased tubular reabsorption of sodium as a result of decreased aldosterone secretion. A new steady state is achieved only when the filtered sodium load is reduced by the subsequent development of hyponatremia. The development of the syndrome is dependent on water retention: when large doses of ADH are administered chronically to normal subjects during a period of fluid restriction, the only discernible metabolic abnormality that develops is the excretion of a hypertonic urine.[20] A recently recognized manifestation of the syndrome is hypouricemia, which occurs in conjunction with an in-

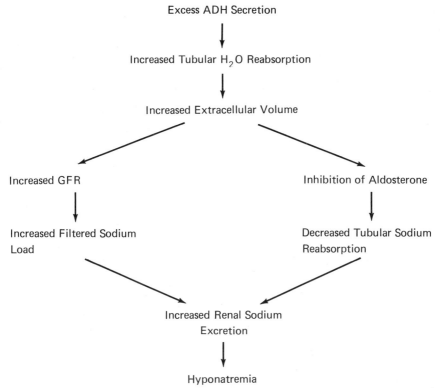

Figure 8-1.   *The pathogenesis of the metabolic abnormalities seen in SIADH.*

creased renal clearance.[21] Hypouricemia accompanies SIADH regardless of etiology, but is not found in patients with hyponatremia attributable to other causes.

A wide variety of disorders have now been reported to cause SIADH (Table 8-5). Neoplasms are the most frequent cause of SIADH,[22,23] and, in one recent review, 50 percent of cases were associated with neoplasms.[23] SCC has accounted for the vast majority of reported cases: 20 of the first 26 reported cases were associated with bronchogenic carcinoma (always SCC when the histology was specified).[19,24-37] The other 6 cases all involved cerebral metastases, and therefore may have been caused by another mechanism. Isolated case reports of SIADH associated with tumors of the esophagus,[23] head and neck,[38] lung (non-SCC),[33,38] duodenum,[39] ureter,[40] and pancreas,[41] have appeared but many of these cases were atypical,[33,41] and ADH assays in serum and tumor tissue were reported in only 2

Table 8-5
Causes of SIADH

A. Tumors with aberrant production of ADH
   1. Small cell carcinoma of the lung
   2. Non-small cell lung cancer
   3. Carcinoma of duodenum (1 case report)
   4. Carcinoma of pancreas (1 case report)
   5. Carcinoma of ureter (1 case report)
   6. Carcinoma of prostate (1 case report)
   7. Carcinoma of esophagus (1 case report)
   8. Thymoma
 	
B. SIADH from endogenous ADH
   1. Trauma
   2. Pulmonary disease
     a. Pneumonia
     b. Tuberculosis
     c. Fungal disease
     d. Positive-pressure breathing
   3. Central nervous system disorders
     a. Meningitis
	b. Head injury
	     c. Brain abscess
	     d. Encephalitis
	     e. Guillain-Barré syndrome
	     f. Subarachnoid hemorrhage
	     g. Acute intermittent porphyria
	     h. Peripheral neuropathy
	     i. Delerium tremens
	     j. Psychosis
	     k. Brain metastases
	   4. SIADH in endocrine disease
	     a. Addison's disease
	     b. Myxedema
	     c. Hypopituitarism
	   5. "Idiopathic" SIADH
	
	C. SIADH from drugs
	   1. Oxytocin
	   2. Vincristine, Vinblastine
	   3. Chlorpropamide
	   4. Thiazides
	   5. Clofibrate
	   6. Nicotine
	   7. Phenothiazines
	   8. Cyclophosphamide

cases.[38] It can be safely stated that SIADH rarely exists in association with any neoplasm other than SCC.

Schwartz et al.[19] postulated in 1957 that tumors produce SIADH by synthesizing and secreting ADH or ADH-like substances in an unregulated manner. Substantiation of this hypothesis has proven technically difficult, since reliable assays for ADH have been developed only recently. Amatruda et al.[25] first demonstrated ADH activity in tumor tissue from a patient with SCC, using a bioassay in which acetone-dried tumor tissue was injected into rats and antidiuretic response was measured. This observation was subsequently confirmed by several other investigators.[26,42–48] The activity in tumor tissue could be abolished with thioglycollate,[24,42,45] which suggested that this material, like ADH, contained disulfide bonds. Lee et al.[42] showed high urine and serum levels of ADH activity in a patient with SIADH. Vorherr et al.[41] studied 10 patients with SIADH, also using a biologic assay to detect ADH. Only 4 of 10 patients were found to have increased levels of ADH activity in tumor extracts.. Of these 4 patients, only 3 were shown to have increased serum ADH activity, and the levels in these 3 were only slightly elevated. The authors postulated that slight increases in serum ADH, perhaps beyond the sensitivity of their assay, could produce SIADH.

The first demonstration of ADH synthesis by tumor tissue was in 1972,[46] when ^{3}H-phenylalanine was shown to be incorporated into a substance with ADH-like activity after incubation with SCC tumor cells. Further evidence for ADH synthesis and secretion by tumor cells was provided by Pettengill et al.,[15] who succeeded in establishing a tissue-culture cell line from SCC bone marrow metastases. ADH was detected within the cells in culture by immunoperoxidase labeling, and increased levels of ADH were also measured in the medium surrounding the tumor cells. Of special interest in this study was the fact that a population of cells in culture did not stain positive for ADH by the immunoperoxidase method and apparently did not contain ADH.

The development of a reliable radioimmunoassay for ADH in 1972[47,48] has led to further rapid advances in the understanding of this syndrome. Morton et al.[49] studied 19 patients with bronchogenic carcinoma, and determined ADH concentration by radioimmunoassay in tissue from primary tumor and metastases. In 10 SCC patients with clinical SIADH, ADH was detected in all primary tumors and all metastases tested. The concentration of ADH found, however, was less than one-tenth of the concentrations found in normal pituitary tissue. Three SCC patients with no clinical evidence of SIADH were studied; plasma ADH levels were not measured, but tissue from two of three primary sites showed ADH (one at low levels). No ADH was found in tumor samples from 6 patients with non-small cell lung cancer. In light of the accumulated evidence, it is accepted that SIADH associated with SCC is caused by synthesis and secretion of ADH (or ADH-like material) by the tumor cells. Both biologic and immunologic studies indicate that the tumor product resembles very closely or is identical to ADH found in the pituitary.

In spite of its appeal, the concept of a tumor secreting large amounts of ADH in a random and unregulated fashion and thereby producing SIADH is overly simplistic. Robertson et al.[38,50] have recently measured serum ADH levels during hypertonic saline infusions in both normal subjects and in patients with SIADH. Since hypertonicity is a potent stimulus for ADH secretion, normal subjects all showed a linear rise in ADH. In all normals ADH levels began to rise when serum osmolality rose above 280–

290 mOsm, and these subjects experienced thirst at 290–300 mOsm. When SIADH patients were tested, four distinct response patterns were observed. Twenty percent of patients showed random variations in ADH unrelated to serum osmolality—the expected pattern in a completely autonomous tumor. The other three response patterns all showed preserved response, albeit abnormal, to serum osmolality. Thirty-five percent of patients showed linear increases in ADH levels during saline infusion, but showed initial rises at the 250–260-mOsm range and complained of thirst at 260–270 mOsm. This response suggests a "resetting" of the osmostat; such patients will therefore maintain a hypotonic serum when normally hydrated. The pathophysiologic mechanism for this response pattern in SCC patients is unclear. It has been suggested that tumor secretion of ADH may be dependent in some cases on serum osmolality. Another patient group (35 percent) showed a basal hypersecretion of ADH, coupled with a linear rise similar to that seen in normal subjects. The final pattern (10 percent) was characterized by suppressed ADH levels, which showed no rise until the plasma osmolality exceeded the normal threshold level. This pattern is the most difficult to reconcile with other studies, which have shown consistently elevated ADH levels in patients with SCC and SIADH. Robertson has reported one patient with SCC who had no detactable ADH at basal conditions and who responded to hypertonic saline infusions with ADH rise only when normal plasma osmolality was reached.[38] This patient consistently showed inappropriate concentration of his urine and failed to dilute his urine with water loading, even though his plasma ADH levels were maximally suppressed. We have seen a similar patient who had normal plasma ADH levels as measured by radioimmunoassay, despite having all the other characteristics of SIADH. This situation must be very rare in association with SCC (to our knowledge these are the only two cases), and suggests production of an unrecognized antidiuretic substance.

The availability of the radioimmunoassay for ADH has also permitted a more precise definition of the frequency of SIADH in SCC. The incidence of clinically recognized cases has varied in reported series, but has usually been in the range of 5–10 percent.[10,51–53] However, a much larger percentage of patients fail to excrete maximally dilute urine when standard water-loading tests are performed. Ginsberg et al.[52] found abnormal responses in 27 of 40 patients with SCC (66 percent). Thirteen of 15 patients with extensive-stage disease were abnormal, compared to 4 of 11 with limited-stage disease. Similarly, 34 of 49 patients (69 percent) tested by Gilby et al.[54] showed abnormal water load test results. When ADH levels were measured on these same 49 patients, 17 (35 percent) were

Table 8-6
Incidence of Inappropriate ADH Secretion in Patients
with Small Cell Carcinoma of the Lung

Investigators	Criterion	% Abnormal	
Barjon et al.[56]	Water load	2/6	(33%)
Ginsberg et al.[52]	Water load	27/40	(66%)
Haefliger et al.[57,*]	Basal urinary ADH	15/23	(65%)
Odell and Wolfsen[5,*,†]	Basal serum ADH	17/41	(41%)
Gilby et al.[54,55]	Water load	34/49	(69%)
	Basal serum ADH	17/49	(35%)

*No water load-testing performed.
†Type of lung cancer unspecified.

found to have persistently high values. These patients also had hypotonic serum and inappropriately concentrated urine, but "most" were asymptomatic (no further details given). The higher percentage of abnormal results seen with water loading is intriguing and may define a group of patients with normal basal ADH levels but abnormal ADH suppression with water loading. A summary of work in this area appears in Table 8-6.

Because serum ADH levels are elevated in 30–40 percent of patients with SCC, there has been recent interest in using ADH as a tumor marker to assist in treatment of SCC patients. Related work has been done using neurophysins—polypeptides that act as binding proteins for ADH. Neurophysins can also be detected by radioimmunoassay, and current data indicate that their synthesis, storage, and secretion parallels that of ADH.[58,59] North et al.[59] found elevated levels in 11 of 26 patients with SCC (42 percent), and noted a "good correlation" between serum levels and response to chemotherapy when levels were serially monitored in 5 patients. At present, however, there does not appear to be any advantage to measuring neurophysins rather than ADH.

The treatment of SIADH in SCC patients has been problematic, since the syndrome is usually present at the time of diagnosis (occasionally SIADH precedes the diagnosis by as much as several months) and persists throughout the untreated course of the disease. In the 5–10 percent of patients who are symptomatic, hyponatremia is usually severe, with serum values in the range of 105–120 mEq/liter. Fluid restriction alone can correct the hyponatremia and hypoosmolality, but patients often find it difficult to comply with the necessary 500–750 cc/day restriction.

Recent interest has focused on the use of lithium[60] and demeclocycline[61–63] in the treatment of SIADH. Both of these agents produce a nephrogenic diabetes insipidus by interfering with the action of ADH on the renal collecting duct.[64,65] Maximal urine concentrating ability is impaired, causing a diuresis which corrects the hyponatremia and hypoosmolality within 4–7 days of starting the drug. Demeclocycline has been shown to be more reliable than lithium in producing nephrogenic diabetes insipidus,[66] and is associated with fewer side effects. For these reasons, it is the preferred agent. However, reversible declines in renal function (usually mild to moderate) have been reported with demeclocycline[67,68]; the mechanism of this impairment is not clear.

Combination chemotherapy is now the definitive treatment of SIADH. Aggressive treatment schedules produce objective tumor regressions in most patients,[69] and most recent reports indicate equal efficacy in causing resolution of SIADH.[53,70] Cohen et al.[70] reported 7 patients with SIADH who achieved either partial or complete tumor responses with chemotherapy; serum sodium values rose to greater than 128 mEq/liter within 14 days after beginning treatment. Conflicting data have been reported by Gregor et al.,[71] who found that 5 of 6 patients with SIADH failed to respond to chemotherapy. However, the treatment regimen used was less intensive than others currently in use.

Fourteen patients with SCC and SIADH have been treated with intensive combination chemotherapy at Vanderbilt University Medical Center during the last 3 yr (Table 8-7). Thirteen of 14 attained a normal serum sodium within 3–6 wk of starting treatment, despite unrestricted fluid intake. Serial ADH measurements were obtained in 4 of these patients. The levels were initially elevated in all 4, and became normal in 3 patients coincident with resolution of hyponatremia. Levels remained elevated in the fourth patient, who had persistence of his SIADH, in spite of a partial tumor response on chest x-ray. In the Vanderbilt series, 12 patients have had recurrence of tumor after varying periods of response, and, in 8 of 12, SIADH recurred coincident with disease progression. Serum ADH levels also rose in the single patient in whom serial measurements were obtained. Surprisingly, 4 of the 12 patients showed no recurrence of their SIADH as they relapsed and died from their tumor. Unfortunately, serial ADH levels were not available on these patients during relapse. Although the explanation for the permanent resolution of SIADH in these patients is unknown, it seems likely that not all tumor cells produce and secrete ADH, and that the recurrent neoplastic populations in these 4 patients did not have this capacity. The work of Pettengill et al.[15] provides indirect experimental evidence for this hypothesis: immunoperoxidase staining of cultured SCC cells showed that only some of the cells contained ADH. Further studies using immunoperoxidase stains on tumor tissue from similar patients may help to explain the apparent change in tumor biology.

Table 8-7
Vanderbilt Series of Patients with Small Cell Carcinoma
and SIADH: Results of Treatment with Chemotherapy*

Initial serum sodium range was 103–128 mEq/liter.
11/14 had extensive disease.
All were treated with combination chemotherapy (cytoxan, adriamycin, vincristine, some also with methotrexate and radiotherapy).
13/14 had complete resolution of hyponatremia in 3–6 wks.
ADH levels were measured serially in 4 patients and correlated with clinical response.
12/14 patients have had tumor recurrence, 8/12 had recurrence of SIADH.

*Total of 14 patients.

In summary, SIADH is characterized by hyponatremia with hypoosmolality of the serum, and by less than maximally dilute urine with continued sodium excretion. These abnormalities are caused by persistently elevated ADH levels, and are manifest only with normal volume status. SCC is the single most common cause of this syndrome, and accounts for the vast majority of cancer-related cases. ADH is synthesized and secreted by tumor cells in an uncontrolled (or abnormally controlled) fashion. Five to 10 percent of patients with SCC will have the clinical syndrome, usually manifest at the time of diagnosis of tumor, while an additional 40–50 percent will have subclinical abnormalities in either urinary dilution capacity or elevated serum ADH levels, or both. Current chemotherapy is effective definitive treatment in most cases. Demeclocycline and fluid restriction are valuable adjuncts before remission is obtained, and also in recurrent cases resistant to chemotherapy. Serial ADH measurements may be useful in monitoring response to therapy and in predicting relapse.

Adrenocorticotropin

In 1928, Brown[72] described a woman who developed truncal obesity, hirsutism, hyperpigmentation, and diabetes. At autopsy an "incidental" lung tumor was found. The pathogenesis of the syndrome was not clear at the time; in fact, it was not until 4 yr later that Cushing described this syndrome in association with pituitary adenoma.[73] Although it was subsequently recognized that Cushing's syndrome occasionally occurred in association with a "nonendocrine" tumor, it was not until the early 1960s that several series were published stressing clinical differences between these patients and those with pituitary or adrenal Cushing's syndrome.[74,75] The first major advance in the understanding of this syndrome occurred in 1962, when Meador et al.[76] demonstrated elevated ACTH activity in plasma and tumor tissue from 5 patients, and postulated that the tumor was responsible for the synthesis and secretion of ACTH. Since then, our understanding of both the clinical and biochemical aspects of tumor-related Cushing's syndrome has improved.

Unlike SIADH, which occurs almost exclusively in association with SCC, ectopic ACTH secretion has been reported with a wide variety of tumors. Early reports included many different tumor types; however, Azzopardi and Williams demonstrated in 1968 that many of these cases were poorly documented pathologically.[77] These investigators identified four groups for which good documentation existed: (1) SCC; (2) endocrine tumors of the foregut (includes islet cell tumors; carcinoids of the bronchus, stomach, and pancreas; thymoma; and medullary carcinoma of the thyroid); (3) pheochromocytoma and related tumors; and (4) certain ovarian tumors (arrhenoblastoma). The authors noted that all of these tumors except SCC were "endocrine associated": recent evidence indicates that SCC is also endocrine related, perhaps arising from APUD cells as do the above-mentioned tumor types. Single case reports (which seem to be well documented) of ectopic ACTH secretion in other tumors not included in these categories include non-small cell lung cancer, squamous carcinoma of the larynx, adenocarcinomas of the salivary glands, stomach, gallbladder, kidney, colon, and prostate, and melanoma. However, SCC accounts for the majority of reported cases (Table 8-8).

The incidence of Cushing's syndrome associated with ectopic ACTH production in SCC has varied widely in reported series depending on the criteria used to establish the diagnosis. Severe clinical symptoms occur in only 3–7 percent of patients with SCC.[51,55,79,80] Good evidence exists, however, that higher percentages of patients have mild, clinically unrecognized hypercortisolism. Gilby et al.[81] found elevated midnight cortisol levels with resistance to suppression by dexamethasone in 22 of 43 patients with SCC (51 percent). Several investigators have found high incidences of elevated ACTH levels in the plasma of SCC patients,[9,81–85] as summarized in Table 8-9. Although detection of ACTH-like products having low biologic activity may account for some of the measured elevations, ectopic ACTH production is clearly underdiagnosed clinically in SCC.

The clinical and laboratory features of Cushing's syndrome associated with SCC differ in many respects from those of Cushing's syndrome of other etiologies (Table 8-10). The disease occurs predominantly in males over 50 yr of age, although the incidence in females can be expected to increase as lung cancer in females becomes more common. Only rarely do

Table 8-8
Nonendocrine Tumors and Ectopic ACTH Production

Tumor Type	% of Cases
Small cell carcinoma of the Lung	60
Thymic tumors	15
Islet cell tumors	10
Carcinoids	4
Miscellaneous	11

Uncommon types: Pheochromocytoma, medullary carcinoma of the thyroid, neurogenic tumors, arrhenoblastoma.

Rare types (single case reports): Adenocarcinomas of the prostate, kidney, parotid, gallbladder, colon, stomach; testicular; melanoma squamous carcinoma of the esophagus.

Modified from Amatruda.[78]

patients exhibit the "classic" findings of centripetal obesity, moon facies, easy bruisability, striae, and hirsutism. Imura et al.[86] reported that none of 15 patients with SCC and ectopic ACTH production had these features: similarly, only 1 of 8 patients in Friedman's series appeared "Cushingoid."[87] Although the chronic effects of hypercortisolism on fat and protein metabolism are absent, the acute metabolic effects of severe cortisol excess are marked. Severe weakness is universal, and weight loss rather than weight gain is usually seen. Glucose intolerance is more common than in other types of Cushing's syndrome, and is often severe. Mineralocorticoid excess produces edema (30–40 percent), hypertension (30–60 percent),[4,86] and hypokalemia. Hyperpigmentation is more common than in other types, and occurs in 25–30 percent.[86] It is evident that the clinical

Table 8-9
Incidence of Elevated Serum ACTH Levels in Patients with Bronchogenic Carcinoma

Investigator	No. of Patients	Incidence (%)
Yalow[82,*]	136	44
Odell et al.[83,*]	61	72
Gilby et al.[81,†]	36	11
Hansen et al.[9]	73	30
Krauss et al.[84,85]	66	40

*Includes all histologic types of lung cancer.
†Includes previously treated patients.

Table 8-10
Clinical and Laboratory Features of Patients with Small
Cell Carcinoma and Ectopic ACTH Production

"Classic" Cushing's syndrome is rarely present.

Weight loss, severe weakness in almost 100%.

Glucose intolerance, 60–70%.

Mineralocorticoid excess more frequent: edema, 30–40%; hypertension, 30–60%

Hyperpigmentation, 25–30%.

Metabolic abnormalities often severe—hypokalemic alkalosis present in
70–90%.

Urinary 17-OHCS levels markedly elevated.

Serum ACTH levels >200 pg/ml in 65%.

Dexamethasone produces suppression very rarely.

symptoms and signs are nonspecific and overlap those of the underlying malignancy, hence the diagnosis is often overlooked.

Several laboratory features are also distinctive. Severe hypokalemic alkalosis (potassium < 3.0 mEq/liter, bicarbonate > 35 mEq/liter) is common only in Cushing's syndrome associated with ectopic ACTH production. Bagshawe found that all 23 cases in the literature with potassium levels of less than 3.0 mEq/liter were associated with tumor.[74] The incidence of these abnormalities in patients with SCC and ectopic ACTH production is 70–90 percent.[87,88] Urinary 17-hydroxycorticosteroids are usually greatly elevated, and plasma ACTH levels exceed 200 pg/ml in 65 percent of patients.[89] Dexamethasone produces no suppression in cortisol levels in the vast majority of cases.

Although some of the more indolent tumors associated with ectopic ACTH production can be occult at the time that Cushing's syndrome becomes manifest, this situation rarely occurs with SCC. Sophisticated tests to elucidate the cause of Cushing's syndrome are therefore almost never needed and will not be discussed here.

During the last 10 years, major advances have been made in our understanding of the biosynthesis of ACTH and related products by tumors. A knowledge of the normal biosynthesis of ACTH and related peptide hormones by the pituitary provides a necessary background. As shown schematically in Figure 8-2, several peptides appear to be synthesized from a common precursor with a molecular weight of at least 31,000 daltons.[11] The structure of this precursor molecule has not been characterized completely. The function of the amino-terminal portion (comprising approximately one-half of the molecule) is unknown. ACTH contains 39

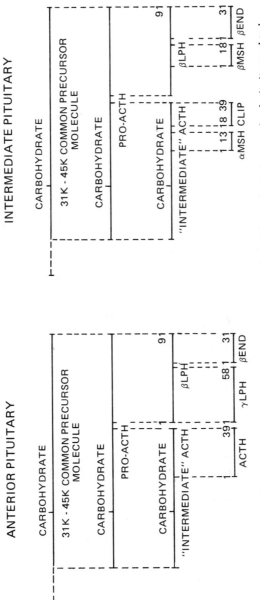

Figure 8-2. A schematic representation of ACTH and related peptide products in an animal pituitary gland.

amino acids and occupies a central position in the precursor molecule. Beta-lipotropin is a 91-amino acid molecule that has γ-lipotropin as its 1–58 sequence, β-melanocyte stimulating hormone (β-MSH) as its 41–58 sequence, and the endogenous opiate peptide β-endorphin as its 61–91 sequence. The biologic functions of these peptides are poorly understood. Fragments of $ACTH_{1-39}$ have also been found; these are the corticotropinlike intermediate lobe peptide (CLIP, 18–39ACTH), and α-MSH (acetyl-1–13ACTH-NH_2). As shown in Figure 8-2, these various fragments are synthesized in different areas of the pituitary; as the adult human pituitary does not contain an intermediate lobe, certain of these peptides (α-MSH, β-MSH, CLIP) are not normally present.

All the peptides found in the pituitary (including those not present in the adult human pituitary) have been identified in tumors, in various combinations. It is well established that many tumor types (Table 8-8) produce ACTH that is identical biologically, immunologically, and chemically to pituitary ACTH ($ACTH_{1-39}$).[4,90] SCC tissue-culture cells have been shown to secrete immunoreactive ACTH into culture medium in vitro.[91] A single patient with a carcinoid tumor has been shown to secrete $ACTH_{2-38}$[92]; the authors postulated the existence of different cleavage enzymes in the tumor cells.

In 1971, a peptide that cross-reacted immunologically with ACTH but had a much higher molecular weight, was described in an extract of a thymoma.[92] This peptide, called "big ACTH," has since been found in many tumors, in the culture media of SCC cells in vitro,[91] and in small concentrations in the pituitary.[94] "Big ACTH" may be pro-ACTH; it is a glycoprotein with a molecular weight of 20,000 daltons.[95] It possesses less than 4 percent of the biologic activity of $ACTH_{1-39}$, but can be converted to fully active $ACTH_{1-39}$ by trypsin.[96] Big ACTH accounts for most (70–80 percent) of the ACTH activity detected in tumor tissue and also in the plasma of patients with ectopic ACTH production.

Several investigators have found elevated immunoreactive ACTH levels in the tumor extracts of 60–80 percent of patients with lung cancer of all types.[97,98] A large number of these patients were also found to have elevated plasma ACTH levels (presumably mostly big ACTH) in the absence of clinical evidence of hypercortisolism. However, recent data indicate that patients with SCC or carcinoid lung tumors have higher immunoreactive and bioactive levels of tumor ACTH than do patients with other types of lung cancer.[99] Interpretation of reports demonstrating increased plasma ACTH levels in large percentages of lung cancer patients is difficult, since multiple factors may complicate the findings. These include patient stress, sampling at inappropriate times of day, and interference of plasma proteins with the radioimmunoassay.

Lipotropins have also been found in tumor extracts and plasma of patients with the ectopic ACTH syndrome.[100,101] The frequency of association appears to be quite high; plasma lipotropins were elevated in 36 percent of patients with lung cancer in a recent series.[102] The biologic significance of the lipotropins is not clear; they may have melanotropic activity, but their potency as compared to MSH is controversial. Alpha-MSH[103] and β-MSH[100] have also been identified in tumor tissue, but question exists as to whether the "α-MSH" activity was due to cross-reaction with ACTH or other fragments.

Several ACTH fragments have also been demonstrated in tumor tissue. Using separate radioimmunoassays for the C-terminal and N-terminal ends of ACTH, Orth et al.[90] demonstrated large excesses of both C- and N-terminal fragments without ACTH-like bioactivity. The N-terminal fragments had some MSH activity; the C-terminal fragments had no detectable activity. These fragments may have been CLIP ($ACTH_{18-39}$); this peptide was identified in extracts from a carcinoid tumor by other investigators.[104]

Finally, corticotropin-releasing factor (CRF) has been isolated from ectopic ACTH-producing tumors.[105] This substance has been shown to stimulate ACTH release in rat models; it is chemically distinct from ADH, which also has some CRF activity. Yamamoto et al.[106] found CRF activity in 7 of 12 ACTH-producing tumors. It has been postulated that CRF, rather than ACTH, is responsible for producing hypercortisolism in the rare patient who shows cortisol suppression with dexamethasone. At present, however, the role of CRF in producing Cushing's syndrome is undefined, since all tumors from which it has been isolated have also produced ACTH.

The prognosis of patients with Cushing's syndrome associated with SCC has traditionally been very poor. Ross reported on 9 patients who survived an average of 24 days after diagnosis.[107] Bornstein et al.[75] had an average survival of 3 months in 17 patients, with no survivors past 6 months. Severe metabolic abnormalities produced by the hypercortisolemia were responsible for many deaths, rather than direct tumor effects. Immediate management of the metabolic abnormalities is difficult. The hypokalemia is often refractory and requires large amounts of potassium replacement. Occasional successes have been reported using metyrapone to block adrenal synthesis of cortisol,[108] but the majority of patients have not responded well. To date, there have been no reported series of patients treated with combination chemotherapy. Our experience with 5 patients indicates that they can be expected to respond similarly to patients with SIADH; a majority will achieve remission within 3–6 weeks of initiating chemotherapy. As in SIADH, the syndrome frequently recurs with subsequent tumor progression.

In summary, Cushing's syndrome associated with neoplasms is caused by tumor synthesis and secretion of ACTH. SCC is the most common cause of this syndrome, accounting for approximately 60 percent of cases. The majority of remaining cases are also produced by tumors in the APUD group. Severe clinical symptoms occur in 3–7 percent of patients with SCC (similar to the incidence of SIADH), but abnormal cortisol secretion has been demonstrated in 50–60 percent. Clinical presentation differs from Cushing's syndrome of other causes, with severe metabolic abnormalities (hypokalemia and alkalosis), and very high plasma ACTH levels. Although the biochemical details are still incomplete, tumor synthesis of ACTH employs precursor molecules and enzymes similar to those utilized by the pituitary. Most of the peptides derived from the ACTH precursor molecule in the pituitary have also been identified in tumor tissue. Tumor synthesis, probably proceeds in an uncontrolled manner, however, and current evidence indicates that an individual tumor has only some of the normal pituitary enzymes present. For this reason, large amounts of precursors and ACTH fragments with little or no biologic activity are secreted, and the quantity and types of peptides secreted vary from tumor to tumor. Currently unexplained is the frequent finding of "big ACTH" in tumor types that are only rarely associated with ectopic ACTH production. These tumors may be unable to synthesize and/or secrete biologically active ACTH; alternatively (and seemingly less likely), the substance being detected may not really represent an ACTH precursor. Prognosis and treatment have both been poor; however, early evidence indicates that effective combination chemotherapy can produce remissions in most patients. The utility of ACTH and related products as tumor markers in SCC awaits clarification.

Calcitonin

Calcitonin is a 32-amino acid peptide hormone that was first identified in the parathyroid gland of several lower animals and from the ultimobronchial glands of fish, amphibians, reptiles, and birds.[109] In man, calcitonin is produced in the parafollicular cells (C cells) of the thyroid gland. C cells are derived from the neural crest and are probably remnants of the ultimobronchial glands of lower animals.

Calcitonin inhibits the resorption of bone and is a physiologic antagonist of parathyroid hormone. The mechanism of this action is poorly understood, but calcitonin can inhibit bone resorption even in the presence of circulating parathyroid hormone. The effect of calcitonin secretion is very rapid (much more rapid than the onset of parathyroid hormone activity), but the duration of action is very short. Elevated plasma calcium causes immediate calcitonin secretion. Calcitonin, therefore, seems to protect against acute hypercalcemic situations, whereas parathyroid hormone governs calcium homeostasis on a chronic basis.

The utility of calcitonin as a tumor marker was first recognized in association with medullary carcinoma of the thyroid.[110,111] Although these patients do not exhibit any metabolic abnormalities, a majority have elevated basal serum calcitonin levels which fall to normal with successful surgical treatment. When calcitonin release is stimulated with calcium or pentagastrin infusions, 100 percent of patients with medullary carcinoma are abnormal.[112-114] These tests can identify patients with very small tumors and with "C cell hyperplasia," and are used to screen families with multiple endocrine adenomatosis type II.

Calcitonin was initially thought to be a specific tumor marker for medullary carcinoma of the thyroid. However, with improvement and more widespread use of the calcitonin radioimmunoassay[115] several patients were reported during the early 1970s with elevated calcitonin levels from tumors other than medullary carcinoma.[116-119] Silva et al.[117] demonstrated calcitonin production by SCC using selective venous catheterization: venous concentrations (draining from the tumor) were 1900 pg/ml, whereas thyroidal vein concentrations were only 200 pg/ml (also of interest in this patient was the fall in serum calcitonin from 1250 to 50 pg/ml following chemotherapy with cyclophosphamide and methotrexate). Subsequently, tissue culture cells from an "undifferentiated" lung cancer were shown to produce calcitonin even after 18 mo in culture.[120]

Since these initial case reports, hypercalcitoninemia has been associated with a wide variety of tumor types. Milhaud et al.[121] found hypersecretion in a number of tumors in the APUD group, including carcinoid, pheochromocytoma, insulinoma, melanoma, and SCC. Non-APUD tumors, including breast carcinoma and non-small cell lung cancer, also frequently have elevated plasma calcitonin. Coombs et al.[122] found elevated plasma levels of calcitonin in 8 of 8 patients with breast cancer; calcitonin was detected in tumor extracts from 7 of these patients.[123] The same investigators also demonstrated release of calcitonin into culture medium in tissue culture lines from 8 to 15 patients with breast cancer.[124] Schwartz et al.[125] recently found elevated levels in patients with lung (38 percent), pancreas (42 percent), breast (38 percent), gastric (30 percent), and colon (24 percent) cancers. These results show much higher frequencies than those previously reported and are probably explained by the use of calcitonin levels of 150 pg/ml, rather than the previously used 400 pg/ml, as the upper limit of normal.

Although it is evident that plasma calcitonin levels are frequently elevated in association with tumors, these elevations in some cases are caused by increased thyroidal secretion rather than by tumor production. Silva et al.[126] reported a patient with adenocarcinoma of the lung who had a plasma calcitonin level of 630 pg/ml (normal value being less than 350 pg/ml); catheterization of the right middle thyroidal vein showed a concentration of 4100 pg/ml. Similarly, catheterization of 6 patients with lung cancer showed thyroidal origin of calcitonin in 4 of 6 patients (in 1 of 4 with SCC) and tumor origin of calcitonin in only 2 of 6 patients (both with SCC).[127] It was initially suspected that the presence of bone involvement with tumor could stimulate thyroidal calcitonin production; however, the incidence of elevated plasma calcitonin levels has been shown to be unaffected by bone metastases.[128] At present, the relative frequency of thyroidal versus tumor origin of elevated calcitonin levels in patients with cancer is not known. It is likely, however, that the hypercalcitoninemia associated with the APUD-related tumors is usually caused by tumor secretion, given the propensity of this tumor group to produce ectopic products.

Most of the recent interest in calcitonin has focused on its potential use as a tumor marker in lung cancer patients. Calcitonin levels have been elevated in 38–67 percent of patients with lung cancer,[84,85,125,127–129] with most series showing an incidence of 55–65 percent. SCC has consistently been the histologic type most frequently associated with hypercalcitoninemia (60–70 percent), followed by adenocarcinoma, epidermoid, and large cell carcinoma in descending order of frequency. Tumor calcitonin measurements have not been performed in most of these series, so the mechanism of calcitonin production may not always be tumor related. SCC is generally associated with higher calcitonin levels than are the other types; in one series 25 percent of SCC patients had calcitonin levels in the medullary carcinoma range (greater than two times the normal).[130] Krauss et al.[84,85] found higher incidences in patients with extensive disease (83 percent with extensive SCC versus 55 percent with limited disease), but other series have not confirmed this finding.[127,130] Although limited biochemical work has been done, one group has reported that circulating calcitonin in patients with lung cancer is composed of predominantly high-molecular-weight forms (20,000–30,000 daltons), whereas medullary carcinomas secrete seven different forms (molecular weight 2500–30,000 daltons) in approximately equal amounts.[131]

The reliability of serial calcitonin measurements in reflecting response to therapy has been assessed in only small numbers of patients. Silva et al.[127] reported decreasing calcitonin levels coincident with either chemotherapy or surgical therapy in 12 of 16 lung cancer patients (all types). Subsequent calcitonin measurements in these patients were concordant with changes in disease activity in 67 percent of instances. Krauss et al.[84,85] followed serial calcitonin levels in 6 patients with SCC, and found that levels decreased with successful chemotherapy and increased with relapse in all patients. Wallach et al.[132] monitored calcitonin in 8 patients before and after combination chemotherapy, and the hormone levels correlated with disease activity in all patients.

The future usefulness of calcitonin as a tumor marker is currently unclear. The incidence of elevated serum levels in patients with lung cancer is higher than that of any other substance currently known. Thyroid origin of elevated levels in some cases may hinder interpretation; the relative frequency of this occurrence needs to be better defined. Finally, serial calcitonin levels must be measured in larger numbers of patients before reliability in mirroring tumor activity can be adequately assessed.

Other Tumor Products

Other peptide hormones, enzymes, and amines have been associated occasionally with SCC, and the importance or potential utility of these associations remains unclear.

Beck and Burger[133] measured immunoreactive growth hormone in 18 primary lung tumors and found elevated levels in 7 tumors, 2 of which were SCC. Gilby et al.[134] noted paradoxical elevations of growth hormone following a glucose meal in 11 of 38 SCC patients (29 percent). They concluded that this was probably a nonspecific finding, since similar responses occur in non-neoplastic conditions.

Baylin et al.[135] measured plasma and tumor histaminase activity in patients with lung cancer. They detected elevated enzyme activity in sera from about one-third of 25 SCC patients and in 4 of 5 tumors, but they found histaminase activity in sera of only 3 of 20 patients with large cell or squamous carcinoma.

A patient with SCC who developed unilateral gynecomastia in association with elevated serum FSH and estradiol levels has been reported.[136]

Gilby et al.[134] detected significant elevations of TSH, LH, or FSH in only 2 of 32 SCC patients. The association of "gonadotropinlike activity" and lung cancer has been described in multiple reports.

Serotonin,[137,138] histamine,[138] and 5-hydroxytryptophan[139] have been detected in sera or tumor tissue of patients with SCC. Gilby et al.[134] found no elevation of 5-hydroxyindoleacetic acid excretion in 14 SCC patients.

Hypercalcemia due to parathyroid-hormone-like activity has been reported very rarely in SCC,[140,141] and concomitant primary hyperparathyroidism should be considered in these patients. Hypercalcemia, even in the presence of bony metastases, is extremely rare in SCC in comparison to other histologic types of lung cancer.[141]

Hauger-Klevene[142] described elevated plasma renin activity in a patient with SCC with hypokalemic alkalosis, normal plasma ACTH and cortisols, and aldosterone secretion that was increased but responsive to changes in sodium intake. Detectable reninlike material was present in tumor tissue at death.

Entwistle et al.[143] reported a patient in whom pure red cell aplasia preceded the diagnosis of SCC by more than 1 yr. The serum of this patient appeared to contain a factor that suppressed erythropoiesis in laboratory animals but was not present after radiotherapy.

Tumor Markers in SCC

A reliable "blood test" for cancer remains elusive. This is partially due to major gaps in our understanding of the physiology and behavior of both normal and neoplastic cells. Whether the low concentrations of a variety of substances detected in tumors or blood of cancer patients represent qualitative or quantitative differences from "normal" is often unknown. In addition, the validity of our methods for identifying many of these peptides as ectopic hormones remains suspect, and until the identities of "normal" and ectopic hormones are proved, we would be more accurate in describing activities of these peptides as "hormonelike." Radioimmunoassays of these substances, often described as "sensitive and specific," may prove to be neither sensitive enough for clinical utility nor adequately specific for identification of immunoreactive materials as hormones in patients with SCC. Despite these difficulties, experience with HCG in choriocarcinoma and HCG and α-fetoprotein in germ cell neoplasms has proved the value of measurements of such substances in diagnosis and management of patients with these neoplasms, and the search continues for biochemical markers in many types of tumors. Ideally, a tumor marker should have the following characteristics:

1. It should be produced only by tumor cells.
2. Its concentration in blood or urine should reflect the extent of disease, and measurement should be sensitive enough to detect microscopic or subclinical disease.
3. The assay technique should be convenient, inexpensive, and accurate.
4. The marker should occur with sufficient frequency to make measurement worthwhile. [134]

No marker meets all of these requirements, and in SCC these ideal properties stand in contrast with the current status of biochemical markers. None of the tumor-associated products is produced exclusively by SCC cells, and some are found in substantial quantities in blood or urine in association with non-neoplastic diseases. Furthermore, despite the higher frequency of positive assays in patients with extensive-stage versus limited-stage disease, there is no firm correlation between quantity of a marker and quantity of disease in individual patients. Many of the assays are cumbersome and expensive and are not widely available for general application.

Early attempts to correlate serial measurements of markers with disease status were confounded by a lack of understanding of the biology of SCC, inadequacy of chest roentgenograms for assessing complete remission status, and inability to attain remissions lasting more than a few months. Our understanding of the natural history of this disease and of the impact of therapy on this natural history is rapidly changing.

In contrast to the other histologic types of advanced lung cancer, the therapy for SCC, albeit somewhat empirically derived, has improved substantially over the past few years. The majority of patients with limited-stage disease attain a complete response to therapy. The problem arises in that small amounts of tumor are not easily detected by modern diagnostic techniques. The development of more effective therapy requires a refined definition of the complete response. This is cogently illustrated by patients with choriocarcinoma in which a biochemical marker that correlates with the amount of neoplastic tissue present (HCG) can be measured and used as a standard by which to continue or stop therapy. We are at the stage in the therapy of SCC where a tumor-associated product or products might aid substantially in further improving therapy. A need remains for a more sensitive method that will reflect the presence of neoplastic tissue and indicate growth or regression following therapy. The potential usefulness of tumor-associated products may be viewed in several areas, including (1) initial detection and diagnosis, (2) prognostic indication for determination of recurrent or relapsing disease, (3) evaluation of response, and (4) better understanding of the biochemical expression of malignancy and the changes that occur during the natural course or the treated course of the disease.

Reliable tumor-associated products or markers would improve the therapy of patients with SCC by increasing the sensitivity of detecting occult metastases and monitoring the disease course during therapy. The biologic characteristics of SCC, mainly its putative origin from "neuroendocrine" precursor cells and its frequent association with measureable peptide products, with or without ectopic hormone syndromes, make it an ideal tumor in which to correlate tumor-associated peptide products with the amount of neoplastic tissue detectable by other methods. In the evaluation of therapy based on the measurement of peptide products, it must be recognized that most patients with SCC probably have a heterogeneous tumor, some cells expressing product or marker activity and others not. The metastases from these tumors similarly may or may not express the biologic markers expressed by the primary tumor. Therefore, circulating tumor-associated products or markers may not necessarily correlate with the neoplastic disease activity. Added to this problem is the fact that the peptide hormones are not specific or unique products of SCC, and elevations may result from normal or abnormal secretions from the pituitary gland, thyroid gland, and other tissues.

With the limitations in mind, we began a study to evaluate the usefulness of plasma ADH and calcitonin as markers in SCC. From March 1978 to October 1979, we measured plasma ADH and calcitonin by radioimmunoassay every 6 wk on a group of patients who were currently undergoing therapy and on several new patients both before and during therapy. All patients were treated with intensive combination chemotherapy, with or without radiotherapy. A total of 87 patients had plasma samples measured on at least one occasion. The preliminary results are illustrated in Table 8-11. Fifty-four patients had both hormones measured before therapy. Of these, 17 percent (9 patients) had elevated ADH (> 8 pg/ml), 40 percent (22 patients) had elevated calcitonin (> 200 pg/ml), and 11 percent (6 patients) had an elevation of both hormones. Therefore, 57 percent of the patients had elevated levels of either ADH or calcitonin.

A total of 65 patients had serial measurements during the course of their disease and following therapy. From this group, correlations were made between the quantity of the hormone level and the disease status or activity as determined by standard clinical and laboratory methods. In 42

Table 8-11
ADH and Calcitonin as Small Cell Carcinoma Markers:
Preliminary Results

Number of Patients	87	
Patients with pretreatment values	54	
Patients with no pretreatment values	33	
Patients with serial values	65	
Patients with a single value only	22	
Patients with pretreatment values	54	
Elevated ADH	9	(17%)
Elevated calcitonin	22	(40%)
Elevated ADH and calcitonin	6	(11%)
Neither value elevated	23	(43%)
Patients with serial values	65	
Positive correlation of value with disease activity		
ADH	11	
Calcitonin	23	
Both	6	
Negative correlation of value with disease activity	2	
ADH	1	
Calcitonin	1	
Normal values consistently throughout course unrelated to disease activity	23	

of the 65 patients (65 percent) either one or both hormones were elevated during the course of therapy. Many of these patients are currently being followed and have not relapsed. Correlations of disease regression and progression were made with the hormone values over time. There was a positive correlation of the hormone values with the disease status in 40 patients (11 with ADH, 23 with calcitonin, 6 with both hormones). Thus far, an increased hormone value has been detected in 6 patients who were in remission and correctly predicted a clinical relapse in all 6 occasions. The time from the elevated value to relapse has ranged from 4 to 18 wk. Two patients have shown a negative correlation—an elevated value corresponding with decreasing disease activity (1 with ADH, 1 with calcitonin). Twenty-three patients had consistently normal values throughout their treatment course and follow-up, regardless of the status of the disease. Several of these patients are still being observed. From our preliminary findings, it appears that both ADH and calcitonin may provide a valuable guide to therapeutic management. A more detailed analysis of these data and serial measurements of ACTH is in preparation. Longer follow-up on a greater number of patients will be necessary to determine the reliability of these or other markers in defining their quantitative relationship with tumor volume.

Neurologic Syndromes

Several neurologic syndromes are associated particularly with SCC.[144-146] None of these paraneoplastic syndromes are related solely to SCC, but most of the neurologic syndromes to be discussed occur more frequently in conjunction with SCC than with other cancers. The association with SCC can not easily be explained by chance alone.

To assert that all SCC paraneoplastic syndromes will eventually be found to be attributable to substances directly produced by the tumor is presumptuous. There are undoubtedly other causative mechanisms. For the purpose of discussion, the idea of relating particular tumor products to the paraneoplastic syndromes provides a useful framework, but should not be looked upon as rigid or absolute. Many of the clinical syndromes in which a tumor product has not been recognized may be caused by some other factor related to the neoplastic disease, such as an immunologic effect (see Chapter 14, this monograph) or an infection. In addition, tumor products that are found in association with some of the clinical syndromes may not necessarily be related to the pathogenesis of the syndrome. Further study may demonstrate that some of these syndromes are caused by relatively independent events. For example, progressive multifocal leukoencephalopathy, a neurologic disease associated with several neoplasms,[147] has been clearly demonstrated to be caused by a virus.[148] Regardless of the pathogenic mechanisms, better recognition and characterization of the various clinical neurologic syndromes have practical importance.

The Carcinomatous Neuromyopathies

The carcinomatous neuromyopathies are paraneoplastic syndromes referred to and popularized by Brain and co-workers.[149-152] They are clinical disorders of the central nervous system, peripheral nerves, neuromuscular junction, or muscle, that are not due either to direct invasion or to metastases to these sites. These syndromes are viewed as remote effects of cancer on the neuromuscular system.[152]

A variety of pathologic changes occur in the central nervous system, peripheral nerves, and muscles. The classification outlined in Table 8-12

Table 8-12
Neurologic Paraneoplastic Syndromes

Encephalopathy	Myasthenic syndrome
Cerebral	Peripheral neuropathy
Brainstem	Sensory
Optic nerve	Sensorimotor
Cerebellum	Myopathy
Myelopathy	Polymyositis/dermatomyositis
Anterior horn cell degeneration	
Necrotizing myelopathy	

is a combination of pathologic and clinical features. The clinical manifestations are very diverse and depend on the location and extent of lesions.

The true incidence of carcinomatous neuromyopathies is difficult to determine. In a large series, 162 of 1465 patients with various neoplasms had carcinomatous neuromyopathies.[153] In a smaller series of neurologic disorders associated with cancer,[154] 66 of 696 patients had a carcinomatous neuropathy. The majority of the disorders were either peripheral neuropathies or myopathies, the central nervous system complications being relatively rare. Of 250 patients with lung cancer reported by Croft and Wilkinson,[155] 40 had these syndromes. However, the true incidence with cancer is difficult to pinpoint, since similar clinical disorders of the neuromuscular system appeared to occur as frequently in a group of men with chronic non-neoplastic lung disease.[156] Many types of neoplasms have been reported in association with carcinomatous neuromyopathies, but SCC appears to be found with these syndromes more often than any other neoplasm.[144-146] Therefore, it is very unlikely that the association with SCC is by chance alone.

A tumor-related "mediator" has not been identified in any of these syndromes. However, a SCC patient may have one of these neurologic disorders, or any of the other paraneoplastic syndromes, in conjunction with an elevated plasma level of one or more tumor-associated products.

Toxic, infectious, metabolic, nutritional, and autoimmune etiologies have been postulated as potential causes of the carcinomatous neuromyopathies.[145,146] As mentioned, one disorder previously classified as a "paraneoplastic syndrome," progressive multifocal leukoencephalopathy, has been shown to be caused by a viral agent. Other infectious agents could be responsible for some of the carcinomatous neuromyopathies.

There is no evidence at present to support an infectious agent in any of the other syndromes, however, and the etiology of these complications remains unexplained.

Accurate recognition of the type of nervous system dysfunction in patients with cancer can be difficult. The neurologic complications of cancer take several forms, including: lesions caused by metastases; concomitant but unrelated neurologic diseases; lesions produced by cancer chemotherapeutic agents or radiotherapy; and syndromes attributed to the remote effects of cancer. In the presence of nervous system impairment in a patient with cancer, it is important that one investigate the more common possibilities of metastases, metabolic problems, or iatrogenic lesions first, before seriously entertaining the diagnosis of carcinomatous neuromyopathies.

The occurrence of the carcinomatous neuromyopathies is generally not related to the size of the tumor, presence of metastases, or length of time the tumor has been present. The syndrome may be diagnosed months or years before the discovery of the neoplastic disease, although their simultaneous occurrence is most common. There has been no constant correlation between the response to treatment of the cancer and improvement of the neuromyopathy. This may be related to the fact that therapy for the neoplasm was simply not effective enough, since more recent reports indicate that some of the carcinomatous neuromyopathies respond to successful treatment of the neoplasm.[157,158] The frequent association of carcinomatous neuromyopathies with SCC suggests that the neoplasm is, in some fashion, either producing a neuropathic or myopathic factor or allowing the proper environment for the development of these syndromes. The increased incidence of carcinomatous neuromyopathy in patients with SCC should stimulate further investigation of these syndromes in this neoplastic disorder. Therapy for SCC is now more effective than before, and detailed observation of the clinical course of the associated neurologic disorders following therapy will be important to document. Further study of the immunologic and neuroendocrinologic aspects of SCC may lead to important clues vital to our understanding of the neurologic paraneoplastic syndromes.

Only a minority of patients can be rigidly classified into one syndrome as outlined in Table 8-12. The majority of patients have overlapping clinical pictures related to the central nervous system, peripheral nerves, and muscles. This overlap suggests that there may be a common etiologic factor. Keeping in mind that many of the syndromes are often overlapping, a brief discussion of each of the clinical disorders are now presented.

Encephalopathy

The clinical presentation of the encephalopathic syndromes may involve the cerebrum, brainstem, optic nerves, and cerebellum.[145] Any one anatomic area may dominate, but pathologic lesions are usually found in all areas. Dementia is the most common cerebral manifestation related to carcinomatous encephalopathy. Dementia is quite variable in presentation and may fluctuate from a slight confusional state to a severe organic brain syndrome. The onset may be acute or insidious. There are often variations in mood from depression to euphoria. Dementia may predate the clinical recognition of the neoplasm by many months but more commonly occurs simultaneously. Laboratory studies are often nonspecific, with the spinal fluid often showing an elevated protein level and, occasionally, a slight to moderate pleocytosis. The electroencephalogram is often diffuse and slow. Radiographic studies of the brain are normal. There are usually no other neurologic signs, unless there is an overlapping syndrome (brainstem, optic nerves, spinal cord). Brain biopsy or postmortem examination of the brain may reveal no discernible changes, but often there are areas of lymphocytic infiltration in the brain substance and perivascular areas, or degeneration of the thalamus, hippocampus, and amygdaloid nuclei. Inflammatory lesions may also be found in the brainstem, optic nerves, spinal cord, and meninges, although these lesions may have been clinically silent. Electron microscopy has not demonstrated evidence of the presence of a virus.

The pathologic findings in patients developing a syndrome predominantly involving the brainstem or cranial nerves is similar to the cerebral lesion, but demyelination may also be present. Signs representing brainstem involvement include opthalmoplegia, ataxia, vertigo, nystagmus, and bulbar palsies. These are part of the encephalopathy with major lesions and clinical findings originating from the brainstem. The brainstem may be involved with a degenerative and inflammatory process. Extensive demyelination may also extend to the optic nerves, producing either unilateral or bilateral optic neuritis, associated with decreased visual acuity, papilledema, and scotomas.

Cerebellar degeneration has been the most frequently reported central nervous system paraneoplastic syndrome.[145] As in most of these syndromes, SCC is the predominant neoplasm accompanying this disorder.[144] The signs of cerebellar degeneration may come on acutely or subacutely and are usually bilateral and symmetrical. Trunkal and extremity ataxia may impair movement significantly. Dysarthria and tremors are quite severe, and, rarely, vertigo and nystagmus are present. Examination of the cerebrospinal fluid is often normal but occasionally shows elevation in protein content and lymphocytosis. In the past, the course has been rapid and disability occurs within a few weeks or months. However, patients can improve with effective therapy of the underlying neoplastic disease.[157] Pathologically, there is severe degeneration of the Purkinje cells and perivascular inflammation deep in the cerebellum. There is usually no inflammation in the cortex, but the degeneration is diffuse as opposed to focal as in alcoholic cerebellar degeneration. Occasionally, the brainstem is also involved, emphasizing the rather diffuse nature of these disorders pathologically.

Myelopathy

The myelopathies are characterized by an anterior horn cell degeneration and a necrotizing myelopathy.[146] The anterior horn cell degeneration is similar to amyotrophic lateral sclerosis. Presently there is no good evidence supporting the separation of this syndrome from amyotrophic lateral sclerosis, although Brain felt that its course may be more "benign" than "classic" disease.[146] It is essentially a motor neuron disease with normal sensory findings, normal mental status, and normal cerebrospinal fluid findings. There are progressive signs related to degeneration of the corticobulbar and corticospinal tracts. Muscle weakness, weight loss, muscular atrophy, spasticity, fasciculations, hyperactive reflexes, and extensor plantar responses characterize the disorder. There is some question as to whether amyotrophic lateral sclerosis may be an independent disease in patients with cancer without a causal relationship. In only one patient has the syndrome reversed after successful therapy of the neoplasm; in several other patients there was no improvement.[146]

Necrotizing myelopathy is also a very rare disorder characterized by rather acute paraplegia that is initially spastic but becomes flaccid. Usually the pathology shows necrosis of the spinal cord in the thoracic region. Lesions above the thoracic cord are uncommon. Cerebrospinal fluid protein is usually markedly elevated. The most commonly associated neoplasm is carcinoma of the lung[159] (histologic types not specified).

Peripheral Neuropathy

Peripheral neuropathies are the most common of the neurologic para-neoplastic syndromes.[144,146,155] A pure sensory neuropathy associated with lung cancer was first described by Denny-Brown in 1948.[160] The patients develop decreased sensation and parasthesia. Overlapping problems related to myopathy and signs of central nervous system involvement are commonly observed. Pathologically, there appears to be destruction of neurons in the dorsal root ganglia associated with a patchy inflammatory reaction. The peripheral nerves show loss of myelin and axis cylinder, and occasionally lymphocytic infiltration and segmental demyelination are present. Patients who have symptoms confined to peripheral nerves often have an inflammatory reaction in the spinal cord, brainstem, limbic system, and cerebral cortex. These findings suggest a common pathogenesis. Degeneration of dorsal root ganglia has been noted in many patients with neoplastic diseases who have not had the clinical symptoms and signs related to sensory neuropathy. This suggests that the pathogenesis is on-going and may need to reach a certain threshold before it is clinically relevant. Most of the neoplasms associated with sensory neuropathy and de-generation of dorsal root ganglia arise in the lung or mediastinum.[146] The majority are lung cancer, but others have been thymoma, esophageal carcinoma, laryngeal carcinoma, and mediastinal lymphomas.[146]

Antibodies directed against brain tissue have been demonstrated in the sera and cerebral spinal fluid of some patients with sensory neuropathy.[161,162] Other studies suggest that there are antibodies directed against neurons throughout the central nervous system in many of these patients.[163] Detection of these antibodies are interesting and may help in eventually finding the cause of paraneoplastic neuropathy. However, these antibodies may be an associated phenomenon rather than a causative agent. Indeed, there is not a pathologic resemblance of sensory neuropathy and the well-known autoimmune diseases allergic encephalomyelitis and polyneuritis.

Treatment of the neoplasm has not generally correlated with improvement; however, effective antineoplastic therapy for the underlying neoplasm has not been available in the past. Steroid therapy has been reported to be effective in some patients,[144] but the fact that neuropathy may spontaneously remit makes this difficult to determine. There have been no well designed trials comparing therapies. Sensorimotor neuropathies are also found in association with SCC. The clinical presentation is not spe-

Table 8-13
Myasthenia Gravis and the Myasthenic Syndrome

	Myasthenia Gravis	Myasthenic Syndrome
Sex and age	Young females	Males over age 40
Associated tumors	Thymoma in 50%	Malignant neoplasms in 75%—usually small cell lung cancer
Primary location of weakness	Bulbar and ocular muscles	Proximal extremities
Lesions at neuromuscular junctions	Impaired release of acetylcholine	Unknown? Antibodies against acetylcholine receptors
Electromyography	Fatigue with a decrease of evoked muscle potential	Facilitation with an increase of evoked muscle potentials
Anticholinesterase	Effective	Ineffective
Guanidine	Ineffective or poor effect	Effective

Modified from Hildebrand.[166]

cific. There are many causes of peripheral neuropathy, and there is a legitimate question as to whether sensorimotor neuropathy is a remote effect of tumor or the result of other causes that are frequently present in patients with cancer.

Myasthenic Syndrome

The Eaton-Lambert syndrome or the myasthenic syndrome is intimately related to SCC.[164,165] The majority of patients with this entity have this neoplasm. The myasthenic syndrome is different from myasthenia gravis (Table 8-13). It is usually seen in males with SCC who are over 40 yr of age. The proximal muscles are weak and fatigue easily, and the lower limbs are often predominately involved. There are gait abnormalities and difficulty in rising to a sitting position or in climbing stairs. Often, strength may be transiently increased by repetitive movements. Bulbar signs are rare. The myasthenic syndrome may also be found together with other carcinomatous neuromyopathies. Patients have a marked sensitivity to curarelike medications. The electromyogram is definitive and unique for this disease. There is a facilitation of the muscular potentials with continued stimulation. This is occasionally detected clinically when the grip becomes stronger with effort. The pathogenesis of the myasthenic syndrome is not clear; however, there does appear to be a defect in neuromuscular transmission at the neuromuscular junction. Patients do not respond to treatment with anticholinesterases. Pathological changes have been nonspecific. The myasthenic syndrome usually resolves when effective cytotoxic therapy is given for the neoplasm.[158,167] Guanidine increases the release of anticholinesterases and may be effective, but it is an indirect therapy with a number of side effects[168] and should be reserved for patients not responding to cytotoxic therapy or for patients who develop the syndrome in relapse.

Myopathy

Polymyositis and dermatomyositis are inflammatory diseases of muscle and, in dermatomyositis, of the skin as well. The clinical pattern of these disorders that occurs in association with neoplastic disease is similar to the pattern occurring in patients without cancer. There is proximal muscle weakness, progressing over weeks or months, often with spontaneous exacerbations and remissions. Muscular tenderness, muscular swelling and pain, dysphagia, and Raynard's phenomena are frequent. Serum creatine phosphokinase and aldolase are frequently elevated, and muscle biopsy usually shows severe inflammation. Pure muscle involvement occurs in approximately half of the patients. In the other half there are also other forms of carcinomatous neuromyopathies present. The fact that polymyositis occurs with the other neurologic paraneoplastic syndromes favors the idea that dermatomyositis and polymyositis are remote effects of the neoplasm and, thus, are true paraneoplastic syndromes. The incidence of neoplasms in patients with polymyositis and dermatomyositis range from 15 to 30 percent.[169] The incidence of cancer in men over the age of 50 is common, and polymyositis in this group usually predates the development of cancer. There may be no basic difference between dermatomyositis and polymyositis, except for the presence or absence of the skin rash.

Summary

SCC is associated with a variety of paraneoplastic syndromes. Several of the endocrinologic syndromes are mediated by tumor-associated hormones or hormonelike products. Even though only a minority of patients have a hormone-mediated syndrome, a majority have either measurable ACTH, ADH, or calcitonin in their plasma. The utility of these products as markers of neoplastic disease activity is currently being explored and may prove useful in patient management.

In addition to the hormones and their relationship to SCC, there are several poorly understood neurologic syndromes that occur more frequently with SCC than with any other neoplasm. Whether these syndromes are related to "mediators" released from tumor cells or to other mechanisms is currently a matter for speculation. It is important to recognize these syndromes, because the therapy for the underlying neoplasm is now more successful. Eventually, a more detailed understanding of the various paraneoplastic phenomena may provide insights to the more basic mechanisms of neoplastic growth.

References

1. Hall TC: Introductory remarks, in Hall TC (ed): Paraneoplastic Syndromes. New York, Annals of the New York Academy of Sciences, 1974 p 5
2. Tischler AS: Small cell carcinoma of the lung: cellular origin and relationship to other neoplasms. Semin in Oncol 5:244–252, 1978
3. Liddle GW, Island D, Meador CK: Normal and abnormal regulation of corticotropin secretion in man. Recent Prog Horm Res 18:125–166, 1962
4. Liddle GW, Nicholson WE, Island DP, et al: Clinical and laboratory studies of ectopic humoral syndromes. Recent Prog Horm Res 25:283–314, 1969
5. Odell WD, Wolfsen AR: Hormonal syndromes associated with cancer. Annu Rev Med 29:379–406, 1978
6. Rees LH: The biosynthesis of hormones by non-endocrine tumors— A review. Endocrinol 67:143–175, 1975
7. Omenn GS: Pathobiology of ectopic hormone production by neoplasms in man. Pathobiol Annu 3:177–202, 1973
8. Primack A, Broder LE, Diasio RB: Production of markers by bronchogeneic carcinoma: A review, in Straus MJ (ed): Lung cancer: Clinical Diagnosis and Treatment. New York, Grune & Stratton, 1977, pp 33–47
9. Hansen M, Hummer L: Ectopic hormone production in small cell carcinoma, in Muggia F, Rozencweig M (ed): Lung Cancer: Progress in Therapeutic Research. New York, Raven Press, 1979, pp 199–207

10. Richardson RL, Greco FA, Oldham RK, Liddle GW: Tumor products and potential markers in small cell lung cancer. Semin Oncol 5:253–262, 1978

11. Mains RE, Eipper BA: Biosynthesis of ACTH in mouse pituitary tumor cells. J Biol Chem 251:4115–4120, 1976

12. Braunstein GD, Rasor J, Wade ME: Presence in normal human testes of a chorionic-gonadotropin-like substance distinct from human lutinizing hormone. N Engl J Med 293:1339–1343, 1975

13. Bertagna XY, Nicholson WE, Sorenson GD, et al: Corticotropin, lipotropin and β-endorphin production by human non-pituitary tumor in culture: Evidence for a common precursor. Proc Natl Acad Sci USA 75:5160–5164, 1978

14. Bertagna XY, Nicholson WE, Pettengill OS, et al: Ectopic production of high molecular weight calcitonin and corticotropin by human small cell carcinoma cells in tissue culture: Evidence for separate precursors. J Clin Endocrinol Metab 47:1390–1393, 1978

15. Pettengill OS, Faulkner CS, Wurster-Hill LH, et al: Isolation and characterization of a hormone producing cell line from human small cell anaplastic carcinoma of the lung. J Natl Cancer Inst 58:511–518, 1977

16. Fer MF, Rogers LW, Oldham RK, et al: The intermediate subtype of small cell lung cancer—A frequently unrecognized neoplasm. Clin Res 27:384A, 1979

17. Nathanson L, Hall TC: Lung tumors: How they produce their syndromes, in Hall TC (ed): Paraneoplastic Syndromes. New York, Annals of New York Academy of Sciences, 1974, pp 367–377

18. Winkler AW, Crankshaw OF: Chloride depletion in conditions other than Addison's Disease. J Clin Invest 17:1–12, 1938

19. Schwartz WB, Bennett W, Curelop S, Bartter FC: A syndrome of renal sodium loss and hyponatremia probably resulting from inappropriate secretion of ADH. Am J Med 23:529–542, 1957

20. Leaf A, Bartter FC, Santos RF, et al: Evidence in man that urinary electrolyte loss induced by Pitressin is a function of water retention. J Clin Invest 32:868–878, 1953

21. Beck LH: Hypouricemia in the syndrome of inappropriate secretion of ADH. N Engl J Med 301:528–530, 1979

22. Bartter FC, Schwartz WB: The syndrome of inappropriate secretion of ADH. Am J Med 42:790–806, 1967

23. DeTroyer A, Demanet JC: Clinical, Biological and Pathogenic features of the syndrome of inappropriate secretion of ADH. Q J Med 45:521–531, 1976.

214   Greco et al.

24. Schwartz WB, Tassel D, Bartter FC: Further observations on hypo-
     natremia and renal sodium loss probably resulting from inappro-
     priate secretion of ADH. N Engl J Med 262:743–748, 1960
25. Amatruda TT, Mulrow PJ, Gallagher JC, et al: Carcinoma of the lung
     with inappropriate antidiuresis: demonstration of ADH-like activ-
     ity in tumor extract. N Engl J Med 269:544–549, 1963
26. Bower BF, Mason DM, Forsham PH: Bronchogenic carcinoma with
     inappropriate antidiuretic activity in plasma and tumor. N Engl J
     Med 271:934–938, 1964
27. Ivy HK: Renal sodium loss and bronchogenic carcinoma. Arch Int
     Med 108:47–55, 1961
28. Claxton CP Jr, McPherson HT, Sealy WC, et al: Hyponatremia from
     inappropriate ADH elaboration in carcinoma of the lung. J Thorac
     Cardiovasc Surg 52:331–339, 1966
29. Dossetor JB, Venning EH, Beck JC: Hyponatremia associated with
     superior vena cava obstruction. Metabolism 10:149–161, 1961
30. Portwood RM, Verner JV, Menefee EE: Abnormal water retention
     associated with carcinoma of the lung. North Carol Med J 21:106–
     109, 1960
31. Lindsey DC, Barnes RN: Hyponatremia probably due to inappro-
     priate secretion of ADH associated with bronchogenic carcinoma.
     South Med J 55:337–340, 1962
32. Ross EJ: Hyponatremia syndromes associated with carcinoma of the
     bronchus. Q J Med 32:297–320, 1963
33. Schwartz E, Fogel RD, Chokas WV, et al: Unstable osmolar homeo-
     stasis with and without renal sodium wastage. Am J Med 33:39–53,
     1962
34. Williams RT: Carcinoma of the bronchus with hyponatremia and
     dermatomyositis. Br Med J 1:233–236, 1963
35. Turner P, Williams R: Unexplained steatorrhoea in the syndrome of
     hyponatraemia and carcinoma of the bronchus. Br Med J 1:287–290,
     1962
36. Roberts HJ: The Syndrome of hyponatremia and renal sodium loss
     probably resulting from inappropriate secretion of ADH. Ann Int
     Med 51:1420–1426, 1959
37. Thorn NA, Transbol I: Hyponatremia and bronchogenic carcinoma
     associated with renal excretion of large amounts of antidiuretic ma-
     terial. Am J Med 35:257–268, 1963
38. Robertson GL: Cancer and inappropriate antidiuresis, in Rudden
     RW (ed): Biological Markers of Neoplasia: Basic and Applied As-
     pects. New York, Elsevier, 1978, pp 277–293

39. Lebacq E, Delaere J: Hyponutrémie avec diluhon plasmatique, par sécrétion inadequate de vasopressive, dans un cas de tumeur duodenale. Rev Med-Chir mal Foie 46:169, 1965

40. Mellinger LC, Petermann FL, Jurgenson JC: Hyponatremia with low urinary aldosterone occurring in an old woman. J Clin Endocrinol Metab 34:85–94, 1972

41. Vorherr H, Massry SG, Utiger RD, Kleeman CR: Antiduiretic principle in malignant tumor extracts from patients with inappropriate ADH syndrome. J Clin Endocrinol Metab 26:970–974, 1966

42. Lee J, Jones JJ, Barraclough MA: Inappropriate secretion of vasopressin. Lancet 2:792–793, 1964

43. Utiger RD: Inappropriate antidiuresis and carcinoma of the lung: detection of arginine vasopressin in tumor extracts by immunoassay. J Clin Endocrinol Metab 26:970–974, 1966

44. Barraclough MA, Jones JJ, Lee J: Production of vasopressin by anaplastic oat cell carcinoma of the bronchus. Clin Sci 31:135–144, 1966

45. DeSousa RC, Delaers J, Berde B: Inappropriate secretion of vasopressin. Lancet 1:436–438, 1965

46. George JM, Capen CC, Phillips AS: Biosynthesis of vasopressin in vitro and ultrastructure of a bronchogenic carcinoma. J Clin Invest 51:141–148, 1972

47. Robertson GL, Mahr EA, Athar S, et al: Development and clinical application of a new method for the radioimmunoassay of arginine vasopressin in human plasma. J Clin Invest 52:2340–2357, 1973

48. Husain MK, Fernando N, Shapiro M, et al: Radioimmunoassay of arginine vasopressin in human plasma. J Clin Endocrinol Metab 37:616–625, 1973

49. Morton JJ, Kelley P, Padfield PL: Antidiuretic hormones in bronchogenic carcinoma. Clin Endocrinol 9:357–370, 1978

50. Robertson GI, Shelton RL, Athar S: The osmoregulation of vasopressin. Kidney Int 10:25–37, 1976

51. Eagan RT, Maurer LH, Forcier RJ, et al: Small cell carcinoma of the lung: Staging, paraneoplastic syndromes, treatment, and survival. Cancer 33:527–532, 1974

52. Ginsberg S, Comis R, Miller M: Syndrome of inappropriate ADH secretion in oat cell carcinoma of the lung. Clin Res 26:435A, 1978

53. Greco FA, Richardson RL, Hande KR, et al: Treatment of inappropriate secretion of ADH in small cell lung cancer. Clin Res 27:385A, 1979

54. Gilby ED, Bondy PK, Fosling M: Impaired water excretion in oat cell lung cancer. Br J Cancer 34:323–324, 1976

55. Gilby ED: Ectopic hormone products of bronchial neoplasms. Br J Dis Chest 70:282, 1976

56. Barjon P, Michel FB: Recherche systématique d'une sécrétion inappropriée d'hormone antidiurétique au cours du cancer bronchique primitif. Sem Hop Paris 48:3305–3309, 1972

57. Haefliger JM, Dubied MC, Vallotton MB: Excrétion Journaliére de L'hormone antidiurétique Lors Carcinome bronchique. Schweiz Med Wochenschr 107:726–732, 1977

58. Hamilton BPM, Upton GU, Amatruda TT: Evidence for the presence of neurophysin in tumors producing the syndrome of inappropriate antidiuresis. J Clin Endocrinol Metab 35:764–767, 1972

59. North WG, LaRochelle FT Jr, Melton J, et al: Human neurophysins as potential tumor markers for small cell carcinoma. Clin Res 26:536A, 1978

60. White MG, Fetner CD: Treatment of the syndrome of inappropriate secretion of ADH with lithium carbonate. N Engl J Med 292:390–392, 1975

61. DeTroyer A, Demanet JC: Correction of antidiuresis by Demeclocycline. N Engl J Med 293:915–918, 1975

62. Cherrill DA, Stote RM, Birge JR, et al: Demeclocycline treatment in the syndrome of inappropriate ADH secretion. Ann Int Med 83:654–656, 1975

63. DeTroyer A: Demeclocycline: Treatment for syndrome of inappropriate ADH secretion. JAMA 237:2723–2726, 1977

64. Singer I, Rotenberg D, Puschett JB: Lithium-induced nephrogenic diabetes insipidus: In Vivo and In Vitro studies. Ann Int Med 79:679–683, 1973

65. Wilson DM, Perry HO, Sams WM Jr, et al: Selective inhibition of human distal tubular function by Demeclocycline. Curr Ther Res 15:734–740, 1973

66. Forrest JN Jr, Cox M, Hong C, et al: Superiority of Demeclocycline over lithium in the treatment of chronic syndrome of inappropriate secretion of ADH. N Engl J Med 298:173–177, 1978

67. Oster JR, Epstein M, Ulano HB: Deterioration of renal function with Demeclocycline administration. Curr Ther Res 20:794–801, 1976

68. Danovitch GM, LeRoith D, Glick S: Renal function during treatment of inappropriate secretion of ADH with Demeclocycline. Isr J Med Sci 14:852–857, 1978

69. Greco FA, Oldham RK: Small Cell Lung Cancer. N Engl J Med 301:355–358, 1979

70. Cohen MH, Bunn PA, Ihde DC, et al: Chemotherapy rather than demeclocycline for inappropriate secretion of ADH. N Engl J Med 298:1423–1424, 1978

71. Gregor A, Morgan PGM, Morgan RL, et al: Small cell carcinoma: Combined approach to treatment. Thorax 34:789–793, 1979

72. Brown WH: A case of Pluriglandular syndrome: Diabetes of bearded women. Lancet 2:1022–1023, 1928

73. Cushing H: The basophil adenomas of the pituitary body and their clinical manifestations (Pituitary Basophilism). Bull Johns Hopkins Hosp 50:137–195, 1932

74. Bagshawe KD: Hypokalaemia, carcinoma and Cushing's syndrome. Lancet 2:284–287, 1960

75. Bornstein P, Nolan JP, Brnanke D: Adrenocortical hyperfunction in association with anaplastic carcinoma of the respiratory tract. N Engl J Med 264:363–371, 1961

76. Meador CK, Liddle GW, Island DP, et al: Cause of Cushing's syndrome in patients with tumors arising from "Nonendocrine" tissue. J Clin Endocrinol Metab 22:693–703, 1962

77. Azzopardi JG, Williams ED: Pathology of "Nonendocrine" tumors associated with Cushing's syndrome. Cancer 22:274–286, 1968

78. Amatruda TT Jr: Nonendocrine secreting tumors. Duncan's Diseases of Metabolism (ed 6). Philadelphia, W. B. Saunders, 1969, pp 1227–1244

79. Azzopardi JG, Freeman E, Poole G: Endocrine and metabolic disorders in bronchogenic carcinoma. Br Med J 4:528–529, 1970

80. Kato Y, Ferguson TB, Bennett DE, et al: Oat cell carcinoma of the lung: Review of 138 cases. Cancer 23:517–524, 1969

81. Gilby ED, Rees LH, Bondy PK: Ectopic hormones as markers of response to therapy in cancer. Exc Med 375:132–138, 1975

82. Yalow RS: Ectopic ACTH in carcinoma of the lung, in Muggia FM, Rozencweig M (eds): Lung Cancer Progress in Therapeutic Research. New York, Raven Press, 1979, pp 209–216

83. Odell W, Wolfen A, Yoshimoto Y, et al: Ectopic peptide synthesis: A universal concomitant of neoplasia. Clin Res 25:525A, 1977

84. Krauss S, Macy S, Ichiki AT: A study of immunoreactive calcitonin and adrenocorticotropic hormone in lung cancer and other malignancies. Proc Am Association Can Res 21:144, 1980

85. Krauss S: Personal communication

86. Imura H, Matsukura S, Yamamoto H, et al: Studies on ectopic ACTH-producing tumors. Cancer 35:1430–1437, 1975

87. Friedman M, Marshall-Jones P, Ross EJ: Cushing's syndrome: Adrenocortical hyperactivity secondary to neoplasms arising outside the pituitary–adrenal system. Q J Med 35:193–213, 1967

88. O'Neal IW, Kipnis DM, Luse SA, et al: Secretion of various endocrine substances by ACTH-secreting tumors: Gastrin, melanotropin, norepinephrine, serotonin, parathormone, vasopressin, glucagon. Cancer 21:1219–1232, 1968

89. Ratcliffe JG, Knight RA, Besser GM, et al: Tumor and plasma ACTH concentrations in patients with and without the ectopic ACTH syndrome. Clin Endocrinol 1:27–44, 1972

90. Orth DN, Nicholson WE, Mitchell WM, et al: Biologic and immunologic characterization and physical separation of ACTH and ACTH fragments in the ectopic ACTH syndrome. J Clin Invest 52:1756–1759, 1973

91. Ellison ML, Hillyard CJ, Bloomfield GA, et al: Ectopic Hormone production by bronchial carcinomas in culture. Clin Endocrinol 5 (Suppl):397–406, 1976

92. Lowry PJ, Rees IH, Tomlin S, et al: Chemical characterization of ectopic ACTH purified from a malignant thymic carcinoid tumor. J Clin Endocrinol Metab 43:831–835, 1976

93. Yalow RS, Berson SA: Size heterogeneity of immunoreactive human ACTH in plasma and in extracts of pituitary glands and ACTH-producing thymoma. Biochem Biophys Res Commun 44:439–445, 1971

94. Gewirtz G, Yalow RS: Ectopic ACTH production in carcinoma of the lung. J Clin Invest 53:1022–1032, 1974

95. Orth DN, Nicholson WE: High molecular weight forms of human ACTH are glycoproteins. J Clin Endocrinol Metab 44:214–217, 1977

96. Gewirtz G, Schneider B, Krieger DJ, Yalow RS: Big ACTH: conversion to biologically active ACTH by Trypsin. J Clin Endocrinol Metab 38:227–230, 1974

97. Ayvazian LF, Schneider B, Gewirtz G, Yalow RS: Ectopic production of big ACTH in carcinoma of the lung. Am Rev Respir Dis 111:279–287, 1975

98. Wolfsen AP, Odell WD: Early diagnosis of lung cancer using peptide markers. Clin Res 25:502A, 1977

99. Bloomfield GA, Holdaway IM, Corrin B, et al: Lung tumors and ACTH production. Clin Endocrinol 6:95–104, 1977

100. Hirata YS, Matsukura H, Imura M, et al: Size heterogeneity of Beta-MSH in ectopic ACTH-producing tumors: Presence of Beta-LPH-like peptide. J Clin Endocrinol Metab 42:33–40, 1976

101. Tanaka K, Nicholson WE, Orth DN: The nature of the immunoreac-

tive lipotropins in human plasma and tissue extracts. J Clin Invest 62:94–104, 1978

102. Odell WD, Wolfsen AR, Bachelot I, et al: Ectopic production of lipotropin by cancer. Am J Med 66:631–637, 1979

103. Abe K, Island DP, Liddle GW, et al: Radioimmunologic evidence for Alpha-MSH (melanocyte Stimulating Hormone) in human pituitary and tumor tissues. J Clin Endocrinol Metab 27:46–52, 1967

104. Ratcliffe JG, Scott AP, Bennett HPJ, et al: Production of a corticotrophin-like intermediate lobe peptide and of corticotropin by a bronchial carcinoid tumor. Clin Endocrinol 2:51–55, 1973

105. Upton GV, Amatruda TT, Jr: Evidence for the presence of tumor peptides with corticotropin-releasing-factor-like activity in the ectopic ACTH syndrome. N Engl J Med 285:419–424, 1971

106. Yamamoto H, Hirata H, Matsukura S, et al: Studies in ectopic ACTH-producing tumors. Acta Endocrinol 82:183–193, 1976

107. Ross EJ: Endocrine Syndromes of Non-endocrine origin: Cancer and the adrenal cortex. Proc R Soc Med 59:335–338, 1966

108. Jeffcoate WJ, Rees LH, Tomlin S, et al: Metyrapone in long-term management of Cushing's disease. Br Med J 2:215–217, 1977

109. Copp DH: Calcitonin—Ultimobronchial hormone. Proc Int Union Phys Sci 6:15–36, 1968

110. Tashjian AH Jr, Hewland BG, Melvin KEW, et al: Immunoassay of human calcitonin: Clinical measurement, relation to serum calcium, and studies in patients with medullary carcinoma. N Engl J Med 283:890–895, 1970

111. Deftos LJ, Bury AE, Hahener JF, et al: Immunoassay for human calcitonin: Clinical studies. Metabolism 20:1129–1137, 1971

112. Hennessy JF, Gray TK, Cooper CW et al: Stimulation of thyrocalcitonin secretion by pentagastrin and calcium in two patients with medullary carcinoma of the thyroid. J Clin Endocrinol Metab 36:200–203, 1973

113. Hennessy JF, Wells SA, Ontjes DA, et al: A comparison of pentagastrin injection and calcium infusion as provocative agents for the detection of medullary carcinoma of the thyroid. J Clin Endocrinol Metab 39:487–495, 1974

114. Sizemore GW, Go VEW: Stimulation tests for diagnosis of medullary thyroid carcinoma. Mayo Clin Proc 50:53–56, 1975

115. Silva OL, Snider RH, Becker KL: Radioimmunoassay of calcitonin in human plasma. Clin Chem 20:337–339, 1974

116. Kaplan EL, Sizemore G, Hill BJ: Calcitonin in non-thyroid tumors in man. Clin Res 20:724, 1972

117. Silva OL, Becker KL, Primack A, et al: Ectopic production of calcitonin. Lancet 2:317, 1973

118. Silva OL, Becker KL, Primack A: Ectopic secretion of calcitonin by oat-cell carcinoma. N Engl J Med 290:1122–1124, 1974

119. Cattan D, Vesin P, Reugier P, et al: Hyperthyrocalcitoninaemia, Schwartz-Bartter syndrome, and oat-cell carcinoma. Lancet 1:938, 1974

120. Ellison M, Weedhouse D, Hillyard C, et al: Immunoreactive calcitonin production by human lung carcinoma cells in culture. Br J Cancer 32:373–379, 1975

121. Milhaud G, Calmette C, Taboulet J: Hypersecretion of calcitonin in neoplastic conditions. Lancet 1:462–463, 1974

122. Coombes RC, Greenberg PB, Hillyard C, MacIntyre I: Plasma-immunoreactive-calcitonin in patients with non-thyroid tumours. Lancet 1:1080–1083, 1974

123. Hillyard CJ, Coombes RC, Greenberg PB, et al: Calcitonin in breast and lung cancer. Clin Endocrinol 5:1–8, 1976

124. Coombes RC, Ellison ML, Casty GC, et al: The ectopic secretion of calcitonin by lung and breast carcinomas. Clin Endocrinol 5 (Suppl): 387S–396S, 1976.

125. Schwartz KE, Wilfsen AR, Forster B, Odell WD: Calcitonin in nonthyroidal cancer. J Clin Endocrinol Metab 49:438–444, 1979

126. Silva OL, Becker KL, Primack A: Hypercalcitonemia in bronchogenic cancer: Evidence for thyroid origin of the hormone. JAMA 234:183–185, 1975

127. Silva OL, Broder LE, Doppman JL, et al: Calcitonin as a marker for bronchogenic cancer. Cancer 44:680–684, 1979

128. Silva OL, Becker KL, Primack A, et al: Increased serum calcitonin levels in bronchogenic cancer. Chest 69:495–499, 1976

129. Abe K, Adachi I, Miyakawa S, et al: Production of calcitonin, adrenocorticotropic hormone, and Beta-MSH in tumors derived from amine precursor uptake and decarboxylation cells. Cancer Res 37:4190–4194, 1977

130. Hansen M, Hummer L: Ectopic hormone production in small cell carcinoma, in Muggia F, Rozencweig M (eds): Lung Cancer: Progress in Therapeutic Research. New York, Raven Press, 1979, pp 199–207

131. Becker KL, Snider RH, Silva DL, Moore CF: Calcitonin heterogeneity in lung cancer and medullary thyroid cancer. Acta Endocrinol 89:89–99, 1978

132. Wallach SR, Royston I, Taetle R, et al: Plasma calcitonin as a marker

of disease activity in patients with small cell carcinoma of the lung during chemotherapy. Clin Res 28:56A, 1980

133. Beck C, Burger HG: Evidence for the presence of immunoreactive growth hormone in cancers of the lung and stomach. Cancer 30:75–79, 1972

134. Gilby ED, Rees LH, Bondy PK: Ectopic hormones as markers of response to therapy in cancer, in Maltoni C (ed): Biological characterization of human tumors. New York, American Elsevier, 1975, pp 132–138

135. Baylin SB, Abeloff MD, Wieman KC, et al: Elevated histaminase (diamine oxidase) activity in small-cell carcinoma of the lung. N Engl J Med 293:1286–1290, 1975

136. Fairlamb D, Boesen E: Gynaecomastia associated with gonadotrophin-secreting carcinoma of the lung. Postgrad Med J 53:269–271, 1977

137. Horai T, Nichihara H, Tateishi R, et al: Oat-cell carcinoma of the lung simultaneously producing ACTH and serotonin. J Clin Endocrinol Metab 37:212–219, 1973

138. Majcher SJ, Lee ER, Reingold IM, et al: Carcinoid syndrome in lung cancer. Gastroenterology 48:832, 1965 (Abst)

139. Gowenlock AH, Platt DS, Campbell ACP, et al: Oat-cell carcinoma of the bronchus secreting 5-hydroxytryptophan. Lancet 1:304–306, 1964

140. Omenn GS, Ross SI, Baker WH: Hyperparathyroidism associated with malignant tumors of nonparathyroid origin. Cancer 24:1004–1012, 1969

141. Bender RA, Hansen H: Hypercalcemia in bronchogenic carcinoma. A prospective study of 200 patients. Ann Intern Med 80:205–208, 1974

142. Hauger-Klevene JH: High plasma renin activity in an oat cell carcinoma: A renin-secreting carcinoma? Cancer 26:1112–1114, 1970

143. Entwistle CC, Fentem PH, Jacobs A: Red-cell aplasia with carcinoma of the bronchus. Br Med J 2:1504–1506, 1964

144. Dayan AD, Croft TB, Wilkinson M: Association of carcinomatous neuromyopathy with different histological types of carcinoma of the lung. Brain 88:435–448, 1965

145. Joynt RJ: The brain's uneasy peace with tumors, in Hall TC (ed): Paraneoplastic Syndromes. New York, Annals of the New York Academy of Science (vol 230). 1974, pp 342–347

146. Tyler HR: Paraneoplastic syndromes of nerve, muscle and neuromuscular junction, in Hall TC (ed): Paraneoplastic Syndromes. New

York, Annals of the New York Academy of Science (vol 230). 1974, pp 348–357

147. Richardson EP: Our evolving understanding of progressive multifocal leukoencephalopathy, in Hall TC (ed): Paraneoplastic Syndromes. Annals of the New York Academy of Science (vol 230) 1974, pp 358–364

148. Walker DL: Progressive multifocal leukoencephalopathy: An opportunistic viral infection of the central nervous system, in Vinken PJ, Bruyn GW (eds): Handbook of Clinical Neurology (vol 34). Amsterdam, North Holland, 1978, pp 307–329

149. Brain WR, Henson RA: Neurological syndromes associated with carcinoma: The carcinomatous neuromyopathies. Lancet 2:971–975, 1958

150. Brain WR: The neurological complications of neoplasms. Lancet 1:179–184, 1963

151. Brain WR, Croft PB, Wilkinson M: Motor neurone disease as a manifestation of neoplasm. Brain 88:478–500, 1965

152. Brain WR, Norris FH (eds): Remote Effects of Cancer on the Nervous System. New York, Grune & Stratton, 1965

153. Croft PB, Wilkinson M: The incidence of carcinomatous neuromyopathies in patients with various types of carcinoma. Brain 88:427–434, 1965

154. Hildebrand J: Preface, in Hildebrand J (ed): Lesions of the Nervous System in Cancer Patients. New York, Raven Press, 1978, pp V–VII

155. Croft PB, Wilkinson M: Carcinomatous neuromyopathy: its incidence with patients with carcinoma of the lung and of the breast. Lancet 1:184–188, 1963

156. Wilner EC, Brody JA: An evaluation of the remote effects of cancer on the nervous system. Neurology (Minneap) 18:1120–1124, 1968

157. Paone JF, Jeyasingham K: Remission of cerebellar dysfunction after pneumonectomy for bronchogenic carcinoma. N Engl J Med 302:156, 1980

158. Bunn PA, Nugent JL, Matthews MJ: Central nervous system metastases in small cell bronchogenic carcinoma. Sem Oncol 5:314–322, 1978

159. Mancall EL, Rosales RK: Necrotizing myelopathy associated with visceral carcinoma. Brain 87:639–656, 1964

160. Denny-Brown DE: Primary sensory neuropathy with muscular changes associated with carcinoma. J Neurol Neurosurg Psychiat 11:73–87, 1948

161. Croft PB, Henson RA, Urich H, et al: Sensory neuropathy with bronchial carcinoma: A study of four cases showing serological abnormalities. Brain 88:501–514, 1965

162. Wilkinson PC: Serological findings in carcinomatous neuromyopathy. Lancet 1:1301–1303, 1964

163. Wilkinson PC, Zeromski J: Immunofluorescent detection of antibodies against neurones in sensory carcinomatous neuropathy. Brain 88:529–538, 1965

164. Lambert EH, Rooke ED: Myasthenic state and lung cancer in Brain WR, Norris FH Jr (eds) The Remote Effects of Cancer on the Nervous System. New York, Grune & Stratton, 1965, pp 67–80

165. Satoyoshi E, Kowa H, Fukuna GAN: Subacute cerebellar degeneration and Eaton-Lambert syndrome with bronchogenic carcinoma. Neurology (Minneap) 23:764–768, 1973

166. Hildebrand J: Carcinomatous neuromyopathies, in Hildebrand J (ed): Lesions of the Nervous System in Cancer Patients. New York, Raven Press, 1978, pp 121–143

167. Norris FH, Izzo AJ, Garvey PH: Brief report. Tumor size in Lambert-Eaton syndrome, in Brain WR, Norris FH (eds): The Remote Effect of Cancer on the Nervous System. New York, Grune & Stratton, 1965, pp 81–82

168. Oh, SJ, Kim KW: Guanidine hydrochloride in Eaton-Lambert syndrome. Neurology (Minneap) 23:1084–1090, 1973

169. Bohan A, Peter JB: Polymyositis and dermatomyositis. N Engl J Med 293:344–347; 403–407, 1975

9

THE GROWTH CHARACTERISTICS OF SMALL CELL CARCINOMA OF THE LUNG

Stanley E. Shackney
Marc J. Straus
Paul A. Bunn, Jr.

Over the past 20 years, it has become clear that rapidly growing human tumors are often responsive to chemotherapy and that complete responses in such tumors are often quite durable. In contrast, complete clinical responses are less frequent in slowly growing human tumors, and most patients with slowly growing tumors eventually succumb to their disease, whether or not they respond to therapy initially.[1] Early reports of short tumor doubling times[2,3] and high tritiated thymidine (^{3}HTdR) pulse-labeling indices[4,5] in small cell carcinoma of the lung (SCC) had suggested that this is a rapidly growing tumor. This impression was in keeping with the finding that SCC is responsive to chemotherapy. However, more recent data on the growth behavior of SCC have indicated that it is a more slowly proliferating tumor than had been supposed initially. The purpose of this chapter is to review the data on the growth characteristics of SCC and their possible relationship to responsiveness to treatment.

The Clonal Nature of SCC

The ability of a single transplanted viable tumor cell to multiply and produce a lethal body burden of tumor has been demonstrated in many experimental tumor systems. In such experimental systems, cure is achieved only when the last viable tumor cell has been eradicated. Recent flow cytometry studies have demonstrated aneuploidy in approximately 80 percent of SCC,[6,7] and it is likely that in the remaining cases there were cytogenetic abnormalities too slight to be detected by flow cytometry. Continuous cell lines of SCC have been established in tissue culture, and aneuploidy has been present in every case[8] (see also Chapter 4, this monograph). The clonal nature of small cell carcinoma implies that the malignancy begins with a single aneuploid cell whose progeny proliferate to produce clinical disease. It follows that in order to achieve clinical cure of this disease, the last aneuploid malignant cell must be eradicated.

The Growth Curve of SCC in Man and Its Therapeutic Implications

The human tumor growth curve can be divided into subclinical and clinical stages of growth (Fig. 9-1). The minimum detectable body burden of tumor in man is generally of the order of 1×10^9 cells (approximately 1 g of tissue) or more, when the tumor cell population has already undergone about 30 doublings. Generally, a lethal body tumor burden is reached when tumor cell mass approaches or exceeds 1 kg or 1×10^{12} cells (40 doublings). Tumors undergo progressive growth retardation with increasing size. In the clinically observable range of tumor growth, one can estimate tumor doubling time from serial measurements of tumor size.[9]

Estimates of tumor growth rate in *subclinical* stages of growth are based on the "period of risk" method first introduced by Collins and co-workers.[10,11] The period of risk method requires two assumptions: (1) that in human tumors a single cell is all that is required to produce a lethal body burden of tumor cells, and (2) that the growth rate patterns of individual tumors are characteristic and reproducible. It would follow that the time of regrowth from a single cell to clinical recurrence following therapy is the maximum time to relapse. This is an estimate of the period of risk. In patients who do not relapse during the period of risk, the last tumor cell can be presumed to have been eradicated.

Because of interpatient and intrapatient biological variation, the period of risk cannot be defined with precision. However, in several human

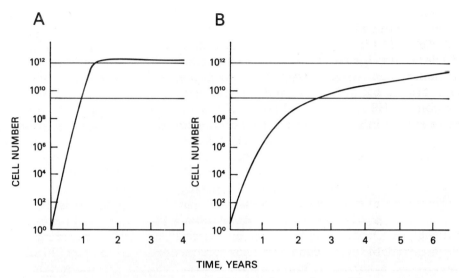

Figure 9-1. *Schematic representation of the growth curve in a rapidly growing human tumor (A) and in a slowly growing human tumor (B). For discussion, see text.*

tumors, particularly in the rapidly growing ones, one can identify a period of risk such that *most* patients with residual disease who relapse will do so within this period, and *very few* patients will relapse beyond this period. Assuming that there are about 30 doublings from a single cell to tumor recurrence, average subclinical tumor doubling time can be calculated from such estimates of the period of risk.[1]

In rapidly growing tumors, short subclinical doubling times may persist through the early clinically detectable range, as shown schematically in Figure 9-1, panel A. Indeed, an operational definition for rapidly growing human tumors might be that the short doubling times obtained from serial tumor volume measurements in clinically apparent disease are close to the average subclinical doubling time estimated from the period of risk. On the other hand, in slowly growing human tumors, significant growth retardation will have occurred long before clinical tumor detection (Fig. 9-1, panel B). The doubling times for the last five to ten subclinical doublings are likely to be longer than those in very early subclinical disease, approaching the long doubling times observed in clinically detectable stages of tumor growth.

Published values for clinical tumor doubling times in SCC are given in Table 9-1. It is readily apparent that the range of doubling times is very broad in this disease (17–264 days). Whereas some patients have tumors

Shackney et al.

Table 9-1
Tumor Doubling Times in Small Cell Carcinoma of the
Lung

Mean (or Median) Tumor Doubling Time (days)		Range (days)	No. of Cases	Reference No.
23.5		23–24	2	2
39		17–71	3	3
91	(mean)			
81	(log mean)	25–160	12	12
77	(median)			
68		17–264	46	13

with relatively short doubling times (< 30 days), in the majority of cases the doubling time exceeds 2 mo.

A comparison of clinical tumor doubling times in carcinoma of the lung by histologic cell type is given in Table 9-2. Log mean clinical tumor doubling times are similar in SCC, large cell carcinoma, and squamous cell carcinoma. The log mean tumor doubling time in adenocarcinoma is significantly longer than that of squamous cell carcinoma ($p < 0.001$) and SCC ($p < 0.01$). (Distributions of tumor doubling times tend to be skewed to the right, whereas distributions of the logarithms of tumor doubling time are more symmetric.[1] Thus, for purposes of statistical analysis, logarithms of tumor doubling time and log means were used.)

Quantitative estimates of subclinical tumor doubling times in SCC have not been available until recently. Early estimates of the period of risk for SCC had been in the range of 2 yr, in keeping with the belief that this tumor was a rapidly growing one. However, if one assumes that the average tumor doubling time during the last 10 subclinical doublings (between 1×10^6 cells and 1×10^9 cells) is not very different from the average clinical doubling time of 2–3 mo, then patients with residual body bur-

Table 9-2
Tumor Doubling Times in Non-Small Cell Lung Cancer

Cell Type	Log Mean Doubling Time (days)	Range (days)	No. of Cases	Reference No.
Large cell carcinoma	85	48–115	3	2,13
Squamous cell carcinoma	87	24–381	72	Cited in 1
Adenocarcinoma	134	17–960	36	Cited in 1

Table 9-3
³HTdR Labeling Indices (LI) in Small Cell Carcinoma of
the Lung

Mean or Median LI	Range	No. of Patients	Method of Labeling	Reference No.
0.15	0.07–0.24	12	In vivo, intratumor	4
0.24	0.19–0.30	5	In vitro	5
0.11	0.02–0.28	14	In vitro	16
0.09	0.06–0.14	6	In vivo, intravenous	17

dens of tumor of 1×10^6 cells could remain clinically disease free for 2 yr or longer and then relapse. Thus, one could predict that patients with still smaller body burdens of tumor (from 1 to 1×10^6 cells) could remain clinically disease free for much longer than 2 yr (say, 4–5 yr) and still relapse.[12] This prediction has been borne out in a recent study of long-term survivors with SCC.[15] Among 20 patients who survived longer than 2½ yr and later died of tumor recurrence, 8 died within 30–33 mo of diagnosis, 10 had tumor recurrences within 36–51 mo of diagnosis, and 2 had tumor recurrences at 8 and 9 yr, respectively.

From a practical standpoint, it would seem reasonable to consider the period of risk for SCC to be about 5 yr. In patients with disease-free survivals exceeding 5 yr, the likelihood of tumor recurrence would be small. Tumors that recur within 1 to 2 yr might be considered early recurrences in which the residual body tumor burden after treatment was relatively large. Tumor recurrences after 4 yr would suggest that initial therapy had been successful in reducing body tumor burden to very low levels (perhaps approaching one cell). Treatment protocols that produce large numbers of such patients might be subject to improvement simply by increasing the number of courses of treatment.

Cell Cycle Characteristics of SCC

Tritiated thymidine pulse-labeling indices in SCC are summarized in Table 9-3. There is considerable variability in the labeling index (LI), with values ranging from 0.02 to 0.3 among patients in different studies. In retrospect, early estimates of the average labeling index in SCC[3] were somewhat high, and representative values probably lie in the range of 0.1–0.2. The mean fraction of cells in DNA synthesis (S) as determined by flow cytometry is 0.18–0.20 (Raber et al.[7] and Bunn PA, unpublished observations).

For comparison, the [3]HTdR labeling indices for the different histologic types of bronchogenic carcinoma of the lung are given in Table 9-4. The ranges and average values for the [3]HTdR labeling index appear to be similar in SCC, large cell carcinoma, and squamous cell carcinoma. In adenocarcinoma, average labeling indices appear to be lower than in the other cell types, and the range is much narrower.

Fractions of cells in S by flow cytometry have been found to be similar among all the histologic cell types of carcinoma of the lung, including adenocarcinoma (Raber et al.[7] and Bunn PA, unpublished observations).

A single case of SCC has been studied by the percent labeled mitosis (PLM) method.[4] A well-defined wave of labeled mitoses was observed during the first 24 hr after labeling, but no clear second wave was seen. The initial wave of labeled mitoses did not achieve 100 percent labeling, and the subsequent PLM curve segment did not fall to zero percent labeling during the 44-hr observation period. These PLM curve features indicate a considerable degree of cell cycle time heterogeneity. The PLM curve features of SCC do not differ substantially from those obtained in other cell types of lung carcinoma.[19,20] The PLM data suggest that, in the various histologic cell types of bronchogenic carcinoma, the more rapidly proliferating cells have cell cycle times in the range of 24–72 hr.

The discrepancy between the short cell cycle times of the rapidly proliferating cell fraction and the long tumor doubling times in carcinoma of the lung is attributable either to the presence of slowly proliferating cells not detected by the PLM curve method or to cell loss, or both. At present, there are insufficient kinetic data available to distinguish between these alternatives or to estimate the relative importance of each.

Overview and Conclusions

SCC is not as rapidly growing a tumor as had once been supposed. Clinical tumor doubling times in SCC usually exceed 2 mo, and are similar to those of large cell carcinoma and squamous cell carcinoma. In contrast, the mean clinical doubling time in adenocarcinoma of the lung is significantly longer than that of SCC.

Malaise et al.[21] showed that the LI—a measure of the fraction of cells actively synthesizing DNA, and therefore an index of the rate of cell production—is high in human tumors with short doubling times and low in slowly growing human tumors. Although calculated rates of cell loss were highest in the most rapidly growing tumors, short population doubling

Table 9-4
Comparison of the ³HTdR Labeling Index (LI) in Lung
Cancer by Cell Type

Cell Type	Mean or Median LI	Range	No. of Patients	Reference No.
Small cell carcinoma	0.15	0.08–0.24	12	4
	0.24	0.19–0.30	5	5
	0.11	0.02–0.28	14	16
	0.09	0.06–0.14	6	17
Large cell carcinoma	0.10	0.04–0.18	5	18
	0.11	0.02–0.26	29	16
	0.11	—	6	17
Squamous cell carcinoma	0.03	0.03–0.04	3	5
	0.04	0.01–0.10	6	18
	0.08	0.01–0.26	38	16
	0.08	—	6	17
Adenocarcinoma	0.03	—	2	5
	0.04	0.03–0.05	5	18
	0.05	0.01–0.21	18	16
	0.03	—	2	17

times did in fact reflect high rates of cell production, whereas long population doubling times were associated with low rates of cell production.

If this general observation applies to the various histological cell types
of carcinoma of the lung, then adenocarcinoma of the lung, with its long
average clinical doubling time and low labeling index, would have relatively low rates of cell production and correspondingly low rates of cell
loss. The poor clinical responsiveness of tumors of this cell type to chemotherapy might be accounted for in large part by the kinetic resistance of
slowly proliferating cells to the lethal effects of cytotoxic drugs.

Clear-cut kinetic distinctions among SCC, large cell carcinoma, and
squamous cell carcinoma have not been demonstrated to date. The greater
responsiveness of SCC to therapy could be explained on kinetic grounds if
all of the following conditions prevail during clinical stages of tumor
growth:

1. The cell cycle time distribution is clustered about relatively short
   values (resulting in high rates of tumor cell production).
2. The rate of cell death (defined as the loss of the capacity to reproduce)
   is high.
3. The clearance rate of end-stage cells is relatively low, resulting in a

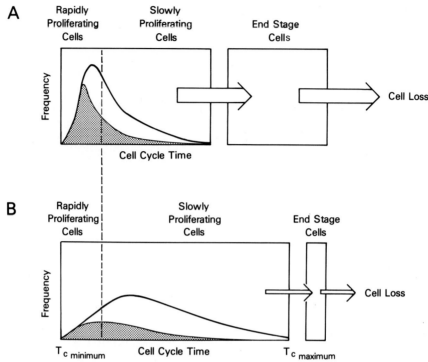

Figure 9-2. *(A) Schematic representation of a tumor with high rates of cell production and cell loss, and a large pool of end-stage cells owing to a low clearance rate of these cells. (B) Schematic representation of a tumor with low rates of cell production and cell loss, and a high clearance rate of end-stage cells. Shaded regions represent labelled cell fractions. For discussion, see text.*

large pool of end-stage cells during steady state or near steady-state growth.

Under these conditions, tumor doubling would be long and the LI would be relatively low, but the viable tumor cell compartment would consist predominantly of rapidly proliferating cells that might be especially responsive to chemotherapy. These conditions, which might be representative of SCC, are shown schematically in Figure 9-2, panel A.

If the cell cycle time distribution is broad, if the rate of cell death is low, and if the clearance rate of end-stage cells is relatively high, as shown in Figure 9-2, panel B, tumor doubling time and LI might be comparable to those in Figure 9-2, panel A, but the tumor would contain many more slowly proliferating, drug-resistant viable cells. These conditions might be representative of non–small cell lung cancer.

It should be emphasized that, although the schematic representations shown in Figure 9-2 are consistent with the available kinetic data and with clinical observations, their validity has not been definitively established. It may be possible to obtain more detailed information regarding cell death rates and rates of clearance of end-stage cells in the future from studies of lung cancer cell lines grown *in vitro* or in nude mice.

It should also be borne in mind that many factors other than the kinetic characteristics of the tumor may be important in determining tumor responsiveness to chemotherapy (e.g., intrinsic biochemical susceptibility or resistance and drug pharmacokinetics). Again, the relative contributions of these factors can be studied in tissue culture and in the nude mouse system.

At present, there is no information on the magnitude and time course of the effects of chemotherapeutic agents on the growth behavior of SCC in man. Information on the transient kinetic changes induced by drugs in situ will be of critical importance for the rational design of clinical drug treatment schedules in the future.

References

1. Shackney SE, McCormack GW, Cuchural GJ: Growth rate patterns of solid tumors and their relation to responsiveness to therapy. Ann Intern Med 89:107–121, 1978

2. Meyer JA: Growth rate vs. prognosis in resected primary bronchogenic carcinoma. Cancer 31:1468–1472, 1973

3. Chahinian P: Relationship between tumor doubling time and anatomoclinical features in 50 measurable pulmonary cancers. Chest 61:340–345, 1972

4. Muggia FM, Krezoski SK, Hansen HH: Cell kinetic studies in patients with small cell carcinoma of the lung. Cancer 34:1683–1690, 1974

5. Livingston RB, Ambus U, George SL, et al.: *In vitro* determination of thymidine-^{3}H labeling index in human solid tumors. Cancer Res 34:1376–1380, 1974

6. Bunn P, Schlam M, Gazdar A: Comparison of cytology and DNA content analysis by flow cytometry (FCM) in specimens from lung cancer patients. Proc Am Assoc Cancer Res 21:40, 1980

7. Raber M, Barlogie B, Farquhar D: Determination of ploidy abnormality and cell cycle time distribution in human lung cancer using DNA flow cytometry. Proc Am Assoc Cancer Res 21:40, 1980

8. Gazdar AF, Carney DN, Russel EK, et al.: Small cell carcinoma of the lung: Establishment of continuous, clonable, tumorigenic cell lines having amine precursor uptake and decarboxylation properties. Cancer Res: 40:3502–3507, 1980

9. Schwartz M: A biomathematical approach to clinical tumor growth. Cancer 14:1272–1294, 1961

10. Collins VP, Loeffler RK, Tivey H: Observations on growth rates of human tumors. Am J Roentgenol 76:988–1000, 1956

11. Collins VP: Wilms' tumor; its behavior and prognosis. J La State Med Soc 107:474–480, 1955

12. Brigham BA, Bunn PA Jr, Minna JD, et al.: Growth rates of small cell bronchogenic carcinomas. Cancer 42:2880–2886, 1978

13. Tubiana M, Malaise E: Combination of radiotherapy and chemotherapy: Implications of cell kinetics, in Muggia F, Rozencweig M (eds): Lung Cancer, New York, Raven Press, 1977, pp 51–61

14. Garland LH, Coulson W, Wollin E: The rate of growth and apparent duration of untreated primary bronchial carcinoma. Cancer 16:694–707, 1963

15. Matthews MJ, Rozencweig M, Staquet MJ, et al.: Long-term survivors with small cell carcinoma of the lung. Eur J Cancer 16:572–531, 1980

16. Hainau B, Dombernowsky P, Hansen HH, Bozgeskov S: Cell proliferation and histologic classification of bronchogenic carcinoma. J Natl Cancer Inst 59:1113–1118, 1977

17. Straus MJ, Moran RE: The growth characteristics of lung cancer, in Straus MJ (ed): Lung Cancer: Clinical Diagnosis and Treatment, (ed 2). New York, Grune & Stratton, 1981

18. Muggia FM: Cell kinetic studies in patients with lung cancer. Oncology 30:353–361, 1974

19. Terz JJ, Curutchet HP, Lawrence W Jr: Analysis of the cell kinetics of human solid tumors. Cancer 28:1100–1110, 1971

20. Straus MJ, Moran RE: Cell cycle parameters in human solid tumors. Cancer 40:1453–1461, 1977

21. Malaise EP, Chavaudra N, Tubiana M: The relationship between growth rate, labeling index and histological type of human solid tumors. Eur J Cancer 9:305–312, 1973

10

MORPHOLOGIC CHANGES FOLLOWING THERAPY

Martin D. Abeloff
Joseph C. Eggleston

There is abundant evidence from a large number of studies that small cell carcinoma of the lung (SCC), is, indeed, a distinct clinicopathologic entity.[1] One of the major implications of the diagnosis of SCC has been that surgical removal of the primary tumor is not indicated even in patients in whom the tumor appears localized to one hemithorax.[2] The almost complete elimination of surgery as a therapeutic modality in SCC and the improvement in the diagnostic techniques of bronchoscopy and mediastinoscopy have resulted in our current practice of making the diagnosis of SCC on the basis of a pathologic examination of a small fragment of biopsy, or frequently cytology material.

During the last seven years, patients diagnosed as having SCC have been treated with systemic chemotherapy regimens, often in conjunction with radiotherapy to the primary tumor. These modern therapeutic approaches have resulted in significant improvements in objective response rate and survival for patients with SCC.[3,4] However, the therapy of SCC appears to have reached a plateau in its ability to produce more complete remissions. Impressive reduction in tumor volume is promptly achieved in 70–80 percent of SCC patients undergoing systemic chemotherapy, but complete disappearance of measurable tumor occurs in only 20–30 percent of these patients.[5]

Portions of this work were funded by Grant PDT-108 from the American Cancer Society.

In an attempt to elucidate the causes of resistance to therapy in this tantalizingly responsive neoplasm, detailed studies of the pathology and biology of SCC have been initiated. In this chapter, we describe the morphologic changes in SCC that have been observed during and following modern therapy and discuss their clinical implications.

Pathology Changes at Autopsy

Three autopsy studies[6-8] have recently been published that examine changes in pathology of SCC following modern therapy. The results of these studies are summarized in Table 10-1. Each diagnostic biopsy in these studies contained only SCC. All patients underwent thorough staging evaluation, which included complete history and physical examination; chest radiographs, including tomograms and oblique views when indicated; radioisotope bone and liver scans; and posterior iliac crest bone marrow aspirate and biopsy. The majority of patients were entered into therapeutic protocols (combination chemotherapy with or without radiotherapy to the primary tumor and prophylactic cranial radiotherapy). These patients were then serially monitored to assess therapeutic response.

Brereton and colleagues[6] studied 21 such autopsies of SCC patients entered on therapeutic protocols at the Radiation Oncology Branch of the National Cancer Institute between November 1974 and May 1975. In 5 cases, no tumor was identified at autopsy, and in 11 cases, only SCC was noted. However, 5 patients (Table 10-1) had carcinomas with at least focal squamous differentiation; 3 patients had predominately SCC with foci of squamous carcinoma; and 2 had only squamous carcinoma at autopsy.

Matthews[7] recently presented a more detailed analysis of autopsy material on 91 patients with SCC treated on chemotherapy or combined chemotherapy–radiotherapy protocols of the Radiation Oncology Branch and Veteran's Administration Medical Oncology Branch of the National Cancer Institute and the Working Party for Therapy of Lung Cancer. (This series also contains the patients noted in Brereton's report). As noted in Table 10-1, there was no evidence of identifiable small cell tumor in 5 cases; in three cases, only anaplastic large cells and tumor giant cells were identified. In two cases, disseminated squamous carcinoma was found at autopsy. In 30 out of 91 autopsies, foci of giant cells, tubules, squamous cells, and carcinoid elements were found, in addition to the predominant small cell component. Such morphologic changes were noted as frequently

Table 10-1
Morphological Changes in SCC at Autopsy

Morphologic Changes	Investigators		
	Brereton (21 Autopsies)	Matthews (91 Autopsies)	Abeloff (40 Autopsies)
Squamous carcinoma (no SCC)	2	2	3
Adenocarcinoma (no SCC)	—	—	1
Large cell undifferentiated carcinoma (no SCC)	—	3*	1
Small cell carcinoma with			
Large cell component	—	12*	1
Squamous cell component	3	3	—
Glandular component	—	8	4
Squamous and glandular components	—	3	1†
Carcinoid component	—	4	—
Totals	5	35	11

*Giant cell component.
†Extensive SCC at autopsy and small focus of glandular differentiation in one lung and separate small poorly differentiated squamous carcinoma of the lung.

in patients receiving chemotherapy alone as in those receiving both chemotherapy and radiotherapy.

Stimulated by our interest in the heterogeneity of cancer and the relationship of SCC to the other histologic types of lung cancer, we reviewed 40 consecutive autopsies of patients with SCC seen at The Johns Hopkins Hospital between 1970 and 1978.[8] In 5 of 40 cases (Table 10-1), non-SCC (squamous carcinoma in 3, adenocarcinoma in 1, and large cell undifferentiated carcinoma in 1) but not SCC was seen at autopsy. Six cases were identified in which other histologic patterns of lung cancer were present in addition to SCC. In 4 of 6, the tumor at autopsy was predominantly SCC, but the primary tumor contained small foci of glandular differentiation of the type characteristic of adenocarcinoma. In one case, there was a small focus of tumor that consisted of both SCC and large cell carcinoma in a hilar node, and, in another case, there was extensive SCC with a small focus of glandular differentiation in one lung and a separate small poorly differentiated squamous cell carcinoma in the other lung.

To determine whether these tumors at autopsy were biochemically as well as morphologically distinct from SCC, histaminase and L-dopa decarboxylase were measured in the lung tumor and in mediastinal metastases in 4 of 5 cases in which no SCC was present at autopsy. These enzymes have previously been shown to be increased in SCC tumor tissue.[9] The levels of these enzymes in the tumors were markedly lower than the levels found in SCC and were similar to those found in non-SCC in previous studies.

In our study and in the series of Brereton and Matthews, the incidence of exclusively non-small cell carcinoma at autopsy in patients with biopsy proved diagnoses of SCC ranged from 5.5 to 12.5 percent. The incidence of mixed histologic patterns ranged from 14.3 to 32.9 percent. Pathologic heterogeneity in patients with SCC undergoing modern therapy is, therefore, not a rare event and raises important questions about clinical and biologic aspects of bronchogenic cancer.

Possible Explanations of Morphologic Changes

The pathologic findings noted in these autopsy studies could be explained by: (1) an initial diagnostic biopsy that was not representative of the entire tumor; (2) selective eradication of the small cell component of a mixed tumor with subsequent growth of the initially inconspicuous non–small cell component; (3) cure of the SCC with emergence or development of a second primary tumor; or (4) alteration of cell differentiation of the SCC with either therapy or time, or both.

In the patients who had only a partial response or no response to antitumor therapy, it is possible that the tumors were initially pleomorphic and that the cytotoxic treatment eliminated the more sensitive small cell populations, permitting the emergence of the more resistant squamous carcinoma, large cell carcinoma, or adenocarcinoma. The coexistence of different histologic patterns within the same lung tumor has been well documented in the pathology literature. In an examination of 10,000 lung cancers, Yesner[10] identified 200 (2 percent) examples of combined tumors of which the most common combination was differentiated squamous carcinoma and mucin-producing adenocarcinoma. Yesner comments that numerous examples were seen of transitions between SCC and squamous cell carcinoma and between SCC and adenocarcinoma.

The development of a second primary tumor is a plausible explanation only for those patients in whom complete regression of the initial tumor was achieved. The tendency to develop multiple primary bronchogenic cancers is also documented in numerous reports in the literature. In fact, Azzopardi[11] in his classic description of the histologic characteristics of "oat cell carcinoma of the bronchus" described two cases of double primary lung tumors (squamous and oat cell in each case). Subsequently, the published incidence of these multiple tumors has ranged from 0.5 to 14.5 percent.[12-15] In a meticulous microscopic study of the tracheobronchial tree of each of 255 patients who died of bronchogenic carcinoma, Auerbach and colleagues[12] concluded that at least 3.5 percent of the patients had multiple primary lung cancers and that, with less strict diagnostic criteria, the number might be as high as 14.5 percent. Patients with SCC were included in this study, and the authors commented that the occurrence of multiple carcinomas was not related to the histologic type of the main tumor. Martini and Melamed[13] identified 50 cases of multiple primary lung cancers (0.97 percent) in 5163 patients treated for primary lung cancer at Memorial-Sloan Kettering Cancer Center between 1955 and 1975. Eighteen had synchronous tumors and 32 had metachronous tumors. The intervals between diagnoses of the metachronous tumors ranged from 4 mo to 16 yr. Histologic patterns in the two different carcinomas were the same in 31 patients (most commonly epidermoid) and were different in 19. In no case was the first tumor a SCC; in 2 cases, SCC was the second tumor. It is interesting to note that, of 28 patients with a radiologically occult cancer diagnosed at Memorial-Sloan Kettering, 7 (25 percent) had a second and separate primary lung cancer. Carter and associates[16] report similar findings regarding the incidence of second primaries in patients with a radiologically occult squamous carcinoma in the Early Lung Cancer Detection program at the Johns Hopkins Hospital.

Although lung tumors with mixed histologic patterns and multiple primary bronchogenic cancers are well documented in the literature, the frequency of these changes in tumor morphology at autopsy of patients with SCC seems excessive when compared with reports that antedate the modern therapy of SCC. Matthews[7] has commented that the mixed histologic patterns seen in approximately one-third of her cases must be considered therapy induced for the most part. Therapy-induced changes in cell differentiation have been postulated in germ cell tumors,[17] which, like SCC are exquisitely sensitive to chemotherapy.

Evaluation of Prospective Clinical Studies

The assessment of the relative importance of these potential explanations awaits a more accurate estimate of the incidence of pleomorphic tumors and multiple primary cancers in patients with SCC at initial diagnosis, during the course of treatment, and at autopsy. We have reviewed the clinical–pathology findings in a series of 54 patients with SCC entered onto experimental therapeutic protocols between September 1977 and June 1979. These protocols were designed to evaluate the effectiveness of very intensive induction chemotherapy with cyclophosphamide, doxorubicin (Adriamycin), and VP-16-213 (CAV). The preliminary therapeutic results and toxicity data from these protocols have been previously reported.[5,18] The overall response rate in this study is 78 percent with 26 percent complete responses. The median survival is slightly greater than 1 yr and the projected 2-yr survival is 22 percent. There have been 34 deaths in these 54 cases, and 14 autopsies have been performed. Three cases from this series illustrate different ways in which a non-SCC may occur in a SCC patient.

Case Reports

Case 1.   F.D. was a 65-yr-old man with a 20-pack/yr smoking history who was discovered to have right hilar adenopathy and a mass in the right lower lobe on a routine chest x-ray prior to cataract surgery in April 1978 (Fig. 10-1, panel A). The patient was asymptomatic and physical examination was normal. Bronchoscopy with a transbronchial biopsy was non-diagnostic. Mediastinoscopy biopsy of a right paratracheal node demonstrated metastatic SCC (Fig. 10-1, panel B). The patient was referred to the Johns Hopkins Oncology Center, where a metastatic work-up revealed no evidence of tumor beyond the right hemithorax. The patient was classified as having localized disease and was randomized to intensive chemotherapy alone (without radiotherapy to the primary tumor) with cyclophosphamide, Adriamycin, and VP-16-213 (CAV). The initial course of chemotherapy resulted in a partial remission, and the second course a month later resulted in complete remission (Fig. 10-1, panel C). Monthly chemotherapy was then begun on an outpatient basis, and the patient did well until June 1979, when he complained of left chest, shoulder, and arm pain. Chest x-ray showed a left apical mass (Fig. 10-1, panel D), and CT scan confirmed the presence of this mass and suggested rib erosion. A percutaneous needle biopsy revealed poorly differentiated squamous carcinoma (Fig. 10-1, panel E). Repeat metastatic work-up revealed no evidence of tumor outside of the left lung, and the patient was treated with radiotherapy directed at the second primary tumor. The pain persisted, and, in December 1979, the patient was admitted with clinical signs and symptoms of cervical cord compression, which was documented by myelography. Cervical laminectomy was performed; pathological examination of bone removed showed squamous carcinoma, and cytologic examination of cerebrospinal fluid revealed undifferentiated carcinoma. Biopsy of a

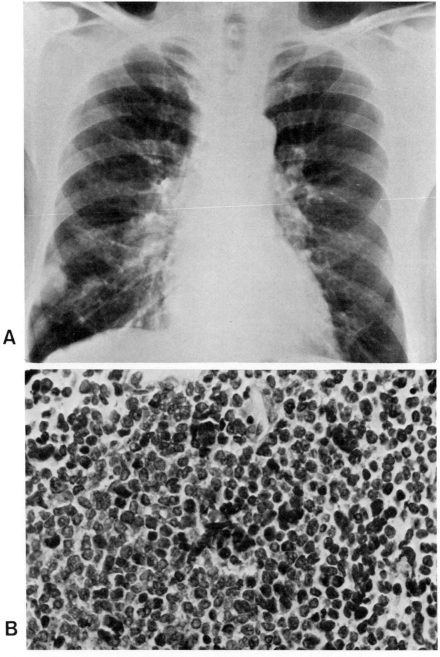

Figure 10-1. *Case 1. (A) Right hilar adenopathy and right lower lobe mass. (B) Mediastinoscopy biopsy of paratracheal node showing SCC.*

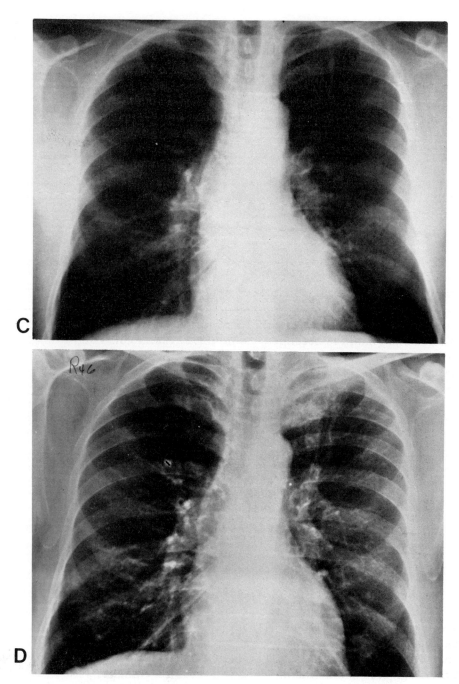

Figure 10-1 *(continued).   (C) Complete resolution of chest tumor. (D) Left apical mass.*

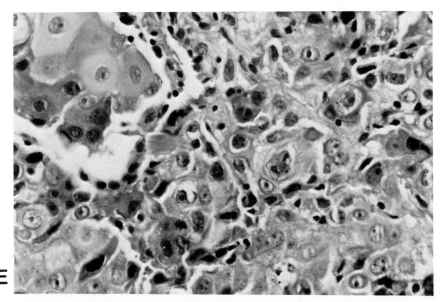

Figure 10-1 *(continued).   (E) Percutaneous needle biopsy of apical mass revealing squamous carcinoma.*

flank mass also demonstrated squamous carcinoma. Biochemical studies of this tumor mass revealed no measurable L-dopa decarboxylase activity and histaminase activity was measured at only 11 units/g wet weight. Median values of L-dopa decarboxylase and histaminase in SCC tissue are significantly higher than the values in this patient's tumor tissue (see Chapter 6, this monograph). The patient developed progressive respiratory deterioration secondary to increasing tumor mass, postobstructive pneumonia, and massive pleural effusion. The patient died in January 1980, 20 mo after the diagnosis of SCC and 6 mo after the diagnosis of a second primary lung cancer. Autopsy revealed squamous carcinoma of the apex of the left lung with endobronchial spread and metastases to left hilar, paratracheal, and carinal lymph nodes. The squamous carcinoma also extended to the left visceral and parietal pleura, the pericardium, and the right ventricular myocardium and had metastasized to the cervical vertebrae, skin of right flank, ileum, and left perirenal soft tissue. There was no evidence of SCC at autopsy.

Case 2. E.H., a 60-yr-old woman with a 120-pack/yr smoking history, was admitted to the hospital in January 1979 because of chest pain. Chest x-ray revealed left hilar and paratracheal masses, a peripheral mass in the lingula, a left pleural effusion, and a few ill-defined infiltrates in the left lung (Fig. 10-2, panel A). Bronchoscopic biopsy of the anterior segment of the left upper lobe revealed SCC (Fig. 10-2, panel B). Staging evaluation documented extensive disease on the basis of abnormal liver functions, filling defects on liver scan, and the left pleural effusion. The patient received induction therapy with two intensive courses of cyclophosphamide, Adriamycin, and VP-16-213 (CAV). The left hilar and paratracheal masses regressed, but there was little change in the lingular mass or liver scan. In March 1979, the patient developed right upper quadrant pain, with further deterioration of hepatic function. Despite further systemic chemotherapy and radiotherapy to the liver, the patient's course was characterized by progressive enlargement of the liver and increasingly abnormal liver function. The lingular mass persisted (Fig. 10-2, panel C), and the coexistence of a second primary tumor was suggested by E.H.'s physician. The patient died of liver failure in August 1979. Autopsy revealed poorly differentiated adenocarcinoma in the lingula with metastases to left lower lobe of lung, diaphragm, liver (which was virtually replaced by tumor), and portal lymph nodes (Fig. 10-2, panel D). Residual SCC was found only in one left hilar lymph node (Fig. 10-2, panel E).

Case 3.   J.B. was a 61-yr-old man with an 80-pk/yr history of cigarette smoking, who presented in November 1977 with chest pain and weight loss. Chest x-ray showed a large right lung mass contiguous to the right hilum (Fig. 10-3, panel A). Bronchoscopy revealed an irregular mucosa in the right main stem bronchus and narrowing of the right middle and lower lobe bronchi. Bronchoscopic biopsy demonstrated SCC (Fig. 10-3, panel B). The metastatic work-up was negative for tumor, and the patient was randomized on the localized disease protocol to CAV, without radiotherapy to the primary tumor. The patient had regression of his chest tumor following the intensive chemotherapy but did not achieve a complete remission. There was no evidence of development of metastases beyond the right hemithorax, so the patient was treated with radiotherapy to the lung tumor in May–June 1978, without prophylactic cranial radiotherapy. Further reduction in tumor mass was achieved, but the response to radiotherapy was less than would be anticipated with a SCC (Fig. 10-3, panel C). Therefore, repeat bronchoscopy was performed in September 1978, and biopsy demonstrated a small fragment of poorly differentiated non-small cell carcinoma. A restaging procedure was performed, and, since there was no evidence of extrathoracic metastases, the patient underwent a thoracotomy in October 1978. Biopsy of mediastinal lymph node and soft tissue revealed mucin-producing adenocarcinoma (Fig. 10-3, panel D).

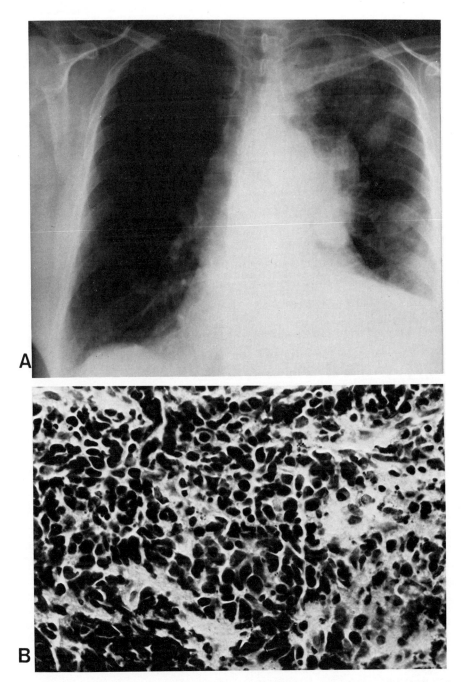

Figure 10-2. *Case 2. (A) Left hilar and paratracheal masses, lingular mass, and pleural effusion. (B) Bronchoscopic biopsy demonstrating SCC.*

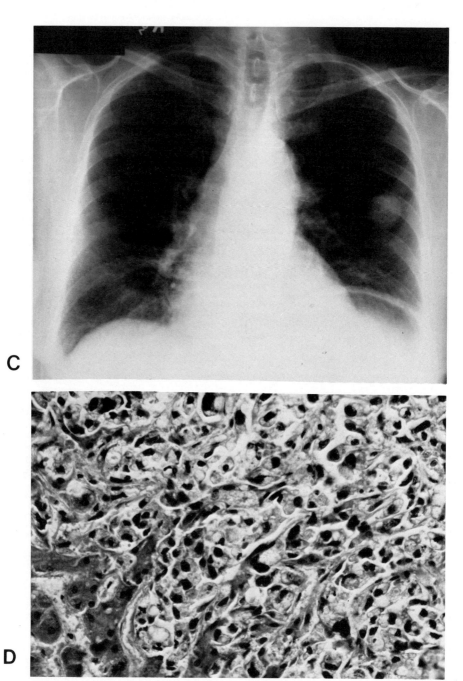

Figure 10-2 *(continued).   (C) Hilar and paratracheal disease resolve, with lingular mass persisting. (D) Adenocarcinoma in liver at autopsy.*

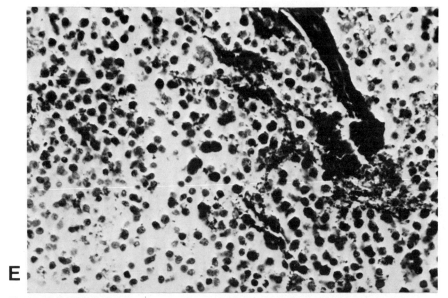

Figure 10-2 *(continued).* *(E) SCC found only in hilar node at autopsy.*

Biochemical studies on the tumor tissue revealed L-dopa decarboxylase activity of 70 units/g wet weight and histaminase of 262 units/g wet weight. These values are comparable to the enzyme activities in SCC tissue (see Chapter 6, this monograph). The tumor was found to be invading the esophagus and was inoperable. Following surgery, the chest tumor appeared to be stable, but in January 1979, the patient developed ataxia and diplopia. CT scan of the head demonstrated cerebellar and cerebral metastases. The patient was begun on cranial irradiation but developed progressive neurologic problems and expired in February 1979. No autopsy was obtained.

Lung cancers other than SCC (documented by biopsy or autopsy, or both) were thus noted in 3 of 54 patients (5.5 percent) on our recent intensive therapy protocol; of the 14 autopsies in this series, 2 (14 percent) had evidence of such tumors. There is convincing evidence in cases 1 and 2 for a second primary tumor. Patient 1 developed a squamous carcinoma of the lung after complete regression of SCC had been achieved, and this patient died as a result of the squamous carcinoma. It is interesting to note that the second tumor in patient 1 was not only morphologically distinct from SCC, but was also biochemically distinguishable from previously studied SCC tissue. In patient 2, the SCC and adenocarcinoma were synchronous

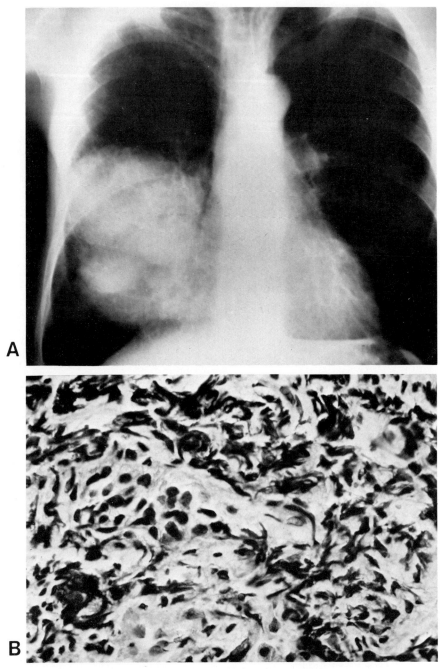

Figure 10-3. *Case 3. (A) Right lung mass. (B) Bronchoscopic biopsy positive for SCC.*

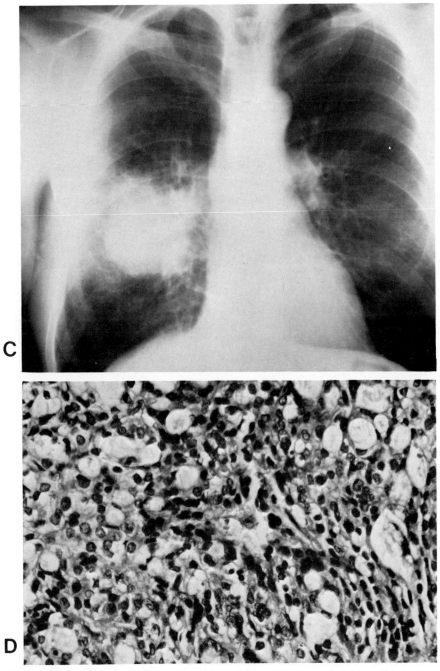

Figure 10-3 *(continued).* *(C) Large mass remaining after chemotherapy and radiotherapy. (D) Adenocarcinoma (mucin positive) biopsied at thoracotomy.*

in their development. The cytotoxic chemotherapy resulted in regression of the more sensitive SCC, so that at autopsy SCC was found in only one hilar node, whereas the chemotherapy-resistant adenocarcinoma resulted in liver failure and death of the patient.

Second primary tumors were suspected on the basis of careful assessment of the clinical findings in cases 1 and 2. In case 3 a biopsy of residual primary tumor was performed because of the failure of the tumor to respond in the expected fashion to chemotherapy or radiotherapy. Pathology examination of the tumor tissue obtained at thoracotomy revealed cells with nuclei similar to those of SCC but with abundant cytoplasm and extensive mucin production. The L-dopa decarboxylase and histaminase levels were in the range reported for previously studied SCC tissue. It appears likely that the change in morphology in case 3 was the result of the effects of cytotoxic therapy, but it is also possible that the tumor may have been pleomorphic at the outset and that the chemotherapy and radiotherapy eliminated the more sensitive small cell population.

In addition to these 3 cases, in which different or altered morphology was detected during or following therapy, we have recently studied 2 patients in whom SCC and another histologic type of lung cancer were detected at the time of diagnosis of SCC. These two patients did not qualify for our research protocols because of the mixed histologic appearance of the tumor in one and the demonstration of a synchronous second (non-SCC) primary tumor in the second. The coexistence of SCC and non-SCC in these two cases could easily have gone unrecognized, as a result either of a sampling error or of a different diagnostic approach.

Case 4.   L.H. was a 67-yr-old man with a smoking history of 150 pack/ yr, who was found to have a right hilar mass and right lower lobe atelectasis on his annual screening chest x-ray (done as part of The Johns Hopkins Early Lung Cancer Study) in June 1978 (Fig. 10-4, panel A). Prior to the x-ray, he had noted the development of cough and a mild increase in dyspnea. Bronchoscopy revealed that the bronchus to the right lower lobe was nearly occluded by a mass and that there was also narrowing of the right middle lobe bronchus. Bronchoscopic biopsy showed in situ and infiltrating bronchogenic carcinoma with features of both SCC and squamous carcinoma (Fig. 10-4, panels B and C). Extensive work-up did not demonstrate any evidence of tumor beyond the right hemithorax. The patient was started on an outpatient modification of CAV in July 1978. Following two courses of CAV, the right hilar mass had regressed, but lower lobe atelectasis persisted (Fig. 10-4, panel D). Repeat bronchoscopy in September 1978 showed marked resolution of the obstruction, but a necrotic lesion was noted in the right lower lobe bronchus. Biopsy revealed

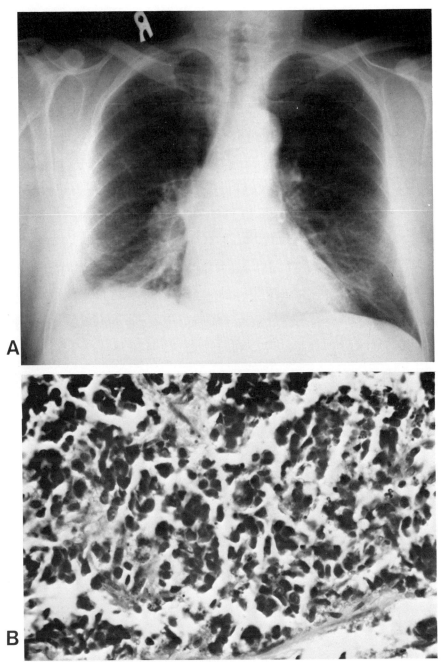

Figure 10-4. *Case 4. (A) Right hilar mass and right lower lobe atelectasis. (B) Initial bronchoscopic biopsy demonstrating SCC.*

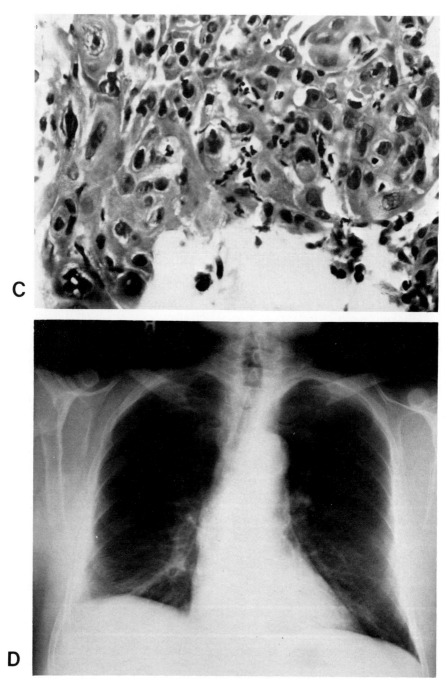

Figure 10-4 *(continued).* *(C) Initial bronchoscopic biopsy demonstrating squamous carcinoma. (D) Regression of right hilar mass.*

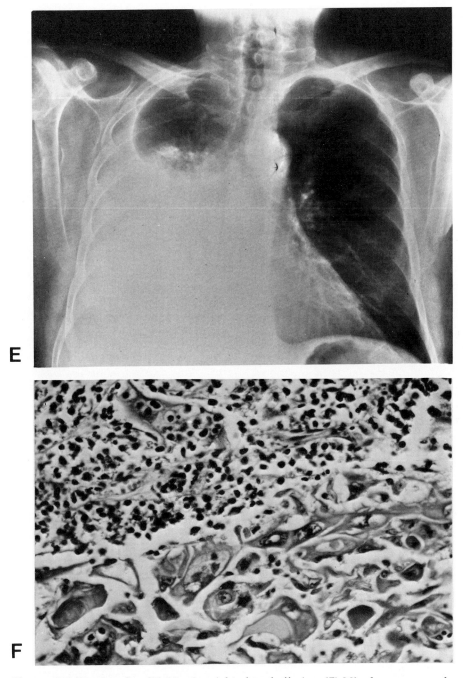

E

F

Figure 10-4 *(continued).* *(E) Massive right pleural effusion. (F) Mixed squamous and SCC in primary site at autopsy.*

only squamous carcinoma, but cytologic examination still showed cells of a SCC. The patient then received radiotherapy to the site of the primary tumor in October–November 1978. Chemotherapy was discontinued in January 1979 at the patient's request. In April 1979, the patient was admitted to the hospital because of development of a right pleural effusion (Fig. 10-4, panel E). Cytologic examination of pleural fluid revealed cells of a SCC. The patient was restarted on chemotherapy but had progressive respiratory deterioration and died in May 1979. At autopsy, the primary tumor was found to be an endobronchial lesion in the right lower lobe, which retained the mixed squamous and small cell characteristics (Fig. 10-4, panel F). The squamous element invaded into the parenchyma of the right lower lobe. The small cell component, however, had spread extensively to right middle, lower, and upper lobes, right paratracheal and hilar lymph nodes, pleurae, chest wall, diaphragm, liver, adrenals, and bone marrow.

Case 5. W.S. was a 61-yr-old man with a 50-pack/yr history of cigarette smoking who presented in July 1977 with increasing cough, anorexia, and weight loss. Chest x-ray and tomography showed a peripheral lesion in the left upper lobe and a left hilar mass (Fig. 10-5, panel A). Bronchoscopy did not show any obstruction, and bronchoscopic and mediastinal biopsy were negative for tumor. A left thoracotomy was performed, and wedge resection of the left upper lobe revealed adenocarcinoma without any evidence of a small cell component (Fig. 10-5, panel B). Biopsy of left hilar nodes revealed only metastatic SCC (Fig. 10-5, panel C). Thus, the patient appeared to have two synchronous separate primaries, with the second primary tumor presumed to be an undetected occult SCC within the lung. There was no other evidence of metastatic disease, so he was treated with outpatient cyclophosphamide, vincristine (Oncovin), methotrexate, and 1,3-bis-(2-chloroethyl)-1-nitrosourea (BCNU)(COMB) as therapy for his SCC. The left hilar mass regressed on chemotherapy (Fig. 10-5, panel D). The COMB regimen was given monthly through April 1978 and was stopped at the patient's request. In September 1978, a new lesion appeared on chest x-ray in the left upper lobe (Fig. 10-5, panel E), and needle biopsy revealed adenocarcinoma. The patient received radiotherapy to the left upper lobe in October–November 1978. He was lost to follow-up, but returned in November 1979 with progressive pulmonary problems. Chest x-ray showed a left pleural effusion and multiple pulmonary nodules. Cytologic examination of sputum and pleural fluid revealed adenocarcinoma cells. The patient deteriorated progressively and died in December 1979. Autopsy was not performed. There was no evidence of recurrent SCC during life.

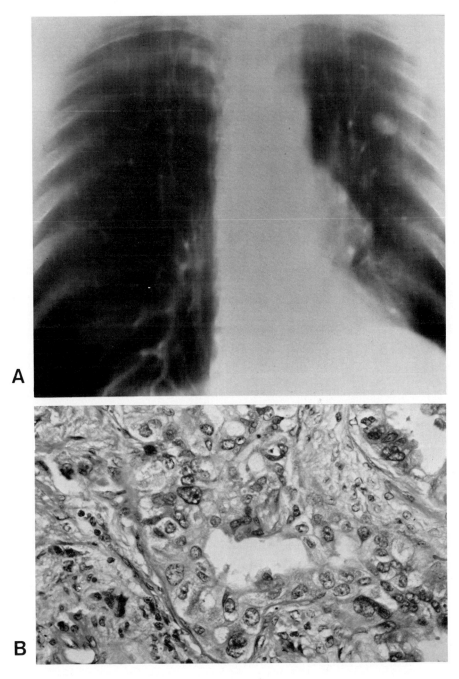

Figure 10-5. *Case 5. (A) Chest tomogram of left hilar mass and left upper lobe lesion. (B) Adenocarcinoma in wedge resection of left upper lobe.*

255

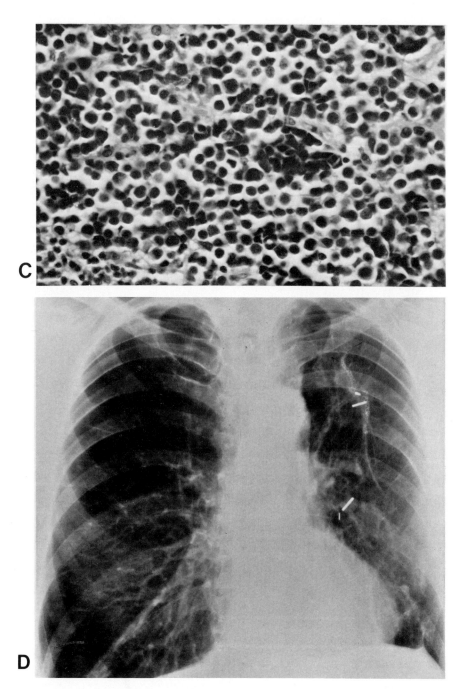

Figure 10-5 *(continued).* *(C) SCC in biopsy of left hilar node. (D) Left hilar mass responding to chemotherapy.*

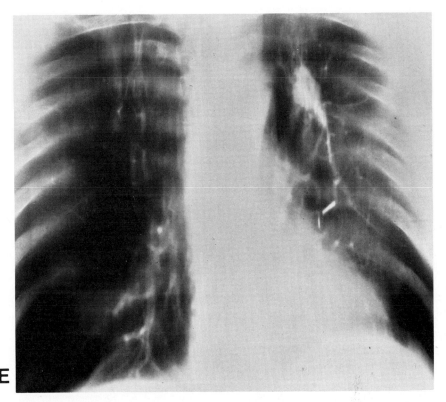

Figure 10-5 *(continued).   (E) New lesion in left upper lobe.*

Clinical Implications

Although the mechanisms for all of the changes in tumor morphologic appearance and mixed pathologic patterns observed in retrospective and prospective studies cannot be firmly determined, the data indicate that it is important to consider the possibility of pathologic heterogeneity when evaluating the newly diagnosed patient with SCC. In their studies of SCC, Minna and co-workers[19] noted that 16 patients had large cell carcinoma mixed with the intermediate subtype of SCC in the diagnostic tumor specimen. These patients were entered onto the intensive chemotherapeutic protocols utilized for patients with SCC. Minna observed that mixed histology large cell–small cell lung cancer has a high objective response rate (88 percent) to combination chemotherapy when compared to non-small cell lung cancer but has a low complete response rate (12.5 percent). These observations in a small number of patients require confirmation by other investigators but emphasize the importance of thorough examination of the diagnostic pathology specimen with appropriate clinical correlations.

In view of the recognition of pathologic heterogeneity in 5.5 percent (clinical series) to 33 percent (autopsy series) of patients with SCC, it would seem reasonable to obtain larger samples of biopsy material, such as biopsy specimens of accessible peripheral lymph nodes, prior to initiation of therapy whenever possible. Rebiopsy of accessible lesions in a patient whose tumor has been resistant to therapy or who has a relapse after an initial response should also be considered. Clinicians must also be vigilant for clues that suggest the development of a second primary tumor.

The identification of morphologic changes in a patient with SCC clearly has therapeutic implications, since the other histologic types of lung cancer are much less responsive to cytotoxic chemotherapy and radiotherapy than is SCC. Obviously, the resistance of tumor to therapy in patients with SCC is generally not accounted for by a change in its histologic appearance. However, biochemical characteristics of SCC (discussed in detail in Chapter 6, this monograph) have been described that reflect properties of lung cancer that are not revealed by the histologic classification and that may prove to be of value in the treatment of such tumors. The usefulness of such biochemical measurements in the management of human cancer is not unprecedented; in human breast cancer, the measurement of estrogen and progesterone receptors in tumor cytosol provides useful prognostic information regarding the natural history of the particular case of breast cancer, as well as a reasonable prediction of the likelihood of response to endocrine therapy. Correlations of biochemical parameters with histologic subtype of lung cancer, extent of disease, response to therapy, and survival may yield similarly useful information.

References

1. Cohen MH, Matthews MJ: Small cell bronchogenic carcinoma: A distinct clinicopathologic entity. Sem Oncol 5:234–243, 1978
2. Fox W, Scadding JG: Medical Research Council comparative trial of surgery and radiotherapy for the primary treatment of small celled or oat celled carcinoma of the bronchus. Ten year follow-up. Lancet 2:63–65, 1973
3. Greco FA, Oldham RK: Current concepts in cancer. Small-cell lung cancer. N Engl J Med 301:355–358, 1979

4. Weiss RB: Small-cell carcinoma of the lung: Therapeutic management. Ann Intern Med 88:522–531, 1978
5. Abeloff MD, Ettinger DS, Khouri NF, et al: Intensive induction therapy for small cell carcinoma of the lung. Cancer Treat Rep 63:519–524, 1979
6. Brereton HD, Matthews MM, Costa J, et al: Mixed anaplastic small-cell and squamous-cell carcinoma of the lung. Ann Intern Med 88:805–806, 1978
7. Matthews MJ: Effects of therapy on the morphology and behavior of small cell carcinoma of the lung—A clinicopathologic study, in Muggia F, Rozencweig M (ed): Lung Cancer: Progress in Therapeutic Research, New York, Raven Press, 1979, pp 155–165
8. Abeloff MD, Eggleston JC, Mendelsohn G, et al: Changes in morphologic and biochemical characteristics of small cell carcinoma of the lung. Am J Med 66:757–764, 1979
9. Baylin SB, Weisburger WR, Eggleston JC, et al: Variable content of histaminase, L-dopa decarboxylase and calcitonin in small cell carcinoma of the lung. N Engl J Med 299:105–110, 1978
10. Yesner R: Spectrum of lung cancer and ectopic hormones. Pathol Annu 13:217–240, 1978
11. Azzopardi JG: Oat-cell carcinoma of the bronchus. J Pathol Bacteriol 78:513–519, 1959
12. Auerbach O, Stout AP, Hammond EC, et al: Multiple primary bronchial carcinomas. Cancer 20:699–705, 1967
13. Martini N, Melamed MR: Multiple primary lung cancers. J Thorac Cardiovasc Surg 70:606–611, 1975
14. Abbey Smith R, Nigam BK, Thompson JM: Second primary lung carcinoma. Thorax 31:507–516, 1976
15. Lehman JA, Cross FS: Bilateral multiple carcinoma of the lung. Cancer 19:1931–1936, 1966
16. Carter D, Marsh BR, Baker RR, et al: Relationship of morphology to clinical presentation in ten cases of early squamous cell carcinoma of the lung. Cancer 37:1389–1396, 1976
17. Hong WK, Wittes RE, Hajdu SI, et al: The evolution of mature teratoma from malignant testicular tumors. Cancer 40:2987–2992, 1977
18. Abeloff MD, Ettinger DS, Khouri NF: Intensive induction therapy for small cell carcinoma of the lung. Proc Am Soc Clin Oncol 20:326, 1979
19. Minna JD, Matthews M, Ihde DC, et al: Identification and combination chemotherapy of mixed histology large cell–small cell (WPL #40/22) lung cancer. Proc Am Soc Clin Oncol 19:397, 1978

11

STAGING PROCEDURES AND PROGNOSTIC FACTORS IN SMALL CELL CARCINOMA OF THE LUNG

Daniel C. Ihde
Heine H. Hansen

Staging procedures that define the extent of tumor dissemination have a number of potential uses in human cancer. When employed prior to definitive therapy, they may guide the selection of treatment modalities and help in establishing prognosis. During therapy, they aid in documenting the completeness of tumor response and may identify certain sites of local, regional, or disseminated disease which are unresponsive to treatment, thus suggesting alternate strategies for tumor eradication. Finally, information derived from their utilization may lead to an increased understanding of the natural history of the neoplasm.

Small cell carcinoma of the lung (SCC) is a rapidly proliferating malignancy with a propensity for early dissemination.[1] Distant metastases are found in 70 percent of patients dying from non–tumor-related causes within 30 days of curative pulmonary resection.[2] At postmortem examination, the tumor is limited to the thorax in only 4 percent of patients. Metastases are found with substantial frequency in almost every organ of the body, with involvement of hilar and mediastinal lymph nodes, liver, adrenals, abdominal lymph nodes, pancreas, bone, contralateral lung, and central nervous system being especially common.[3] Thus, one might expect that pretreatment staging procedures directed at these organs would often yield positive findings.

In view of the long-term disease-free survival enjoyed by a distinct minority of patients receiving current therapies,[1,4] the ability to identify subsets of patients with reasonable prospects for substantial survival prolongation would obviously be desirable. In this chapter we discuss the staging systems currently in use, methods with which evidence of metastases may be sought in various organ systems, and prognostic factors of definite, probable, or uncertain importance in patients treated with combination chemotherapy, with or without radiation.

Staging Systems

The American Joint Committee on Cancer Staging and End Results Reporting proposed a tumor, nodes, metastases (TNM) staging system for lung cancer in 1974.[5] In contrast to other cell types of lung cancer, the prognosis of SCC in this surgically oriented staging system was independent of stage, with 2-yr survivals of approximately 5 percent in all stages. Furthermore, 85 percent of SCC patients presented with stage III disease, defined as extensive or locally invasive primary tumor, mediastinal node involvement, or distant metastases.[5] Even in patients able to undergo surgical resection, preoperative stage had no influence on the median survival of approximately 5 mo, which was similar to the survival of unresected patients.[6] This staging classification, which focuses in great detail on the extent of intrathoracic tumor spread, is thus inappropriate for SCC.

Virtually all recent therapeutic trials in SCC employ the simple two-stage classification of the Veterans Administration Lung Cancer Study Group, in which patients with inoperable lesions were divided into limited and extensive stages. Limited disease was defined as tumor confined to one hemithorax, with or without "local extensions," including mediastinal adenopathy, and with or without ipsilateral supraclavicular nodes. In addition, the tumor was required to be treatable by, and totally encompassed in, a single radiation portal. Extensive stage disease denotes tumor beyond these limits.[7] Median survival of placebo-treated patients with limited and extensive disease was 3.0 and 1.5 mo, respectively,[7] and significant differences between the two stages in the length of survival of chemotherapy- and radiotherapy-treated patients have also been observed in most trials.[1,4]

In actual practice, there has been no strict adherence to a uniform definition of limited disease. Thus, patients with contralateral supraclavicular nodes,[8–10] ipsilateral nodes only,[11–13] and no supraclavicular nodes whatsoever[14,15] have been classified as having limited disease. Ipsilateral

Table 11-1
Frequency of Limited Disease in Large Series of
Systematically Staged Patients with SCC

Reference	No. of Patients	Incidence of Limited Disease		Staging Procedures Employed
		No.	%	
Edmonson[57]	228	44	19	Not reported
Livingston[8]	358	198	30	Chest x-ray, physical exam, bone marrow, liver/brain scans
Lowenbraun[16]	207	61	29	Chest x-ray, physical exam, bone marrow, liver/bone scans
Maurer[9]	225	115	51	Chest x-ray, physical exam, bone marrow, liver/brain/bone scans
Ihde[52]	106	33	31	Chest x-ray, physical exam, bone marrow, liver/brain/bone scans, liver biopsy, bronchoscopy.
Totals	1124	361	32	

pleural effusions have been both included within[14,16] and excluded from[17,18] the limited stage.

An additional source of variation in this staging system is the number and type of staging procedures employed, since more thorough staging will yield a higher frequency of patients with distant metastases. Procedures currently employed in most therapeutic trials include physical examination, chest x-ray, bone marrow examination, and radionuclide scans of the liver, brain, and sometimes of the bones. Table 11-1 lists the percentages of patients with limited disease in several recent studies of 100 or more patients. Approximately one third of cases with SCC will have limited disease at the time of diagnosis.

It is very likely that the current two-stage classification may require modification as more data concerning patients managed with aggressive combination chemotherapy, with or without irradiation, are reported. A wider range of survival expectations, particularly in extensive disease, has recently been observed by some groups, and long-term disease-free survival is noted in both limited and extensive disease.[11,19] The ability to identify in advance those patients with extensive disease who have an increased likelihood for long survival would be likely to lead to revision of the present staging system.

It is important to realize that more extensive utilization of staging procedures in SCC, as in any cancer, will not affect overall therapeutic results (unless certain stage-specific treatment can be demonstrated to be of value). However, thoroughly staged patients will appear to have improved results within individual stages. For example, if 100 patients with SCC have a median survival of 10 mo, minimal staging procedures may identify 50 with limited disease who have a median survival of 12 mo and 50 with extensive disease who have an 8-mo median survival. If more thorough, systematic staging is employed, an additional 20 patients with less obvious (and lesser degrees of) extensive disease might be diagnosed. These 20 "minimally extensive" patients might have a median survival of 10 mo, worse than the 50 original limited cases, but better than the 50 original extensive cases. Transferring them from limited to extensive stage would produce a final tabulation of only 30 patients with limited disease, but the median survival for these 30 might then be 14 mo. Meanwhile the median survival for the 70 patients with extensive disease might be increased to approximately 9 mo. Thus, although the more systematic staging process would not alter overall survival figures, it would increase the apparent median survival in "limited disease" from 12 to 14 mo, and also would result in an apparent improvement in "extensive disease" median survival from 8 to 9 mo. Readers of the literature should be aware of this paradox when evaluating the results of therapeutic trials conducted in only one stage in carefully staged patients.

Intrathoracic Tumor

Staging procedures to be discussed in the remainder of this chapter are listed in Table 11-2. Whether the procedures are currently considered standard screening tests, tests to be employed only in symptomatic patients, or experimental investigations is also indicated. Precise delineation of the extent of intrathoracic tumor dissemination is of little therapeutic importance in SCC, since, with present treatment philosophy, knowledge of whether mediastinal node metastases are present will not affect management except in the rare patient with a peripheral pulmonary nodule who might be a surgical candidate. Nonetheless, intrathoracic tumor will be present and evaluable in most patients, and varied methods by which the degree of therapeutic response can be assessed are available. If, as some recent trials suggest,[11] the primary tumor continues to be a major site of first relapse from complete response, intrathoracic staging procedures may be more commonly utilized during therapy.

A central tumor mass or hilar node enlargement will be present on chest radiograph at the time of diagnosis in 65–80 percent of patients with SCC. Superior mediastinal masses or widening are seen in 13 percent. A

Table 11-2
Staging Procedures Used in SCC

Procedure, by Tumor Type	Current Recommended Use		
	Routine Screening	Symptomatic Patients*	Experimental
Intrathoracic Tumor			
Chest x-ray	×		
Chest tomograms		×	
Computed tomography of thorax			×
Thoracentesis and pleural biopsy		×	
Thoracoscopy			×
Fiberoptic bronchoscopy			×†
Mediastinoscopy			×
Gallium 67 scan			×
Bone Metastases			
Bone marrow aspiration/biopsy	×		
Peripheral blood examination	×		
Radionuclide bone scan	×		
Skeletal x-rays		×‡	
Central Nervous System Metastases			
Radionuclide brain scan		×	
Computed tomography of brain	×§		
Lumbar puncture with cytologic examination		×	
Myelography		×	
Hepatic Metastases			
Biochemical liver function tests	×		
Radionuclide liver scan	×‖		
Percutaneous or peritoneoscopic liver biopsies	×#		
Computed tomography of liver			×
Other Sites			
Computed tomography of abdomen			×
Whole-body gallium 67 scan			×

*Or for specific clinical indication.
†Sometimes used routinely to document complete responses; routine with initial nonevaluable chest X-ray.
‡Or in areas that are positive on bone scan.
§Value of routine screening with CT scan has yet to be established.
‖ If liver biopsy is not to be obtained, and to follow response when positive.
#Preferable if best information concerning liver status considered necessary.

discrete peripheral tumor mass can be appreciated in 20–33 percent, and multiple pulmonary nodules will occasionally be present,[20-21] as will a pleural effusion. Since many patients will have preexisting pulmonary

disease, the requirement of a normal chest x-ray for designation of a complete therapeutic response will often be impossible to fulfill. Thoracic irradiation with subsequent fibrosis further diminishes the value of the chest
x-ray in assessment of response.

Tomograms are sometimes more sensitive than conventional plain radiographs in evaluating intrathoracic disease. Computed tomography
(CT) of the thorax might be expected to be even more efficient in detection
of mediastinal and intraparenchymal masses. It is already being employed
in the design of radiation portals at the National Cancer Institute and at
other centers. According to a preliminary report, in all cell types of lung
cancer the CT scan provided information not apparent in chest x-rays of
several patients, but was associated with 28 percent false-negative findings when compared to mediastinoscopy.[22] Lack of specificity for malignancy in small parenchymal nodules discovered only by CT scan would be
expected to occur as well.

With a combination of pleural biopsy and thoracentesis or, if necessary, repeated thoracenteses, pathologic confirmation of pleural involvement in patients with pleural effusions can be expected in up to 90 percent
of cases.[23] Thoracoscopy with direct visualization and biopsy of pleural
lesions is an even better method for diagnosing pleural tumor masses.
Such knowledge could have therapeutic implications if thoracic radiotherapy is to be employed. Transbronchical biopsy may be of utility in the
occasional patient who presents with the radiographic pattern of lymphangitic carcinomatosis.[24]

Fiberoptic bronchoscopy has recently been employed in the staging
and response evaluation of patients with SCC at several centers. At the
NCI–VA Medical Oncology Branch, over 80 percent of patients have visible endobronchial tumor prior to therapy, and pathologic evidence of cancer can be detected in bronchial washings or biopsy in an additional 10
percent. In 5–10 percent of patients, bronchoscopy will provide the sole
site of evaluable intrathoracic tumor. Bilateral endobronchial tumor may
occasionally be observed. During chemotherapy, bronchoscopy has
proved most useful in identifying a group of patients who, by chest x-ray,
appear to be in complete remission but who, nonetheless, have residual
endobronchial tumor.[25] Approximately 30 percent of cases with complete
radiographic response fall in this category. The prognostic value of postin-
duction therapy bronchoscopy may be considerably less in patients given
chest irradiation.

Hilar and mediastinal lymph nodes contain tumor metastases in up to
96 percent of patients dying of SCC.[3] Even in patients with relatively localized tumor requiring bronchoscopy, mediastinoscopy, or thoracotomy for

diagnosis, malignant tissue can be obtained at mediastinoscopy in 70 percent.[26] At the Finsen Institute, mediastinoscopy has been employed in selected patients to document complete remission prior to discontinuation of chemotherapy.[19]

Radionuclide scanning with gallium 67 almost always reveals uptake in the area of the primary intrathoracic tumor in SCC and is frequently positive in tomographically detected hilar and mediastinal nodes.[27-28] In other types of lung cancer, it is undergoing evaluation as a possible substitute for other methods of identifying mediastinal node metastases. Its usefulness in assessing response and in monitoring for progression of intrathoracic SCC remains to be defined.

Bone Metastases

Bone metastases are present in 35–55 percent of SCC patients at autopsy.[3] Table 11-3 provides the frequency with which several investigators have identified such metastases in staging procedures employed prior to treatment. Many centers assess involvement of bone marrow and bone itself separately, utilizing marrow aspiration/biopsy and radiographic and radionuclide studies of the entire skeleton.

The propensity of SCC for early dissemination to the bone marrow was recognized during the early 1970s.[29,30] Marrow examination revealed malignant cells in over 40 percent of patients in these early studies, and frequently provided the sole evidence that the patient did not have limited disease.[29,30] In recent years, as patients with less advanced disease have entered chemotherapy trials and as more thorough staging evaluations have been employed, the frequency of marrow involvement at diagnosis has declined to approximately 20 percent, and only infrequently is the marrow infiltrated with tumor without there being other evidence of extensive disease.[13,31,32]

When performing bone marrow examinations, needle biopsy with touch preparation of the biopsy, a smear of the aspirate, and sometimes clot section of the aspirate are recommended. The touch preparations are of value since they may provide a rapid means of diagnosis of metastases, particularly when the aspirate is unobtainable because of a "dry tap." In most reports, tumor cells are present in the biopsy as often as, or more often than in the aspirate,[31] but some groups find the aspirate to be more sensitive.[33] It is likely that maximum yield results from utilizing both techniques. The posterior iliac crest is the usual site for screening bone marrow examination, but the sternum has occasionally been employed as

Table 11-3
Sites and Frequency of Distant Metastases in SCC at Diagnosis

Reference	No. of Patients	Bone Marrow	Bone	Brain	Liver	Involvement by Site (%) Other
Eagan[15]	37	47	NR*	14	32	Nodes 55%†, subcutaneous 10%
Reed[18]	279	14	26	12	34	Pleura 10%
Holoye[13]	45	24	NR	11	18	NR
Greco[56]	36	28	33	0	28	Subcutaneous 6%
King[72]	37	11	19	8	27	Nodes 16%, soft tissue 3%
Abeloff[73]	37	31	30	8	27	Nodes 38%, soft tissue 11%, opp. lung 8%
Dombernowsky[48]	157	17	NR	NR	22‡	NR
Ihde[52]	106	21	38	8§	28‡	Nodes 20%, subcutaneous 5%, opp. lung 7%, pleura 24%
Totals	734	19‖ (11–47)	29 (19–38)	10 (0–14)	28 (18–34)	

*NR, not reported.
†Includes ipsilateral supraclavicular nodes.
‡Some or all pathologically confirmed.
§Includes epidural and leptomeningeal metastases.
‖Weighted mean (range).

well.[34] Compared to a unilateral examination, bilateral iliac crest biopsies and aspirates can increase the detection of marrow metastases by up to 30 percent.[35]

Histopathologic evaluation of the marrow biopsy often reveals new bone formation and myelofibrosis associated with the tumor cells of SCC.[31] These changes resemble those found with osseous metastases from prostatic and breast malignancies, and they are rarely seen in other cell types of lung cancer. They are the pathologic correlate of the osteoblastic bone metastases that are sometimes observed radiographically in SCC.[36]

A leukoerythroblastic peripheral blood smear or thrombocytopenia, when present, is highly suggestive of bone marrow involvement in SCC.[31,33] However, even though the mean platelet count is lower in patients with marrow metastases than in patients without them, most patients with marrow involvement will have normal peripheral blood counts except for a mild anemia.[31] Very rarely marrow metastases may be associated with carcinocythemia, or circulating tumor cells in the peripheral blood.[37]

Radionuclide bone scans are much more sensitive in diagnosing skeletal involvement with SCC than are bone x-rays, as is true in most human cancers.[38] At the NCI–VA Medical Oncology Branch, we recently found only 1 patient of 119 with a positive pretreatment skeletal radiograph in the absence of a positive bone scan. The isotopes most commonly used at present for the detection of osseous metastases are ^{99m}technetium polyphosphate and diphosphonate complexes. Bone scans are also more frequently positive than are bone marrow examinations in SCC (Table 11-3), and the two procedures may not be detecting the same tumor sites. In earlier studies of patients with more advanced disease[38] and in more recent investigations, particularly when only patients with extensive disease are considered,[31,39] there was no significant association between the results of the two staging tests. Unlike radionuclide scans of liver and brain, bone scans in SCC[39] and in preoperative staging of all types of lung cancer[40] have a small but definite yield when employed in asymptomatic patients.

Because of the well-known possibility that a positive bone scan in a cancer patient may not be due to osseous metastases, it is important that criteria for scan positivity be carefully defined in published reports so that the implications of a positive bone scan in SCC can be clearly established. Despite the fact that most current trials classify patients into limited or extensive stages on the basis of bone scans, correlations between serial scan changes and tumor response have not been reported. Preliminary data from the NCI–VA group suggest that appropriate improvement or worsening in initially abnormal bone scans accompanies tumor response or progression documented in other sites in over 70 percent of instances. However, there is a definite minority of patients in whom the bone scan worsens with disease remission, or vice versa. The etiology of an initial positive scan and of its subsequent alterations in such cases remains uncertain.

Skeletal x-ray surveys are infrequently positive at the time of diagnosis in SCC.[38] The major value of bone x-rays at present, except in sites of bony symptoms, appears to be in confirming tumor involvement in areas identified by bone scan or in ruling out benign osseous processes as the cause of scan abnormality.

Central Nervous System Metastases

Central nervous system (CNS) metastases, the great majority of which are intracranial, are present in approximately 10 percent of patients with SCC at the time of diagnosis (Table 11-3). At autopsy, from 30 percent to as many as 65 percent of patients will have CNS involvement.[3,41,42] The brain is also the most common area of CNS tumor infiltration at autopsy, but leptomeningeal and epidural metastases also occur.[42] Metastases are frequently present in multiple areas of the neuraxis. In an autopsy series at the NCI–VA Medical Oncology Branch, half of the patients with intracranial tumor and all of those with leptomeningeal or epidural disease had additional metastatic involvement in another distant area of the CNS.[42] At the Finsen Institute, 33 patients with intracranial metastases from SCC were autopsied. In only half of these was disease isolated to a single area of the cranial cavity—either the cerebrum, cerebellum, pituitary, or brainstem. In the remaining patients, multiple intracranial sites were affected. Multiple metastases to different areas of the CNS can also be detected clinically. The NCI–VA group found that 15 of 76 patients with clinically apparent metastases had involvement of more than one area of the neuraxis. All but 1 patient with carcinomatous leptomeningitis and over half of the patients with epidural spinal metastases had simultaneous or subsequent involvement of an intracranial or other CNS site.[42]

Radionuclide brain scans, usually performed with ^{99m}Tc-pertechnetate or other isotopes, are useful in confirming the diagnosis of brain metastases in patients with neurologic symptoms[42] and are often employed to screen for CNS metastases in clinical trials. Several recent reports, however, have confirmed the extremely low yield of this procedure in SCC patients without neurologic symptoms,[39,42-44] and the radionuclide brain scan cannot presently be recommended as a screening procedure in clinical practice. CT of the brain is more sensitive than radionuclide scanning in documenting mass lesions in symptomatic patients. In an early report of a study of asymptomatic lung cancer patients undergoing presurgical evaluation, CT scans detected lesions not apparent on radionuclide scans in 6 percent of cases.[45] Whether this will also prove true in SCC patients prior to and during chemotherapeutic management is under active investigation.

Patients with initial bone marrow or liver metastases are at significantly increased risk for the eventual development of CNS metastases.[42] Age is another factor: younger patients may be at greater risk than those over the age of 70.[41] In the absence of effective prophylactic treatment (such as cranial irradiation), however, the major factor influencing the appearance of CNS disease is the length of survival from diagnosis. In the NCI–VA series, the actuarial cumulative probability of developing a CNS metastases by 24 mo from diagnosis was 80 percent.[42] In an earlier group of patients, who did not receive aggressive chemotherapy, the frequency of brain metastases also increased with lengthening survival.[41]

Infiltration of the leptomeninges with SCC was formerly extremely uncommon but also appears to be diagnosed with increasing frequency as a consequence of improved survival.[42,46,47] Of special clinical importance are the few patients whose sole site of initial relapse from complete remission is in the subarachnoid space.[46] Carcinomatous meningitis is documented by cytologic examination of the cerebrospinal fluid, but can occasionally be diagnosed by myelography. Unfortunately, screening lumbar punctures are of little use in detecting meningeal tumor in asymptomatic patients, as, in the NCI–VA group, they were cytologically negative in 56 consecutive patients subjected to lumbar puncture at the time of diagnosis.[42]

Epidural tumor is demonstrated by myelography. Although this is not employed as a screening procedure because of its morbidity and the expected low yield, it is important that patients in whom the diagnosis of spinal cord compression is suspected undergo myelography at the earliest possible time in order to institute therapy that will hopefully avert progressive neurologic dysfunction.[44]

Hepatic Metastases

The liver is a site that is commonly seeded with metastases from SCC. Up to 60–70 percent of patients will have hepatic involvement documented at autopsy.[3] In pretreatment staging with radionuclide scan (usually employing ^{99m}Tc-sulfur colloid) or biopsy, a 20–30 percent frequency of positive tests will be found (Table 11-3). In two large series, with pathologic confirmation of liver involvement made in most cases, the presence of hepatic metastases was strongly correlated with dissemination to the bone marrow.[31,48]

The most frequently utilized screening test for liver involvement is still the radionuclide scan, despite its definite limitations with regard to accuracy. Biochemical liver function tests, liver biopsy (made either percutaneously or under direct vision at peritoneoscopy), and, occasionally, CT of the liver are other procedures which have been employed.

The radionuclide scan cannot detect lesions less than 1–2 cm in diameter. It only rarely reveals focal defects in uptake in SCC patients in the absence of hepatomegaly or abnormal liver function tests.[39,43] In fact, in an early series in which liver involvement was assessed by direct peritoneoscopic biopsy,[49] pathologic evidence of metastases was obtained only in patients with an elevated serum alkaline phosphatase level. In a larger group of patients studied more recently,[48] hepatic tumor was only occasionally demonstrated unless at least one of three biochemical screening tests was abnormal. In half of the patients with proven hepatic metastases, elevated values were present in all three of the tests—alkaline phosphatase, lactate dehydrogenase, and transaminase (SGOT). It is nevertheless obvious that biochemical abnormalities can be caused by a non-malignant hepatic disorder, so that only procedures that are more specific for the presence of mass lesions or, more preferably, that provide histologic confirmation of liver involvement should be relied upon.

At the NCI–VA unit, the accuracy of radionuclide liver scans in comparison to liver biopsy in 69 SCC patients staged at diagnosis was 87 percent, with approximately equal numbers of false-positive and false-negative scans.[50] Others,[49,51] however, have found lesser degrees of scan accuracy, in the range of 70 percent. There is no question that peritoneoscopic biopsy can document liver metastases in some patients with normal radionuclide scans, liver function tests, and even percutaneous biopsies, and, short of laparotomy, this is the best test to employ if accurate determination of liver involvement is critical. Such accuracy may increase in importance if more data are forthcoming in support of findings in the

Southwest Oncology Group and the NCI–VA unit[52,53] that hepatic metastases are a major adverse prognostic factor in SCC.

Peritoneoscopy does have limitations in addition to its complexity and morbidity. Only lesions on the surface of the liver can be inspected, and the posterior surface is excluded from visualization. The presence of peritoneal adhesions also restricts the ability to inspect the organ fully. Even in patients in whom biopsy cannot be performed because of impaired hemostasis or for technical reasons, macroscopic evidence of liver metastases can sometimes be observed. At the Finsen Institute, tumor could be visually identified on the exposed surface of the liver in 90 percent of patients with positive biopsies.[48]

The value of CT scan of the liver in initial staging of SCC has recently been investigated.[54] Mass lesions in the liver are detected with approximately the same frequency as they are demonstrated with radionuclide scan, and the overall accuracy of the two techniques when compared to the results of hepatic biopsy is similar.[50]

Other Sites

Peripheral lymph nodes and subcutaneous nodules are sites of metastases from SCC that are relatively frequently detected by physical examination at the time of diagnosis (Table 11-3). Special staging procedures to monitor their response to therapy are not required.

Metastases to the pancreas, adrenals, and abdominal lymph nodes are found in 40–55 percent of patients at autopsy.[3] These are the most frequent areas of involvement that cannot be easily assessed with current standard staging procedures. Lymphangiography has not been utilized in SCC patients, but would not be an ideal test for a patient population with a high frequency of compromised pulmonary function. The NCI–VA group has prospectively studied CT scans of the abdomen in 72 untreated patients in an attempt to detect metastases in these retroperitoneal structures. The CT examination revealed mass lesions in 35 percent of patients, including 17 percent with adrenal or retroperitoneal node abnormalites. The remaining abnormal findings were in the liver. Most positive results, however, were found in patients known to have extensive disease by other staging tests; patients otherwise scored as having limited disease had abnormal CT scan only 10 percent of the time. Serial CT examinations demonstrated diminutions and enlargement of retroperitoneal masses that strongly correlated with tumor response and progression in other sites.

However, in only 3 patients did CT scans during therapy provide clinical information that was not suggested by changes in some other test.[50] Abdominal CT scans could play a major role in the treatment of SCC if it becomes critical to identify retroperitoneal metastases, either to construct radiotherapy portals or to ensure that patients have truly "limited" disease.

Ultrasound examination is another procedure which can identify mass lesions in both the retroperitoneum and the liver. There is little or no experience with this technique in SCC as yet, but its absence of toxicity would be a decided advantage if it should prove useful in this disease.

Conflicting results have been reported with the use of whole body radionuclide scans utilizing the "tumor-seeking" isotope gallium 67 in attempts to detect extrathoracic metastases in SCC. Investigators at the University of Chicago observed that gallium scans identified 89 percent of distant metastases found with multiple routine staging procedures in 25 SCC patients.[55] Two additional areas of occult metastases later proven by other means were discovered as well. However, Brereton et al.[27] at the National Cancer Institute reported that, although gallium 67 scans were almost always positive in the primary tumor site, only 2 of 27 extrathoracic metastases found with other radionuclide scanning techniques concentrated gallium. The explanation for this discrepancy is not clear, but could be related to technical factors.

Prognostic Factors

In SCC, as in any other human tumor, knowledge of the pretreatment characteristics of the patients included in a therapeutic trial is essential for critical interpretation of the results. Prognostic factors which have been identified or proposed in SCC are listed in Table 11-4. Stage of disease and initial ambulatory or performance status are probably the dominant factors. Each influences response to therapy, survival, or both, with fully ambulatory patients and those with limited disease more likely to experience superior results[8,9,12,14,56] when identical treatment is administered to all patients regardless of stage. Occasionally, stage of disease has been found to predict only survival, without stage-related response differences being observed.[16,57] Even within a given stage, performance status is an important prognostic variable that affects response rate and survival.[8,9] These two important prognostic characteristics do not occur independently, however, as patients with greater impairment of performance status are more likely to have extensive disease.[8,9,12] At the NCI–VA unit,

Table 11-4
Prognostic Factors in SCC Patients Given Chemotherapy
with or without Irradiation

Definite
   Stage of disease (limited versus extensive)
   Performance status
   Prior chemotherapy

Probable
   Weight loss
   Liver or central nervous system metastases
   Immune status
   Prior radiotherapy

Possible, Uncertain, or Insignificant
   Ipsilateral supraclavicular node metastases and pleural effusion in limited
      disease
   Number of sites of distant metastases
   Bone marrow metastases
   Histologic subtype (lymphocyte-like or "oat cell" versus intermediate or
      fusiform/polygonal)
   Sex
   Age
   Prior pulmonary resection

we have documented that worsening performance status is associated with increasing numbers of sites of distant metastatic disease[52]; this could at least partially explain the major influence of performance status even within disease stage. The finding that patients who have previously failed one chemotherapy regimen do more poorly on subsequent treatment is virtually universal.

Weight loss at the time of diagnosis is known to affect survival negatively in both treated[58] and untreated lung cancer patients[7] of all cell types. Weight loss strongly correlated with inferior performance status in one series of SCC patients,[59] and whether this factor is influential independently of performance status and tumor burden remains to be established.

The prognostic importance of specific sites of metastases in SCC is not clearly defined. The University of Chicago group reported that limited-stage patients with supraclavicular node involvement had inferior outcomes,[60] but, in two large cooperative group studies[9,53] and at the NCI–VA unit, ipsilateral or even contralateral supraclavicular node metastases did not worsen prognosis within limited disease. Limited-stage patients with ipsilateral pleural effusion had prognoses similar to those of patients with limited disease without effusion in the Southwest Oncology Group[61] (see also Chapter 12, this monograph).

Hepatic and CNS metastases bode especially poor outcomes in both treated and untreated lung cancer patients,[7,58] and this is likely to be true in treated SCC as well. Hepatic involvement has been reported to have major adverse prognostic impact by three groups.[13,52,53] Patients with CNS metastases at diagnosis have significantly shortened median survival compared to other patients with extensive disease in many,[42,52] but not all,[62] series. At the NCI–VA unit, bone marrow, bone, and distant soft tissue metastases were without major prognostic influence.[52] The lack of adverse effect of bone marrow involvement on survival, at least in extensive disease, has been noted by other groups.[13,30,38] This was not true, however, in a group of 193 extensive-stage patients treated at the Finsen Institute,[63] especially in those patients presenting with thrombocytopenia. Several centers agree that bone marrow involvement does not significantly worsen the hematologic toxicity of initial cytotoxic chemotherapy.[30,31,63]

The overall tumor burden is the critical determinant of prognosis on chemotherapy in several responsive human cancers, such as testicular carcinoma and diffuse histiocytic lymphoma. At the NCI–VA unit, extensive-stage patients with a single site of distant metastases have survival experiences similar to those with limited disease. Moreover, overall survival is not significantly worse in extensive-stage than in limited-stage disease.[52] Prognosis clearly worsens with increasing numbers of sites of extensive disease, a factor that might be expected to correlate reasonably, but by no means precisely, with total body tumor burden. Two other preliminary studies[18,64] that address the question of whether patients with a single site of extensive disease fare better than those with multiple areas of distant metastases have conflicting results. When this issue is resolved, a more precise staging system that subdivides patients with extensive disease may well be required.

Impaired immune status, as reflected in diminished cutaneous delayed hypersensitivity or in low levels of peripheral blood lymphocytes, has been observed to predict shortened survival[65] and to correlate with more disseminated disease[66] in SCC patients treated surgically. Whether this is also true in patients given aggressive chemotherapy and whether such effects might be independent of stage and performance status remain to be documented. Tumor progression after radiotherapy probably impairs response to subsequent chemotherapy,[57] but this has been analyzed only infrequently.[8]

The histologic subtype of SCC, sex, and previous pulmonary tumor resection have occasionally been reported to influence prognosis on chemotherapy, but contradictory results have been observed for most of these factors. Patients with the lymphocyte-like or oat cell subtype were thought to fare more favorably by some investigators,[67,68] but larger series of patients treated with aggressive chemotherapy suggest that subtype has no influence on response to therapy or survival.[8,69-71] Multiple subtypes are often present in the same patient at different sites at the time of diagnosis.[69] The Eastern Cooperative Oncology Group reported that females with SCC lived longer than males,[57] but this has not been confirmed at the NCI–VA unit, the Finsen Institute,[71] or Indiana University.[12] Most centers[52,57,71] find age has no effect on survival in chemotherapy-treated patients. Primary tumor resection has been said to improve the outcome of subsequent chemotherapy.[57] Confirmation of this observation would support renewed consideration of surgical approaches to local tumor control.

Value of Staging Procedures

Utilization of staging procedures to establish stage of disease and, probably, the extent of dissemination to individual metastatic sites clearly has prognostic value in SCC. However, the staging process would be of greatest use practically if it were to aid in making therapeutic decisions. Whether patients with SCC require stage-specific treatment, such as irradiation to the primary tumor in limited-stage disease, in addition to aggressive combination chemotherapy and, perhaps, prophylactic cranial irradiation is subject to debate in the early 1980s. Several randomized trials are addressing this question, and, although some have had negative results, others are ongoing. If radiotherapy of the primary pulmonary tumor in limited disease is to be included in the standard treatment program, the systematic determination of whether a patient's tumor is of limited stage will become increasingly important.

The impressive therapeutic results of combination chemotherapy in SCC which have resulted in a four- to five-fold prolongation of median survival[1,4] (see also Chapter 15, this monograph), may lead to a renewed interest in staging procedures in the minority of patients with long-term disease-free survival. Careful pathologic restaging has been shown to be of value in determining the length of therapy in patients with Hodgkin's disease and is beginning to play a similar role at the Finsen Institute and other centers, where thorough staging procedures are employed in documenting complete disease remission prior to discontinuation of chemotherapy.[19]

There is no question that employment of staging procedures such as bone marrow examination has been of use in determining why locally directed therapies such as surgery and irradiation fail in most patients with SCC. Utilization of the staging process in the identification of sites of tumor recurrence on current treatment regimens is discussed elsewhere in this monograph. Finally, most physicians today would agree that SCC is a distinct clinicopathologic entity with a remarkably different natural history in comparison to other cell types of lung cancer. Documentation of the extent of tumor dissemination at diagnosis and during the course of therapy has had a major role in establishing the unique characteristics of SCC.

References

1. Bunn PA, Cohen MH, Ihde DC, et al: Advances in small cell bronchogenic carcinoma. Cancer Treat Rep 61:333–342, 1977
2. Matthews MJ, Kanhouwa S, Pickren J, et al: Frequency of residual and metastatic tumor in patients undergoing curative surgical resection of lung cancer. Cancer Chemother Rep (Part 3) 4(2):63–67, 1973
3. Matthews MJ: Problems in morphology and behaviour of bronchopulmonary malignant disease, in Israel L, Chahanian P (eds): Lung Cancer: Natural History, Prognosis, and Therapy. New York, Academic Press, 1976, pp 23–62
4. Greco FA, Einhorn LH, Richardson RL, et al: Small cell lung cancer: Progress and perspectives. Sem Oncol 5:323–335, 1978
5. Mountain CF, Carr DT, Anderson WAD: A system for the clinical staging of lung cancer. Am J Roentgenol 120:130–138, 1974
6. Mountain CF: Clinical biology of small cell bronchogenic carcinoma: Relationship to surgical therapy. Sem Oncol 5:272–279, 1978
7. Zelen M: Keynote address on biostatistics and data retrieval. Cancer Chemother Rep (Part 3): 4 (2):31–42, 1973
8. Livingston RB, Moore TN, Heilbrun L, et al: Small cell carcinoma of the lung: Combined chemotherapy and radiation. Ann Intern Med 88:194–199, 1978
9. Maurer LH, Tulloh M, Weiss RB, et al: A randomized combined modality trial in small cell carcinoma of the lung: Comparison of combination chemotherapy–radiation therapy versus cyclophosphamide–radiation therapy, effects of maintenance chemotherapy and prophylactic whole brain irradiation. Cancer 45:30–39, 1980
10. Hansen HH, Dombernowsky P, Hansen M, et al: Chemotherapy of advanced small cell anaplastic carcinoma: Superiority of a four-drug combination to a three-drug combination. Ann Intern Med 89:177–181, 1978

11. Cohen MH, Ihde DC, Bunn PA, et al: Cyclic alternating combination chemotherapy for small cell bronchogenic carcinoma. Cancer Treat Rep 63:163–170, 1979

12. Einhorn LH, Bond WH, Hornback W, et al: Long term results in combined modality treatment of small cell carcinoma of the lung. Sem Oncol 5:309–313, 1978

13. Holoye PY, Samuels ML, Lanzotti VJ, et al: Combination chemotherapy and radiation therapy for small cell carcinoma. JAMA 237:1221–1224, 1977

14. Johnson RE, Brereton HD, Kent CH: "Total" therapy for small cell carcinoma of the lung. Ann Thorac Surg 25:509–515, 1978

15. Eagan RT, Maurer LH, Forcier RJ, et al: Small cell carcinoma of the lung: Staging, paraneoplastic syndromes, treatment, and survival. Cancer 33:527–532, 1974

16. Lowenbraun S, Bartolucci A, Smalley RV, et al: The superiority of combination chemotherapy over single agent chemotherapy in small cell lung carcinoma. Cancer 44:406–413, 1979

17. Petrovich Z, Ohanian M, Cox J: Clinical research on the treatment of locally advanced lung cancer. Cancer 42:1129–1134, 1978

18. Reed RC, Livingston RB: Prognostic significance of pre-treatment variables in small cell carcinoma of the lung. Proc Am Assoc Cancer Res ASCO 18:307, 1977

19. Hansen M, Hansen HH, Dombernowsky P: Long-term survival in small cell carcinoma of the lung. JAMA 244:247–250, 1980

20. Cohen MH, Matthews MJ: Small cell bronchogenic carcinoma: A distinct clinicopathologic entity. Sem Oncol 5:234–243, 1978

21. Miller WE: Roentgenographic manifestations of lung cancer, in Straus MJ (ed): Lung Cancer: Clinical Diagnosis and Treatment. New York, Grune & Stratton, 1977, pp 129–136

22. Underwood GH, Hooper RG, Axelbaum SP, et al: Computed tomographic scanning of the thorax in the staging of bronchogenic carcinoma. N Engl J Med 300:777–778, 1979

23. Salyer WR, Eggleston JC, Erozan YS: Efficacy of pleural needle biopsy and pleural fluid cytopathology in the diagnosis of malignant neoplasm involving the pleura. Chest 67:536–539, 1975

24. Aranda C, Sidhu G, Sasso LA, et al: Transbronchial lung biopsy in the diagnosis of lymphangitic carcinomatosis. Cancer 42:1995–1998, 1978

25. Ihde DC, Cohen MH, Bernath AM, et al: Serial fiberoptic bronchoscopy during chemotherapy for small cell carcinoma of the lung: Early detection of patients at high risk of relapse. Chest 74:531–536, 1978

26. Goldberg EM: Mediastinoscopy in assessment of lung cancer, in Straus MJ (ed): Lung Cancer: Clinical Diagnosis and Treatment. New York, Grune & Stratton, 1977, pp 113–127

27. Brereton HD, Line BR, Londer HN, et al: Gallium scans for staging of small cell lung cancer. JAMA 240:666–667, 1978

28. Mintz U, DeMeester TR, Golomb HM, et al: Sequential staging in bronchogenic carcinoma. Chest 76:653–657, 1979

29. Hansen HH, Muggia FM: Staging of inoperable patients with bronchogenic carcinoma with special reference to bone marrow examination and peritoneoscopy. Cancer 30:1395–1401, 1972

30. Eagan RT, Maurer H, Forcier RJ, et al: Combination chemotherapy and radiation therapy in small cell carcinoma of the lung. Cancer 32:371–379, 1973

31. Ihde DC, Simms EB, Matthews MJ, et al: Bone marrow metastases in small cell carcinoma of the lung: Frequency, description, and influence on chemotherapeutic toxicity and prognosis. Blood 53:677–686, 1979

32. Bagley CM, Roth GJ: Dubious value of marrow biopsy in small cell lung carcinoma. Proc Am Assoc Cancer Res ASCO 17:198, 1976

33. Hirsch F, Hansen HH, Dobernowsky P, et al: Bone marrow examination in the staging of small cell anaplastic carcinoma of the lung with special reference to subtyping: An evaluation of 203 consecutive cases. Cancer 39:2563–2567, 1977

34. Gutierrez AC, Vincent RG, Sandberg AA, et al: Evaluation of sternal bone marrow aspiration for detection of tumor cells in patients with bronchogenic carcinoma. J Thorac Cardiovasc Surg 77:392–395, 1979

35. Hirsch FR, Hansen HH, Hainau, B: Bilateral bone-marrow examination in small cell anaplastic carcinoma of the lung. Acta Path Microbiol Scand Sect A 87:59–62, 1979

36. Napoli LD, Hansen HH, Muggia FM, et al: The incidence of osseous involvement in lung cancer, with special reference to the development of osteoblastic changes. Radiology 108:17–21, 1973

37. Ejeckam GC, Sogbein SK, McLeish WA: Carcinocythemia due to metastatic oat cell carcinoma of the lung. Can Med Assoc J 120:336–338, 1979

38. Hansen HH: Bone Metastases in Lung Cancer: A Clinical Study in 200 Consecutive Patients with Bronchogenic Carcinoma and Its Therapeutic Implications for Small Cell Carcinoma. Copenhagen, Munksgaard, 1974, pp 79; 126

39. Lyman GH, Williams CC: Evaluation of the extent of disease in un-

differentiated small cell bronchogenic carcinoma (USCBC). Clin Res 27:389A, 1979

40. Hooper RG, Beechler CR, Johnson MC: Radioisotope scanning in the initial staging of bronchogenic carcinoma. Am Rev Resp Dis 118:279–286, 1978

41. Burgess RE, Burgess VF, Dibella NJ: Brain metastases in small cell carcinoma of the lung. JAMA 242:2084–2086, 1979

42. Nugent JL, Bunn PA, Matthews MJ, et al: CNS metastases in small cell bronchogenic carcinoma: Increasing frequency and changing pattern with lengthening survival. Cancer 44:1885–1893, 1979

43. Wittes RE, Yeh SDJ: Indications for liver and brain scans: Screening tests for patients with oat cell carcinoma of the lung. JAMA 238:506–507, 1977

44. Bunn PA, Nugent JL, Matthews MJ: Central nervous system metastases in small cell bronchogenic carcinoma. Sem Oncol 5:314–322, 1978

45. Jacobs L, Kinkel WR, Vincent RG: "Silent" brain metastases from lung carcinoma determined by computerized tomography. Arch Neurol 34:690–693, 1977

46. Brereton HD, O'Donnell JF, Kent CH, et al: Spinal meningeal carcinomatosis in small-cell carcinoma of the lung. Ann Intern Med 88:517–519

47. Aisner J, Aisner SC, Ostrow S, et al: Meningeal carcinomatosis from small cell carcinoma of the lung: Consequence of improved survival. Acta Cytol 23:292–296, 1979

48. Dombernowsky P, Hirsch F, Hansen H, et al: Peritoneoscopy in the staging of 190 patients with small-cell anaplastic carcinoma of the lung with special reference to subtyping. Cancer 41:2008–2012, 1978

49. Margolis R, Hansen HH, Muggia FM, et al: Diagnosis of liver metastases in bronchogenic carcinoma. Cancer 34:1825–1829, 1974

50. Ihde DC, Dunnick NR, Johnston-Early A, et al: Abdominal computed tomography in small cell lung cancer: Assessment of extent of disease and response to therapy. Clin Res 28:416A, 1980

51. Van Houtte P, De Jager R: Correlation between liver scintigraphy and peritoneoscopy in small cell carcinoma of the lung. (Unpublished data)

52. Ihde DC, Makuch RW, Cohen MH, et al: Prognostic implications of sites of metastases in patients with small cell carcinoma of the lung given intensive chemotherapy. Proc Am Assoc Cancer Res ASCO 20:264, 1979

53. Weiss RB, Minna JD, Glatstein E, et al: Treatment of small cell undifferentiated carcinoma of the lung: Report on National Cancer Institute meeting. Cancer Treat Rep 64:539–548, 1980

54. Dunnick NR, Ihde DC, Johnston-Early A: Abdominal CT in the evaluation of small cell carcinoma of the lung. Am J Roentgenol 133:1085–1088, 1979

55. Bitran JD, Bekerman C, Pinsky S, et al: Gallium 67 scans in small cell carcinoma. JAMA 241:1106, 1979

56. Greco FA, Richardson RL. Schulman SF, et al: Treatment of oat cell carcinoma of the lung: Complete remissions, acceptable complications, and improved survival. Br Med J 2:10–11, 1978

57. Edmonson JH, Lagakos SW, Selawry OS, et al: Cyclophosphamide and CCNU in the treatment of inoperable small cell carcinoma and adenocarcinoma of the lung. Cancer Treat Rep 60:925–932, 1976

58. Lanzotti VL, Thomas DR, Boyle LE, et al: Survival with inoperable lung cancer: An integration of prognostic variables based on simple clinical criteria. Cancer 39:303–313, 1977

59. Holoye PY, Samuels ML, Smith T, et al: Chemoimmunotherapy of small cell bronchogenic carcinoma. Cancer 42:34–40, 1978

60. Cooksey JA, Bitran JD, Desser RK, et al: Small-cell carcinoma of the lung: The prognostic significance of stage on survival. Eur J Cancer 15:859–865, 1979

61. Livingston RB: Personal communication

62. Eagan RT, Carr DT, Frytak S, et al: VP-16-213 versus polychemotherapy in patients with advanced small cell lung cancer. Cancer Treat Rep 60:949–951, 1976

63. Hirsch FR, Hansen HH: Bone marrow involvement in small cell anaplastic carcinoma of the lung: Prognostic and therapeutic aspects. Cancer 46:206–211, 1980

64. Jacobs SA, Sanitcky MJ, Stoller RG: A comparison of survival in subsets of patients with extensive small cell carcinoma of the lung. Proc Am Assoc Cancer Res ASCO 21:455, 1980

65. Israel L, Mugica J, Chahinian P: Prognosis of early bronchogenic carcinoma: Survival curves of 451 patients after resection of lung cancer in relation to the results of pre-operative tuberculin skin test. Biomedicine 19:68–72, 1973

66. Dellon AL, Potvin C, Chretien PB: Thymus-dependent lymphocyte levels in bronchogenic carcinoma: Correlations with histology, clinical stage, and clinical course after surgical treatment. Cancer 35:687–694, 1975

67. Nixon DW, Murphy GF, Sewell CW, et al: Relationship between survival and histologic type in small cell anaplastic carcinoma of the lung. Cancer 44:1045–1049, 1979

68. Hattori S, Matsudu M, Ikegami H, et al: Small cell carcinoma of the lung: Clinical and cytomorphological studies in relation to its response to chemotherapy. Gann 68:321–331, 1977

69. Carney DN, Matthews MJ, Ihde DC, et al: Influence of histologic subtype of small cell carcinoma of the lung on clinical presentation, response to therapy, and survival. J Natl Cancer Inst (in press)

70. Burdon JGW, Sinclair RA, Henderson MM: Small cell carcinoma of the lung. Chest 76:302–304, 1979

71. Hansen HH, Dombernowsky P, Hirsch FR: Staging procedures and prognostic features in small cell anaplastic bronchogenic carcinoma. Sem Oncol 5:280–287, 1978

72. King GA, Comis R, Ginsberg S, et al: Combination chemotherapy and radiotherapy in small cell carcinoma of the lung. Radiology 125:529–530, 1977

73. Abeloff MD, Ettinger DS, Baylin SB, et al: Management of small cell carcinoma of the lung. Therapy, staging and biochemical markers. Cancer 38:1394–1401, 1976

12

SMALL CELL CARCINOMA: CLINICAL MANIFESTATIONS AND BEHAVIOR WITH TREATMENT

Robert B. Livingston
Christopher J. Trauth
Richard L. Greenstreet

The major focus of this chapter is on the treated course of small cell lung cancer (SSC), especially with reference to a large study carried out by the Southwest Oncology Group from 1974–1976.[1,2] Special consideration is given to the patterns of failure after initial tumor response, because these may provide valuable clues to alterations in future management.

Presentation

The clinical manifestations of SCC at the time of diagnosis have been described in some detail in other reviews.[3,4] It is important to point out that there is no specific grouping of signs or symptoms that is characteristic for SCC as opposed to the other forms of lung cancer. The paraneoplastic syndromes that may be associated with this tumor are diverse and fascinating (see Chapter 8, this monograph), but they are not common, at least as clinical manifestations of the disease. In fact, in most patients, the presenting symptoms and signs are limited to the thorax,[4] with cough, increasing dyspnea, and superior vena caval syndrome as common findings. Hemoptysis is not as common at presentation as it is in patients with tumors that tend to grow exophytically into the bronchial lumen, such as squamous and large cell. Hypercalcemia associated with SCC is distinctly unusual,[5] and its presence should make one think of the possibility of another, coincident cause.

On chest x-ray, the tumor is usually centrally located and is most often seen as a perihilar mass lesion, sometimes with a massive "sunburst" appearance, which reflects its propensity for submucosal spread and regional lymphatic obstruction. Occasionally, there may be only mediastinal widening or bilateral hilar enlargement, symptoms which can be confused with Hodgkin's disease. Peripheral "coin" lesions are rarely SCC, but account for most of the reported cures in this disease from surgery alone.

One feature of clinical manifestations that may be changing has to do with the frequency of limited versus extensive disease (see Chapter 11, this monograph) at the time of presentation. Table 12-1 lists the frequency of limited versus extensive stage in three large, cooperative group studies that were carried out during the mid-1970s.[6–8] One would conclude from these studies that about one-third of patients have limited disease. However, in the most recently completed study by the Southwest Oncology Group (1976–1978), 47 percent of the patients were staged as "limited" by the same criteria which were previously employed.[9] If this trend is real and indicative of general experience, it presumably reflects earlier referral for treatment.

Among patients with limited disease, supraclavicular nodes were clinically positive in 20 percent in the Southwest Group experience[6] and in that of the Cancer and Leukemia Group B.[7] Limited disease at presentation is commonly thought of in terms of "hemithorax only" and "supraclavicular node positive," but there are at least two other categories to consider. One is the group of patients who have undergone complete surgical excision of the evident tumor, with no evidence of active disease at the time that they are started on radiation and/or chemotherapy. In our experience, this is 5 percent of the total. The other group, usually classed as extensive-disease patients, have pleural effusion on the same side of the chest as the primary tumor, and this is their only evidence clinically of metastatic spread. These accounted for 7 percent of our extensive-disease patients. If, however, they were reclassified as "limited," they would account for 16 percent of that category, a frequency almost equal to that of supraclavicular node presentation. There are reasons to consider such a reclassification (see the section on Survival).

Table 12-2 lists the sites of involvement at presentation among patients with extensive disease from the Southwest Group.[6] These proportions are comparable to those reported in the literature for other large se-

Table 12-1

Frequency of Limited versus Extensive Disease in Three
Group-Wide Studies

Group	Period	No. of Patients	Percentage with Limited Disease	Percentage with Extensive Disease
SWOG[6]	1974–1976	375	27	73*
CALGB[7]	1972–1976	225	47	53
SEG[8]	1974–1976	241	30	70*

Abbreviations: SWOG, Southwest Oncology Group; CALGB, Cancer and Leukemia Group
B; SEG, Southeast Group.
*Patients accepted with prior radiation therapy.

ries.[10–12] Liver and bone are commonly involved, and about 1 patient in 7
will have evidence of involvement of "only" one of these systemic sites at
the time of workup. It is noteworthy that 7 percent of our extensive-disease patients had local failure only after irradiation (not necessarily in the
irradiated field), without other evidence of metastatic disease. These represented 24 percent of those who had received prior chest x-ray therapy.
Just over one-third of all patients with extensive disease had clinical evidence of multiple systemic metastases when first seen.

Performance (functional) status was, as one might expect, better in
limited- than in extensive-disease patients. In our study 75 percent of the
limited-disease and 52 percent of the extensive-disease patients were

Table 12-2

Small Cell Lung Cancer—Sites of Involvement at
Presentation Among Extensive-Disease Patients

Site	Percentage of Patients Involved	Percentage of Patients with Isolated Involvement
Liver	32	16
Bone	30	13
Bone marrow	16	5
Brain	14	8
Skin, soft tissue, nodes	16	2
Effusion	15	7
Chest only (prior XRT)	—	7
Other	—	5
Multiple, other than primary	35	—

Source: Southwest Oncology Group, study 7415.[6]
Abbreviation: XRT, X-ray therapy.

found to be fully ambulatory (Karnofsky 8-10 or Zubrod 0-1), basically defined as out of bed during the day and able to carry on most normal activities. Comparable proportions from the large study by Cancer and Leukemia Group B are 70 percent for limited-disease and 55 percent for extensive-disease patients.[7]

Response Characteristics

In the first Southwest Group study, 41 percent of limited-disease and 16 percent of extensive-disease patients achieved a clinical (not broncho-scopically verified) complete response, defined as disappearance of all measurable disease for at least 4 wk. Comparable complete response frequency in limited-disease patients was found in the other major cooperative group study that utilized chest irradiation and chemotherapy combined, with only 10 percent of extensive-disease patients achieving complete response.[7] Complete response was noted in a smaller proportion of patients who received combination chemotherapy alone in the Southeast Group.[8] Pilot studies from single institutions have reported much higher complete response rates in certain instances (see Chapter 15, this monograph). In the Southwest Group, the overall (complete and partial) response rates were 79 percent for limited and 58 percent for extensive disease, in the final analysis of 95 response-evaluable limited-disease and 262 response-evaluable extensive-disease patients (a patient was defined as "response-evaluable" if he had the correct diagnosis and received one day of treatment). Complete response was significantly more likely in fully ambulatory patients with limited disease (48 versus 21 percent, $p < 0.05$), and complete or partial response was more likely in fully ambulatory patients with extensive disease (65 versus 46 percent, $p < 0.01$).

Complete responses were significantly longer than partial responses (medians of 48 versus 29 wk for limited and 39 versus 19 wk for extensive disease, $p = 0.001$). The duration of complete response is plotted graphically in Figure 12-1, which shows an advantage for limited-disease patients of borderline statistical significance ($p = 0.07$ by Gehan's two-tailed test). The relapse rate declines after 18 mo, but failures continue to occur (see Patterns of Failure), such that continuous remission beyond 4 yr is achieved by only 18 percent of limited-disease and 10 percent of extensive-disease patients who obtained an initial complete remission.

Table 12-3 illustrates the median duration of all remissions (complete and partial combined) from four large studies.[6,7,8,13] The range is 3.7–7 mo for extensive and 6.1–8.5 mo for limited disease.

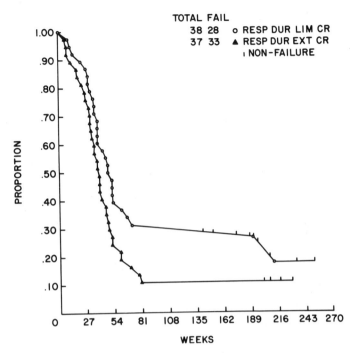

Figure 12-1. *Duration of complete response—limited versus extensive disease.*

Table 12-3
Response Duration in Representative Large Studies

Group	Type of Treatment	Category of Disease	Median Response Duration (mo)
SWOG[6]	CAV + XRT	Limited	8.5
		Extensive	7
CALGB[7]	Chemo (varied) + XRT	Limited	6.1
		Extensive	4.1
SEG[8]	CADIC ± cyclic maintenance (No XRT)	All	4.8
Hansen et al.[13]	CMC (no XRT)	Extensive	3.7
	CMC-V (no XRT)	Extensive	6.1

Abbreviations: SWOG, Southwest Oncology Group; CALCB, Cancer and Leukemia Group B; SEG, Southeast Group; CAV, cyclophosphamide, Adriamycin, and vincristine; XRT, x-ray therapy; CADIC, cyclophosphamide, Adriamycin, and decarbazine; CMC, cyclophosphamide, methotrexate, CCNU; CMC-V, cyclophosphamide, methotrexate, CCNU, vincristine.

Table 12-4
Sites of Relapse in 36 Patients with Limited Disease

Relapse Site	Patients with Complete Response or NED Status (No.)	Patients with Partial Response (No.)
Chest only	13	11
Failure in XRT Port with adequate treatment	(5)	(2)
Liver only	2	1
Brain only	2*	0
Multiple sites	4	2
Extradural only	0	1
Total	21	15

Source: Southwest Oncology Group, study 7415.
Abbreviations: NED, no evidence of disease; XRT, x-ray therapy.
*One patient underdosed (2000 rads) with posterior fossa recurrence; the other refused prophylaxis.

The time to maximal response is an important parameter for which solid data are available only from pilot studies. Almost all responses are evident after two courses of therapy (about 6 wk), including the majority of complete responses.[14–16] With the use of *alternating* combinations in extensive disease, Cohen has reported that almost half of the patients who achieved complete remission did so only after 12 wk (after two courses of the second combination). However, relapse occurred earlier and more often in the group who required 12 wk.[17]

Patterns of Failure

Limited-disease patients in the Southwest Group study had similar patterns of failure, whether they achieved complete or partial response.

Table 12-4 illustrates the specific sites of relapse in 21 complete response or no-evidence-of-disease (NED) patients and 15 partial responders. It bears emphasis that two-thirds of the relapses were initially in the chest alone, and at least 7 of 24 chest relapses were in the irradiated field, after delivery of 4500 rads by a split-course technique (however, the last 1500 rads was delayed by 6 wk following completion of the first 3000). Not shown in Table 12-4 is the fact that 12 of 48 failures after response (25 percent) were *not* from clinical relapse: 9 in the complete response and 3 in the partial response category. Of the 9, 2 had no evidence of tumor at

Table 12-5
Sites of Relapse in 75 Patients with Extensive Disease

Relapse Site	Patients with Complete Response (No.)	Patients with Partial Response (No.)
Chest only	5	13
Single site of prior *metastatic* involvement	7	10
Site(s) of prior involvement and new site(s)	5	10
Multiple sites of prior involvement	5	3
New site(s) only	5	12
CNS, non brain	(0)	(4)
Total	27	48

Source: Southwest Oncology Group, study 7415.

autopsy, after sudden deaths for which a definite cause was not established; 2 died of radiation pneumonitis after overdoses; and 1 developed a second, squamous lung cancer more than 4 yr into the study, which led to his death. The other deaths were related to aspiration pneumonia or other medical diseases. Of the 3 nontumor deaths in the partial response category, 2 had fatal radiation pneumonitis.

Extensive-disease patients also had similar recurrence patterns, regardless of whether complete or partial response was achieved (see Table 12-5). Of the 31 complete and 57 partial responders for whom data were available, 13 (15 percent) died without clinical evidence of recurrent disease. Among those who relapsed, 24 percent failed initially in the chest alone. Failure at a single site (chest or prior metastatic involvement) occurred in 47 percent. Relapse in isolated nonbrain CNS sites (meningeal, epidural) accounted for 5 percent of all and 11 percent of "new" recurrences (i.e., in areas where prior disease had not been identified). A total of 24 patients had documented relapse in multiple sites (32 percent).

In this program, which involved 3000 rads to the primary site and mediastinum over 2 wk after delivery of combination chemotherapy, the occurrence of initial "chest only" relapse was 1 in 4, the same as the incidence of "chest only" presentation in patients who had been given radiation therapy to the primary site before entry on the study. In our most recent study, on the other hand, in which radiation therapy to the chest was not administered to patients with extensive disease, the incidence of "chest only" failure is greater than 50 percent, with comparable response duration (R. Livingston and J. Mira, unpublished data). This may indicate greater ability of the more recent, aggressive chemotherapy to cope with systemic micrometastases, coupled with poor local control because irradiation at the primary site was deleted.

In the analysis of recurrence for patients in the Cancer and Leukemia Group B study,[7] 25 of 43 patients with limited disease (58 percent) had initial failure in the lung, mediastinum, or supraclavicular·lymph nodes. Radiation therapy involved a dose of 3200 rads in 10 treatments over a period of 12 days. Thus, both of the initial, large cooperative group combined-modality studies demonstrated that a majority of patients with limited disease will relapse initially in the chest.

In the pilot study of alternating, cyclic combination chemotherapy by Cohen et al.,[17] 71 percent of limited-disease and 56 percent of extensive-disease complete-response patients relapsed in the chest alone. There was no radiation therapy in their program. In a study that combined radiation to the chest with chemotherapy,[18] McMahon et al. observed that 60 percent of limited-disease and 20 percent of extensive-disease patients had relapse in the chest alone, and that median time to such relapse was twice as long (540 versus 270 days) in patients who received greater than 4000 rads to the chest, compared with those who received only 3000.

The frequency of de novo brain relapse has been markedly reduced in studies which employed elective or "prophylactic" whole brain irradiation.[19] Both limited- and extensive-disease patients demonstrated a higher recurrence rate in brain, in the absence of such treatment.[7] In spite of this, neither *median* survival nor the frequency of brain metastases at autopsy have been as yet altered by elective irradiation of the brain. These observations are explained by the facts that (1) the vast majority of patients still relapse, and do so in systemic sites; and (2) once such relapse has occurred, there is nothing to prevent "reseeding" of the brain and CNS.

Survival

The survival of all patients with limited disease as compared with all patients with extensive disease from the initial SWOG study, updated through March 1, 1980, is plotted in Figure 12-2. The difference is obvious and highly statistically significant ($p = 0.001$ by Gehan's one-tailed test). The change in slope of the survival curves between 1 yr and 18 mo reflects a decreasing hazard of death per unit time, and, indeed, about 10 percent of those with limited and 2 percent of those with extensive disease are long-term survivors. If one looks only at those with complete response (Fig. 12-3), the superiority of limited-disease patients is again apparent,

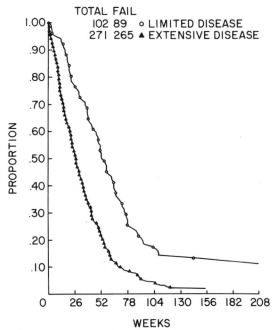

Figure 12-2. *Duration of survival—limited versus extensive disease.*

both graphically and statistically ($p = 0.03$). The "break" in the survival curves appears to be at about 2 yr, after which the hazard rate decreases sharply: one-fourth of limited-disease and one-tenth of extensive-disease patients achieving CR are projected to be alive at 5 yr. Pretreatment performance status is also an important predictor of survival for both limited-disease and extensive-disease patients (Figs. 12-4 and 12-5): the respective p values are 0.006 and 0.001.

The survival of three groups of patients, one usually considered extensive and the others usually considered limited, is plotted in Figure 12-6. In fact, that of the small group with ipsilateral pleural effusion as their only evidence of metastatic spread is no different from the others (supraclavicular nodes clinically positive and "hemithorax only"), and there are no significant differences among the three.

We compared the survival of extensive-disease patients with multiple clinically evident sites of involvement at the time of presentation to that of those who had only one site, or who had chest involvement after previous

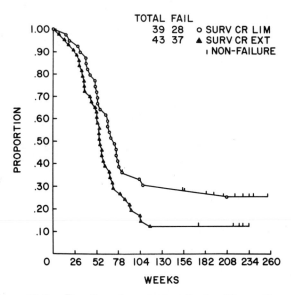

Figure 12-3. *Duration of survival, patients with complete response—limited versus extensive disease.*

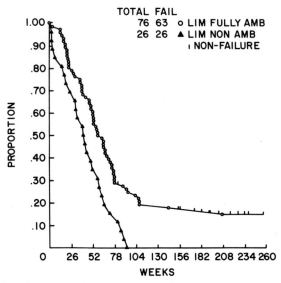

Figure 12-4. *Duration of survival by performance status—limited disease.*

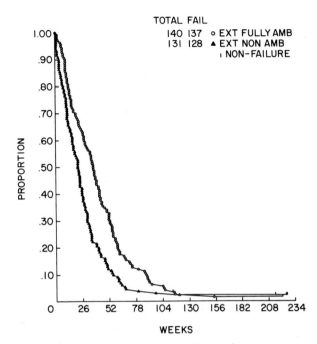

Figure 12-5. *Duration of survival by performance status—extensive disease.*

radiation therapy as the sole manifestation of disease. Although there is no statistical evidence of a difference by Gehan's test ($p = 0.26$, one-tailed test), it is of interest that none of the long-term survivors (3 yr or more) are in the multiple-sites group (see Fig. 12-7).

Survival from the time of relapse is plotted in Figures 12-8 and 12-9. It is clear from these graphs that, once the disease has become clinically recurrent, neither the initial stage nor the quality of response has any impact on survival. Median survivals from the time of relapse were 7–8 wk in these patients, reflecting the lack of effective "salvage" therapy. These results are remarkably similar to the survival figures for patients with extensive disease on supportive care alone.[20]

Overall, the survivals observed, and the importance of stage and performance status are similar to the reports of others for combined modality treatment[7] or chemotherapy used alone.[17] The apparent significance of "pleural effusion only" presentation, the lack of importance of single versus multiple metastatic sites in extensive disease, and the very short documented survival from recurrence are new observations from the SWOG experience.

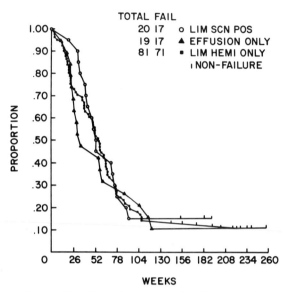

Figure 12-6. *Duration of survival—hemithorax only versus effusion versus supraclavicular nodes positive.*

Conclusions and Implications

Because staging is a maneuver designed to segregate prognostically different groups into comparable subgroups, the data presented here suggest that patients who present with a pleural effusion as their only evidence of metastatic spread should be considered as having limited, rather than extensive, disease. This observation should be confirmed by others before it is widely accepted as fact. There appears to be no need to stratify separately for supraclavicular nodal status, confirming previous reports by others.[7] The tumor–nodes–metastasis (TNM) system presently accepted for the surgical staging of lung cancer has been almost irrelevant to the problem of SCC, since the vast majority of patients, comprising subgroups with very different prognoses, are considered Stage 3. The system may become more relevant, however, if surgery is reintroduced as an effective modality for cytoreduction at the primary tumor site.

It is clear from the data presented and reviewed here that the *clinical* definition of complete response allows one to identify a cohort of patients with distinctly superior prognosis, and that, with rare exceptions, this cohort accounts for the long-term survivors, whether the initial stage was limited or extensive. For considerations relevant to the use of more so-

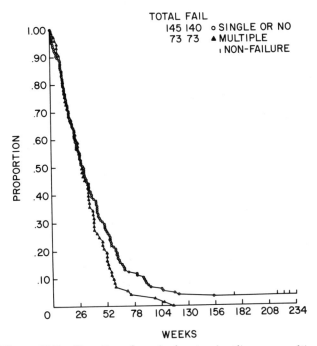

Figure 12-7. *Duration of survival, extensive disease—multiple sites versus other.*

phisticated staging techniques, including repeat bronchoscopy, see Chapter 11 of this monograph.

Analysis of the patterns of relapse reveals that failure to control disease at the primary site is the major problem in limited disease. An obvious approach for improving local control is the attempt to improve radiation therapy. Current efforts in the Southwest Group are focused on the question of "involved field" versus "original extent of tumor" portals after delivery of four courses of combination chemotherapy. Other groups are exploring the role of high—LET (particle) irradiation or the addition of misonidazole to photons. And certain single institutions have begun to explore surgical debulking after delivery of chemotherapy.

In extensive disease, our earlier experience with combined modality therapy indicated that the majority of relapses occurred at systemic sites, although careful analysis reveals that 47 percent failed at a single site of previous known involvement. Both Cohen's experience[17] and our own recent, unpublished experience with intensive, systemic chemotherapy given without chest irradiation, indicate that the relapse rate in the chest

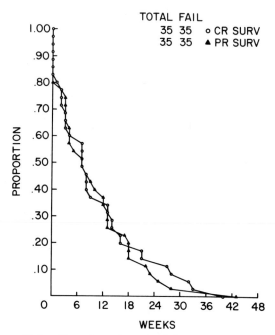

Figure 12-8. *Duration of survival from time of relapse—complete response versus partial response.*

rises to 50 percent or more when x-ray treatment to that site is deleted, with similar time to relapse. In other words, it appears that more effective systemic chemotherapy does delay the appearance of systemic metastases, but cannot prevent the rapid emergence of uncontrolled tumor at the primary site. These observations suggest that "consolidation" radiation therapy should be administered, at least to the chest and possibly (when feasible) to other sites of known, prior bulk disease, at the completion of induction chemotherapy. Other approaches directed toward better control of bulk disease in the chest might include "cytoreductive" surgery.

The role of elective whole brain irradiation in the prevention of relapse isolated to that site has been reviewed elsewhere,[19] and the current analysis of our data only confirms the continued efficacy of this approach: There have been no further brain relapses since the last full-scale analysis in 1977.

The survival data support the contention that a small number of limited-disease patients, and a very few classed as extensive, may have been cured by the therapy reviewed.

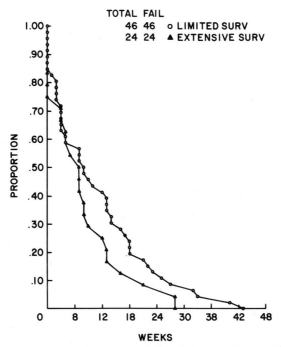

Figure 12-9. *Duration of survival from time of relapse—limited versus extensive disease.*

References

1. Livingston RB, Moore TN, Heilbrun L, et al: Small-cell carcinoma of the lung: Combined chemotherapy and radiation. A Southwest Oncology Group Study. Ann Intern Med 88:194–199, 1978

2. Moore TN, Livingston RB, Heilbrun L, et al: The effectiveness of prophylactic brain irradiation in small cell carcinoma of the lung. A Southwest Oncology Group Study. Cancer 41:2149–2153, 1978

3. Watson W, Berg J: Oat cell lung cancer. Cancer 15:759–768, 1962

4. Kato Y, Ferguson TB, Bennett DE, et al: Oat cell carcinoma of the lung. A review of 138 cases. Cancer 23:517–524, 1969

5. Bender RA, Hansen H: Hypercalcemia in bronchogenic carcinoma. A prospective study of 200 patients. Ann Intern Med 80:205–209, 1974

6. The present series (SWOG).

7. Maurer LH, Tulloh M, Weiss RB, et al: A randomized combined modality trial in small cell carcinoma of the lung. Cancer 45:30–39, 1980

8. Lowenbraun S, Bartolucci A, Smalley RV, et al: The superiority of

combination chemotherapy over single agent chemotherapy in small cell lung carcinoma. Cancer 44:406–413, 1979

9. McCracken J, White J, Reed R, et al: Combination chemotherapy, radiotherapy, and immunotherapy for oat cell carcinoma of the lung. Proc AACR-ASCO 19:395, 1978

10. Hirsch F, Hansen HH, Dombernowsky P, et al: Bone-marrow examination in the staging of small-cell anaplastic carcinoma of the lung with special reference to subtyping. An evaluation of 203 consecutive patients. Cancer 39:2563–2567, 1977

11. Hansen H, Dombernowsky P, Hirsch F: Staging procedures and prognostic features in small cell anaplastic bronchogenic carcinoma. Sem Oncol 5:280–288, 1978

12. Simma EB, Ihde DE, Matthews MJ, et al: Therapeutic implications of bone marrow involvement in small cell carcinoma of the lung. Proc AACR-ASCO 19:393, 1978

13. Hansen HH, Dombernowsky P, Hansen M, et al: Superiority of a four-drug combination to a three-drug combination. Ann Intern Med 89:177–181, 1978

14. Holoye P, Samuels M, Lanzotti V, et al: Combination chemotherapy and radiation therapy for small cell carcinoma. JAMA 237:1221–1224, 1977

15. Cohen MH, Creaven PJ, Fossieck BE: Intensive chemotherapy of small cell bronchogenic carcinoma. Cancer Treat Rep 61:349–352, 1977

16. Cohen MH, Ihde DE, Fossieck BE: Cyclic alternating combination chemotherapy of small cell bronchogenic carcinoma. Proc AACR–ASCO 19:359, 1978

17. Cohen MH, Ihde DE, Bunn P, et al: Cyclic alternating combination chemotherapy for small cell bronchogenic carcinoma. Cancer Treat Rep 63:163–170, 1979

18. McMahon LJ, Herman TS, Manning MR, et al: Patterns of relapse in patients with small cell carcinoma of the lung treated with adriamycin-cyclophosphamide chemotherapy and radiation therapy. Cancer Treat Rep 63:359–362, 1979

19. Livingston RB: Approaches to the control of central nervous system metastases in patients with small cell carcinoma of the lung, in: Rozencweig M, Muggia F (eds): Progress in Cancer Research and Therapy (vol 11) New York, Raven Press, 1978 pp 587–592

20. Zelen M: Keynote address on biostatistics and data retrieval. Cancer Chemother Rep 4:31–34, 1973

13

EXTRAPULMONARY SMALL CELL CARCINOMA

Mehmet F. Fer
Robert M. Levenson, Jr.
Martin H. Cohen
F. Anthony Greco

Since the recognition of small cell lung cancer as a rather distinct clinical and pathologic entity, small cell cancers in various organs other than the lung have attracted attention. Primary small cell cancers of the lung (SCC) and of several extrapulmonary sites may or may not be analogous with respect to their biology, cell(s) of origin, and response to therapy. If all these neoplasms are derived from similar cells found in several locations, such as the amine precursor uptake and decarboxylation (APUD) cells, then the natural history and principles of management of all these neoplasms may be similar. Extrapulmonary small cell carcinoma is rare, and most of the information is in the form of isolated case reports, many of which appeared in the literature before the more routine use of electron microscopy and combination chemotherapy.

Extrapulmonary small cell carcinomas may represent a heterogeneous group of neoplasms, and the similarities in their histologic appearance may not correlate with their biologic behavior. Occasionally it may be difficult to differentiate small cell carcinomas from atypical carcinoid tumors and from poorly differentiated tumors of other histologic varieties, particularly by light microscopy alone. Many of our patients with extrapulmonary small cell cancers, and most cases reported in the literature, were recognized by light microscopy. Further subsets of patients may be

301

defined by the increased use of electron microscopy and the detection of tumor markers in the peripheral blood and in the tumor cells. It is hoped that a better understanding of small cell cancers arising in unusual sites may provide clues to their cells of origin and to improved therapy. In this chapter we report on our experience with extrapulmonary small cell carcinomas seen at two institutions and summarize the other patients reported in the literature.

Review of Patient Experience

Over a period of 6 yr, 400 patients with a histologic diagnosis of small cell carcinoma have been evaluated at Vanderbilt University Medical Center and the National Cancer Institute–Veterans Administration Medical Oncology Branch. Of these, 20 (5 percent) had no detectable pulmonary lesion. In addition to standard chest radiographs, some patients had chest tomography and most had fiberoptic bronchoscopy. In 5 of 6 patients who had an autopsy there was no evidence of a lung primary, and this is relatively strong evidence that the tumor did arise outside the lung. It is possible that some of these patients could have had an occult bronchial primary, but this was detected neither at diagnosis nor at a later date in any of the patients.

The characteristics of the 20 patients who presented with extrapulmonary small cell carcinomas are outlined in Table 13-1. There were 16 males and 4 females, with a median age of 57 yr (range 28–72). The most common presenting sites were in the gastrointestinal system (esophagus in 2, pancreas in 2, stomach in 1) or the head and neck area (neck mass in 4, parotid gland in 1). Two patients had genitourinary tumors (uterine cervix and prostate), and 1 patient presented with a chest wall mass. The remaining 7 patients had metastatic disease without any apparent primary site. Most patients had a staging work-up, including liver scan, bone scan, brain scan, and bilateral posterior iliac crest bone marrow aspirates and biopsies. Twelve patients had disease clinically confined to one anatomic region encompassable in a single radiation port (limited stage), while others had extensive-stage disease. This is unlike patients with lung primaries, two-thirds of whom have extensive-stage disease at initial diagnosis.[1,2] There were no other general differences in the patient characteristics in our study group from those of patients with SCC of the lung. Electron microscopy was performed on tumors from 7 patients, and neurosecretory type granules were seen in each instance.

In general, treatment was similar to that given to the larger group of

Table 13-1
Clinical and Pathological Characteristics of 20 Patients with Extrapulmonary Small Cell Carcinoma

Patient No.	Age	Sex	Presenting Site	Neurosecretory Granules on EM	Metastatic Sites at DX	Therapy*	Response†	Survival (Months after Starting Therapy)	Autopsy
1	55	F	Chest wall	Yes	None	CAPO after complete excision	Not evaluable—lesion recurred at 14 mo	22+	
2	56	M	Esophagus	Not done	R supraclav. nodes	CMC-VAP; Ifosphamide + VP-16	CR—no tumor by esophagoscopy	11	Died in accident; autopsy showed no tumor
3	30	M	Esophagus	Not done	None	Surgery, adjuvant CAV	Not evaluable	6+	
4	60	M	Pancreas	Not done	Liver	CAV; VP-16; Hexamethyl-melamine, MTX	PR—6-mo duration	9	Metastases to liver, brain, lung
5	48	F	Pancreas	Not done	Liver	CAV	PR—3-mo duration	4	No autopsy
6	69	M	Stomach	Yes	None	CAV	PR—7-mo duration	17	No autopsy
7	68	M	Parotid	Not done	None	Excision BX; L rad neck dissection; radiation to local lesion; CCNU	NR	1½	Metastases to mediastinal and abdominal nodes, liver, spleen, adrenals

(continued)

303

Table 13-1 (*continued*)

Patient No.	Age	Sex	Presenting Site	Neurosecretory Granules on EM	Metastatic Sites at DX	Therapy*	Response†	Survival (Months after Starting Therapy)	Autopsy
8	28	F	Uterine cervix	Yes	None	Radiotherapy to local area; CAV later	CR—24 mo duration after RT; NR to CAV	31	No autopsy
9	61	M	Prostate	Not done	Bone	Diethylstilbesterol, cytoxan	PR—3+-mo duration	6+	
10	49	M	Cervical lymph node	Not done	None	Local radiotherapy; CMC-VAP	Not evaluable "adjuvant" chemotherapy; no recurrence	8+	
11	61	M	Neck mass adjacent parotid	Not done	None	Radiotherapy	CR—4 mo duration	4	Died of inflammatory lung disease; no autopsy
12	61	M	Neck mass	Not done	None	CAV	CR—10+-mo duration	11+	
13	62	M	Neck mass	Not done	None	CAV, radiotherapy	CR—8+-mo duration	9+	
14	50	M	Subcutaneous nodules	Yes	None	Radiotherapy to lesion and groin nodes; CMC-VAP; VP-16	PR	9 (57 from DX)	Metastases to left thigh and groin, pleura, abdominal nodes, liver, pancreas, adrenal

15	43	F	Subcutaneous	Yes	Bone	CAV; methotrexate, VP-16, hexamethylmelamine	CR—17 mo duration	24	Brain and liver metastases
16	60	M	Subcutaneous nodules	Not done	None	CAV	PR—6 mo duration	9	Died in accident; no autopsy
17	57	M	Cervical spine epidural spine	Not done	None	Surgery, radiotherapy	CR—23+ mo duration	24+	Small nests of tumor in lungs, bone marrow, vertebral bodies
18	57	M	Widespread metastases at DX—? primary lesion	Not done	Brain, liver, bone marrow	CAPO; whole-brain radiotherapy	NR	2	
19	54	M	Widespread metastases at DX—? primary lesion	Yes	Cervical mass, R and L axiliary nodes, subcutaneous nodule, + liver scan, hepatomegaly	Cranial radiotherapy; CMC-VAP; VP-16	PR—6 mo	8	No autopsy
20	72	M	Widespread metastases at DX—? primary lesion	Yes	Liver, bone	CMC-VAP	NR	4	Tumor found in left upper lobe of lung involving pleura, parenchyma, apical post. bronchus, liver, ant. chest wall, peribronch. hepatic nodes.

*CMC-VAP, Cytoxan, methotrexate, CCNU alternating with vincristine, Adriamycin, and procarbazine[1]; CAPO, cytoxan, Adriamycin, VP-16, and vincristine; CAV, cytoxan, Adriamycin, and vincristine.[3]

†CR, complete response; PR, partial response; NR, no response.

patients with lung primaries. Two patients received local therapy alone, and 18 were given combination chemotherapy. The details of these therapeutic regimens have been described elsewhere.[1,3] Of the 18 patients treated with combination chemotherapy, 3 were treated with chemotherapy on an "adjuvant" basis because they were considered to be at high risk for recurrence. Two of these patients remain free of recurrence at over 6 and 8 mo, respectively, and the third patient relapsed at 14 mo. Of the remaining 15 patients who were evaluable for response, there were 4 complete responses, 7 partial responses, and 4 with no response, for an overall response rate of 73 percent. The median duration of response was 7 mo, and median survival for responders was 9 mo, while all nonresponders died within 4 mo. Several patients are described below in further detail.

Patient 5. M.W., a 48-year-old female, presented with left lower quadrant pain. Physical examination disclosed a large mass in her left abdomen, which had a cystic center as seen by ultrasound. Her chest x-ray was normal. Intravenous pyelogram and barium enema were consistent with an extrinsic mass effect. She had an exploratory laporotomy, which showed that the mass was arising from the tail of the pancreas, with multiple omental implants and liver metastases. Biopsies of the mass revealed small cell carcinoma. A bone scan, brain scan, and bone marrow were normal. Liver scan showed a filling defect compatible with a metastatic lesion. She was treated with cyclophosphamide, doxorubicin, and vincristine, resulting in a partial response. She continues to do well 4 mo after therapy was instituted.

Patient 6. W.B., a 69-year-old man, was hospitalized with a 3-mo history of weight loss and epigastric pain. A radiographic study of the upper gastrointestinal tract revealed prominent gastric folds and a large gastric ulcer was found at endoscopy. Physical examination was unremarkable except for mild cachexia and suggestion of a midepigastric mass. Parenteral nutrition was instituted and he was eventually taken to surgery, at which time a partial gastrectomy was performed. The histology was compatible with small cell anaplastic carcinoma, with involvement of the regional lymph nodes and implants on the omentum. Electron microscopy showed neurosecretorylike granules in the tumor cell cytoplasm. Further evaluation included chest x-rays, bronchoscopy, bone, liver, and brain scans; and bilateral posterior iliac crest bone marrow biopsies, all of which were negative for tumor. He was treated with cyclophosphamide 1000 mg/m^2, doxorubicin 40 mg/m^2, and vincristine 1 mg/m^2. He received three cycles of therapy, during which he felt well and had no evidence of

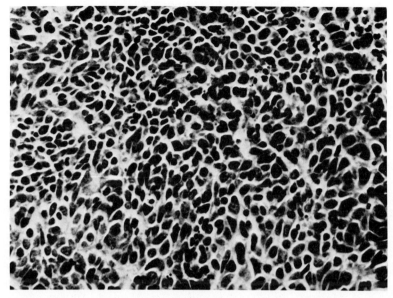

Figure 13-1. *Photomicrograph of cervical biopsy sample demonstrating small cell carcinoma. Hematoxylin and eosin. Original magnification × 250.*

disease progression in his abdomen. He was lost to follow-up for 5 mo, when he was hospitalized in another institution with weakness, confusion, and abdominal pain. He had developed hepatomegaly and a large abdominal mass, which was treated with radiotherapy. His overall condition steadily deteriorated with increasing weakness, diarrhea, and tachypnea, and he died in February 1978.

Patient 8.   G.D., 28-yr-old female, presented with vaginal bleeding during the 25th week of pregnancy, in June 1975. On physical examination, there was a polypoid lesion in the uterine cervix, biopsies of which showed small cell undifferentiated carcinoma (Fig. 13-1). Electron microscopy revealed neurosecretorylike granules in the cytoplasm (Fig. 13-2). Upon her request the therapy of her tumor was deferred until after childbirth. In the 32nd week of pregnancy, a viable infant was delivered by cesarean section, at which time several iliac lymph nodes were removed, and all 15 nodes were free of tumor. Radical surgery was not possible owing to extensive involvement of the vagina. Staging work-up, including chest x-ray, liver function tests, and IVP failed to indicate any distant spread, and she was assessed as stage II-A. Radiotherapy, both externally

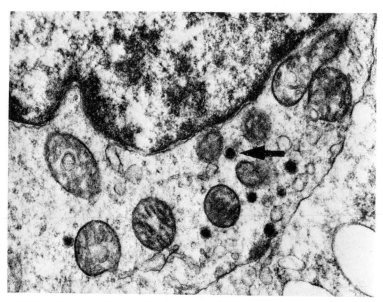

Figure 13-2. *Electronmicrograph of tumor cell from small cell cervical carcinoma, demonstrating dense, neurosecretory type granules (arrow). Original magnification ×26,600. (Courtesy of Alan D. Glick, M.D.)*

and with cesium implants, was given, resulting in complete regression as judged by pelvic examination. She did well until August 1977, when she developed spinal cord compression at the T-7 level, which was treated with laminectomy and radiotherapy. She had a palpable chest wall mass that was also visible on chest x-ray as a pleural-based mass. Biopsies of this mass and tissue obtained at laminectomy were consistent with small cell carcinoma, similar to her primary lesion. In spite of radiotherapy to the chest wall, the lesion progressed and she developed pleural effusion. She was given chemotherapy with cyclophosphamide 1000 mg/m², doxorubicin 40 mg/m², and vincristine 1 mg/m² intravenously every 3 wk without objective benefit. During this period she developed a Cushingoid appearance, hypokalemia, and elevated plasma cortisol levels without any diurnal variation. Twenty-four-hour urinary 17-ketosteroid and 17-hydroxycorticosteroid levels were elevated and were not suppressed by dexamethasone (Table 13-2). Plasma ACTH level was elevated. Immunoperoxidase stains of tumor tissue were positive for intracytoplasmic ACTH (Fig. 13-3). She was started on metyrapone and dexamethasone in an attempt to block her adrenals while supplying physiologic amounts of corticosteroid. Her chest wall mass and pleural effusion progressed in

Table 13-2
Summary of Endocrine Studies—Patient 8, G.D.

Date	Na† (mEq/liter)	K† (mEq/liter)	HCO₃ (mEq/liter)	Plasma Cortisol (μg/dl)*	24-hr Urine 17-OH Corticosteroids (mg/g creatinine)†	24-hr Urine 17-ketosteroids (mg/g creatinine)‡	ACTH (pg/ml)§
11/77	142	3.8	31	37 (6 AM)	—	—	—
2/78	138	3.3	29	46 (6 AM)	9.9 10.0	15.5 13.1	220
2/78 (after dexamethasone 0.5 mg p.o. q-6-hr × 8 doses)	—	—	—	37 (6 AM) 22 (6 AM) 25 (9 PM)	36.9 18.7	23.2 19.5	— —
2/78 (after dexamethasone 2 mg p.o. q-6-hr × 8 doses)	—	—	—	— —	17.3 19.7	11.6 23.0	— —

*Normal values: AM plasma cortisol 5–25 μg/dl, PM plasma cortisol < 9 mg/dl at 12 midnight.
†Normal values: 3–7 mg/g creatinine.
‡Normal values: 4–15 mg/g creatinine.
§Normal values should be < 120 pg/ml in the absence of adrenal insufficiency.

309

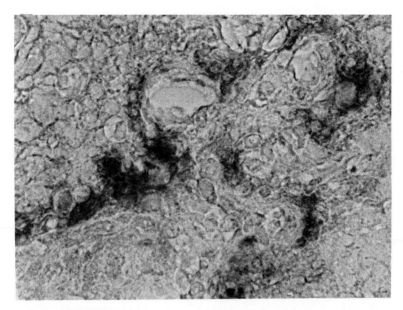

Figure 13-3. *Photomicrograph of immunoperoxidase staining of tumor for ACTH. Areas of dark staining show scattered localization of ACTH. Original magnification × 400. (Courtesy of A.G. Kasselberg, M.D.)*

spite of thoracentesis, chest tube drainage, and trials of VP-16 and hexamethylmelamine. The patient died of respiratory failure in March 1978. Autopsy was not permitted.

Patient 9. H.B., a 61-yr-old man, presented with scrotal and bipedal edema of six wk duration. No other genitourinary or systemic symptoms were present. Physical examination revealed massive enlargement of the prostate, which was hard and fixed. Chest x-ray was normal. There was a 1 × 2 cm right supraclavicular lymph node, and pitting edema over both legs. IVP showed left hydronephrosis. There were multiple areas of increased uptake on the bone scan, in the spine, ribs, and skull, compatible with metastases. A transrectal needle biopsy of the prostate revealed small cell carcinoma. Fiberoptic bronchoscopy was normal. He was treated with diethylstylbesterol 1 mg daily, and cyclophosphamide 500 mg/m² p.o. daily for 5 days every 3 wk, resulting in prompt resolution of his edema and reduction in prostatic size. He has received six cycles of therapy to date and continues to do well 5 mo after diagnosis.

Patient 13. C.S., a 62-yr-old male, presented with a neck mass which had been present for five wk before his evaluation in February 1979. He had no other symptoms and felt well. Physical examination revealed a 6 × 8 cm left cervical mass, and multiple palpable cervical lymph nodes. An incisional biopsy of the mass revealed small cell anaplastic carcinoma of the intermediate cell subtype. Chest x-ray was normal, and sputum cytologies and bronchoscopy were negative for tumor. Staging work-up included brain, liver, and bone scans and bone marrow biopsies, all of which were normal. He was started on chemotherapy with cyclophosphamide 1000 mg/m², doxorubicin 40 mg/m², vincristine 1 mg/m² intravenously every 3 wk, and methothrexate 20 mg/m² i.v. weekly during the first cycle. He responded dramatically to this regimen and achieved complete remission. Therapy was stopped after six cycles, and radiotherapy was given to the left neck, where tumor had been present. He remains free of recurrence.

Patient 15. N.C., a 43-yr-old white female, presented in May 1977 with multiple subcutaneous nodules over her trunk and extremities. She had noticed these nodules three days prior to her evaluation, and had no other symptoms. Physical examination was normal except for multiple subcutaneous nodules over her chest, back, and extremities measuring 2–4 cm in diameter. There were no other masses or visceromegaly. Biopsy of subcutaneous nodules revealed small cell carcinoma. Electron microscopy showed neurosecretory like granules. Chest x-ray was normal. Liver and brain scans and bilateral posterior iliac crest bone marrow biopsies were all normal. Bone scan revealed areas of increased uptake in the left humeral head, temporal bone, and right distal femur. These areas were asymptomatic and x-rays were normal. Barium enema showed a smooth constricting defect in the ascending colon, radiologically felt to be adhesive in nature rather than neoplastic. Colonoscopy was compatible with a smooth circular fold, multiple biopsies were negative for tumor.

Treatment was instituted with cyclophosphamide 1000 mg/m², doxorubicin 40 mg/m², vincristine 1 mg/m² (CAV) intravenously every 3 wk, resulting in prompt disappearance of all subcutaneous tumors. A full reevaluation at the end of four cycles with repeat scans showed normal findings, and her bone scan had improved. Barium enema revealed the circular fold persisting without any change. After two more cycles of CAV, she was maintained on methothrexate, VP-16, hexamethylmelamine, all at attenuated doses owing to poor marrow tolerance, and therapy was stopped after 1 yr. She did well until October 1978, when she presented with right hemiparesis and a solitary mass lesion in the left frontoparietal area. This was surgically removed and the histology was similar to the original lesions. After 3000 rads of whole-brain radiotherapy, she was followed on no specific treatment until May 1979, when she presented with pancytopenia. Bone marrow was hypocellular, with one focus of large immature cells infiltrating the adipose tissue, which were distinctly different from her original tumor cells. Supportive care was given, including blood component therapy, until she died with sepsis in June 1979. At autopsy she had small foci of small cell carninoma in the liver and left frontal lobe of the brain, but no pulmonary neoplasm was identified. Review of marrow and blood specimens was felt to be consistent with an acute undifferentiated leukemia.

Patient 17.   V.A., a 57-yr-old man presented in July 1977 with a 5-mo history of neck and bilateral shoulder pain. A myelogram was done revealing a filling defect. Cervical laminectomy was performed, at which time a tumor mass was found in the epidural space. Histopathologic evaluation revealed small cell carcinoma. His chest x-ray was normal, and there was no overt evidence of tumor in other organ systems. He was given radiotherapy to the cervical spine and referred to Vanderbilt University for further evaluation. His work-up included chest tomograms, sputum cytology, bronchoscopy with brushings and washings, liver, brain, and bone scans, and bone marrow biopsy, all of which were normal. As he had no evaluable lesions or symptoms, it was elected to follow him on no cytotoxic therapy. He has remained well and relapse free.

Review of the Literature

The reports of extrapulmonary small cell carcinoma are discussed according to organ system. These patients are outlined in Table 13-3.

Upper Respiratory Tract

Larynx.   There have been 14 reports of small cell laryngeal cancer[4-16]. The first patient was reported by Olofsson and Van Nostrand in 1972.[4] Although this patient was alive and free of disease 2.5 yr following local therapy alone, later observations indicated that this tumor usually had an aggressive course, with early dissemination. With an increasing awareness of this rare laryngeal tumor and its propensity for early systemic

Table 13-3
Extrapulmonary Small Cell Carcinoma: Literature Survey

Primary Site	No. of Patients	Neurosecretory Granules on EM	Metastases at DX	Metastases at Autopsy	Therapy		Range of Survival
Larynx[4-16]	14	6/6	9/13	12/12	RT Surg Chemo	10/14 12/14 3/14	3–30+ mo; median 10 mo
Trachea[17-23]	7	1/1	4/7	4/6	RT Surg Chemo	5/7 0/3 1/7	2–26 mo
Paranasal sinuses[24]	1	0/0	0/1	0/1	none		Diagnosed at autopsy
Minor Salivary gland[25-26]	14	0/0	3/14	Not listed	RT Surg Chemo	none 12/14 0/14	0–12 yr; median 16 mo
Parotid gland[27]	1	0/1	0/1	0/0	RT, surg, chemo		3+ mo
Esophagus[28-36]	16	7/8	5/16	14/15	RT Surg Chemo	none 14/16 3/16	0–24 mo
Stomach[37,38]	4	2/2	3/4	2/4	RT Surg Chemo	0/4 2/4 0/4	2½–60+ mo
Small bowel[39]	1	1/1	0/1	—	Surg		6+ yr
Colon[40]	4	4/4	3/4	4/4	(?)		0–14 mo
Pancreas[42]	1	0/0	1/1	1/1	none		1/2 mo
Cervix[46-49]	49	6/6	16/48	1/1	RT Surg Chemo	29/49 15/49 1/49	No cumulative data
Prostate[51]	1	1/1	1/1	None	Died after DX		

spread, systemic chemotherapy was tried in some patients with encouraging results.

Of the 14 reported patients with small cell cancer of the larynx, 11 were males, and 3 were females with an average age of 64 yr (range 45–79 yr). Eleven patients were cigarette smokers, and the smoking history was not given in the remaining 3 patients. The most common presenting symptoms were hoarseness, dysphagia, and the presence of a neck mass. Tumors were located in various parts of the larynx with no predilection to any specific area. Electron-microscopic findings were reported in 6 cases, confirming the presence of neurosecretorylike granules in the cytoplasm. One patient had a mixed tumor, with squamous elements at the edge of the small cell carcinoma. None of the patients presented with clinically detectable distant spread, although staging procedures varied in each case, and eventual dissemination of disease was common. All patients had local therapy either by surgery or radiation, or both. Twelve patients had laryngectomy and node dissection, 7 of whom received radiotherapy in addition to surgery either pre- or postoperatively. Three of the 5 patients who had surgery alone developed local recurrence, while there was no local recurrence in those who received surgery and radiotherapy. One patient received radiotherapy as the only therapeutic modality, and, although local disease was apparently controlled, the patient died 4 mo later with progressive disease in his liver and bone marrow. The doses of radiation were usually in the range of 3000–5000 rads. Two patients were given combination chemotherapy as part of the primary therapy. Both achieved complete remission, with one free of recurrence at 15 mo following therapy and the other relapsing at 20 mo. Regional lymph nodes were involved with tumor in 11 of the 14 reported cases at presentation. Of the 12 patients with adequate follow-up information, 3 had no evidence of recurrence at over 4 mo, 15 mo, and 2.5 yr, respectively, whereas 9 had relapsed, 8 of them in distant sites. One patient was lost to follow-up after developing local recurrence. The most common sites of distant spread were liver in 5 patients, lung (multiple nodules) in 3, bone in 2, pleura in 2, adrenals in 1, retroperitoneum in 1, pericardium in 1, and bone marrow in 1.

It appears that smaller tumors give rise to earlier symptoms in the larynx, compared to those in the lung, and more cases may be detected while the tumor is still confined to a limited anatomic region. The consensus of most authors is that these patients may have a significant potential for long-term remission with intensive local therapy followed by combination chemotherapy. The superiority of radiotherapy or surgery in achieving local control is difficult to establish from the sporadic case reports. The tumor is radiosensitive and efforts should be made to preserve vocal cord function if possible, as these patients have a high chance of early systemic spread.

Trachea. Even though small cell carcinoma is most often seen in the proximal bronchial tree, it is rare in the trachea, with only 7 reported patients.[17-23] Five of the 7 patients had involvement in the upper third of the trachea, 4 patients were smokers, and 4 patients presented with metastases to the liver. Two patients were diagnosed postmortem and had been given symptomatic care alone, both having died within 2 months after presenting to their physician. Five patients received radiotherapy and various forms of chemotherapy, all reportedly achieving some short-term palliation. One patient received combination chemotherapy with cyclophosphamide, vincristine and methothrexate leading to marked improvement in respiratory function.[23] After local recurrence, this patient responded to secondary therapy with a repeat course of radiotherapy and an adrimycin-based combination, surviving 26 mo. These limited observations suggest that tracheal small cell cancers may have a similar natural history to their common counterpart arising lower in the bronchi.

Paranasal Sinuses. An oat cell carcinoma involving the paranasal sinuses in the ethmoid area was described in 1965.[24] This patient had erosion of the bones at the base of her skull, and presented with a frontal lobe abscess on the day of her death. Lungs were free of tumor at autopsy, and electron microscopy was not performed.

The Digestive System

Salivary Glands. During a review of 492 minor salivary gland tumors, Koss et al. found 14 small cell carcinomas.[25,26] Remnants of salivary glands were observed in all the tumors. Although the authors stated that this would not be hard enough evidence to confirm the direct derivation of the neoplasm from the salivary glands, this appeared to be the most likely site of origin. A hyaline stroma surrounding the tumor cells, a common finding in minor salivory gland tumors, was often present. Metastases to cervical lymph nodes were present in 7 of the 14 cases, and only one of the patients presented with distant metastases. All received local therapy with surgery, irradiation, or both, and there were 4 long-term survivors, living 6 to 12 yr, with only 2 of these patients dying with recurrent disease. Overall, 8 patients eventually had local recurrence, and 3 reportedly died with disseminated disease. None of the patients in these series had electron-microscopic evidence of neurosecretory granules. Wirman and Battifora later reported a patient with small cell carcinoma arising in the parotid gland, who was studied by electron microscopy that failed to show neurosecretory granules but that revealed evidence for epithelial and myoepithelial differentiation.[27] The authors felt that this would suggest a salivary duct origin and that it would mitigate against a neuroendocrine origin.

Esophagus.   The first case report of a small cell esophageal tumor was by McKeown in 1952[28] and was followed by numerous other reports, mostly from Japan.[29-36] The disease appears to be rare in the Western hemisphere. In their review of 1918 patients with a variety of esophageal cancers, Turnbull et al.[29] found only 1 case of oat cell carcinoma. In contrast, in a Japanese study, 6 of 79 cases of esophageal cancer were classified as small cell type.[34] In a recent review of the literature of 17 esophageal "apudomas" reported before 1978, 13 were from Japan, with only 4 from elsewhere,[36] thus suggesting a difference in the incidence, definition, or recognition of these tumors. Of the patients included in this review, 6 had been studied with electron microscopy, confirming the presence of neurosecretory-type granules, and four of the tumors were associated with ectopic secretion of ACTH. Interestingly, there are at least three cases where the tumors had a mixed histology with squamous features.[28,31,33] Whether these two components are derived from the same cell of origin, with subsequent divergent differentiation, or from different cell types, has not been clarified to date. Clinically, most of the reported patients had lesions in the middle and lower parts of the esophagus, and almost all patients had involvement of the regional lymph nodes at surgery, eventually progressing with widespread metastases and death usually within 1 yr. Experience with the nonsurgical therapy of these neoplasms has been virtually nonexistent. Considering their propensity for early spread, trials of systemic therapy appear reasonable.

Stomach.   In contrast to carcinoid tumors that are common in the gastrointestinal tract, small cell carcinomas have been rare below the esophagus. The stomach is frequently the site for primary lymphomas and carcinoid tumors which may rarely resemble small cell carcinomas in their histologic appearance. Consequently, there are very few well documented cases of gastric small cell cancer. The two patients reported by Matsusaka et al. had tumors which histologically had the oat cell pattern, and consisted of argyrophilic cells.[37] One patient had liver metastases at presentation and died within a year. The second patient had a mixed tumor with an adenocarcinoma component and was free of disease 5 yr. after surgical resection. Two other cases reported by Chejfec et al.[38] were those of undifferentiated gastric cancers, with areas suggesting oat cell patterns. Both had neurosecretorylike granules on electron microscopy, and tumor tissue homogenates contained abnormal levels of vanillylmandelic acid. Both patients had liver metastases at presentation; they died 4 and 10 wk after diagnosis, respectively.

Jejunum.   A small cell tumor of the jejunum was reported in a 17-yr-old girl, who was free of disease 6 yr following resection[39]. Cytoplasmic granules were demonstrated by electron microscopy.

Colon.   Four patients with a light microscopic pattern of oat cell carcinoma in the colon were studied by Gould et al.,[40] and neurosecretory-type granules were shown by electron microscopy. Biochemical analysis of tumor tissue extracts revealed elevated levels of vanillylmandelic acid and catecholamines in all cases, although there were no clinical syndromes in any of the patients resulting from the ectopic production of these substances. Three of the patients died at 9, 11, and 14 mo, and the fourth was diagnosed at autopsy. All had extensive metastases, at the time of death, to the liver, peritoneum, and abdominal lymph nodes, and in 2, metastases to the lung.

Pancreas.   Small cell carcinomas of the pancreas are very rare. In a review of 508 cases of pancreatic cancer, only one was classified as small cell type.[41] This review did not include islet cell and carcinoid tumors, and it is likely that some small cell cancers may have been classified under these groups. Corrin et al.[42] have reported a patient who had clinical, biochemical, and autopsy evidence for ectopic production of ACTH secondary to a small cell carcinoma arising in the pancreatic tail. The patient had presented with extensive liver metastases, as well as multiple metabolic derangements related to her hypercorticism, leading to her rapid demise. At autopsy the lungs were free of tumor, the pituitary normal, and the adrenals hyperplastic. Electron microscopy was not performed.

With the available information it is impossible to determine if these tumors represent part of a spectrum extending from indolent carcinoid tumors to highly malignant small cell anaplastic carcinomas. The natural history of these tumors and more optimal treatment of these patients will have to be determined after more patients are adequately studied and followed.

Genitourinary Tract

Uterine Cervix.   Small cell cancers of the uterine cervix are relatively common tumors that constitute approximately 4–5 percent of all cervical tumors.[43-46] Some authors have suggested that these patients have a worse prognosis than those with squamous carcinomas, if given local therapy alone.[43-45] Wentz et al.[43,45] reported 5-yr survival rates of less than 6 percent (all stages combined) for small cell tumors, compared to 30–45 percent in patients with large cell and keratinizing epidermoid cancers. Van Nagel et al.[46] reported 41 small cell cancers in their series of 1013 cervical neoplasms (4 percent). They confirmed the tendency of the tumor for early spread. 54 percent of their 41 patients died with metastatic disease, most within a year after diagnosis. The common sites of metastasis included the lung, liver, and bones, a pattern similar to small cell cancers of the lung.

In a review of 97 cases of cervical cancer, Tateishi et al.[47] found 5 small cell carcinomas, all of which had electron microscopic characteristics of APUD cells. The same group of authors also demonstrated argyrophylic cells in the normal cervical epithelium in 19 of the 54 patients that they studied, and speculated that these were the cells of origin for the tumors that they described. Since then, there have been at least four other cases of small cell cervical carcinomas that were shown to contain neurosecretory-type granules within the tumor cell cytoplasm (including our Case 1).[48-50]

Prostate.   Wenk et al.[51] described an oat cell carcinoma of the prostate with ectopic production of ACTH. Tumor cells had granules seen on electron microscopy, and intracellular ACTH was demonstrated by immunoperoxidase staining. The patient had no distant metastases at the time of autopsy, 9 mo following the initial diagnosis. There have been at least two other cases of prostatic cancer associated with ectopic ACTH production. The presence of argyrophilic cells have also been shown in normal prostatic tissue, and may well be the source of these tumors.

Other Sites

Thyroid.   Anaplastic carcinoma of the thyroid is subclassified by the Armed Forces Institute of Pathology and the World Health Organization into giant cell, small cell compact, and small cell diffuse carcinomas.[52] The small cell subtypes are often very difficult to distinguish from lymphomas of the thyroid. The origins of these "small cell" carcinomas have not been defined. Ultrastructural studies have not demonstrated any APUD cell characteristics.[53-56] The ultrastructural appearance of these anaplastic thyroid cancers and their occasional association with well-differentiated malignancies of the thyroid have been viewed as evidence for their derivation from the follicular epithelium.[55] It has been emphasized that many "small cell" tumors of the thyroid as judged by light microscopy are in fact lymphomas,[57-59] and electron-microscopic findings have demonstrated this in at least two cases.[58] Realizing this difficulty in the differential diagnosis of these tumors from lymphomas by light microscopy alone, most clinical studies have considered both of these neoplasms to be in the same category.[60] It is generally stated that both small cell anaplastic carcinomas and lymphomas originating in the thyroid gland have a similar natural history, with early systemic spread and rapidly progressive course, although it is impossible to draw any sound conclusions from the available information.

Thymus. Four cases of thymic oat cell carcinomas were recognized by Rosai et al.[61] All these patients presented with mediastinal masses and, at autopsy, had no bronchial primary tumor. The authors emphasized that all mediastinal oat cell carcinomas should be regarded as a lung primary, unless proven otherwise. Carcinoid tumors and normal argentaffin cells have also been described in the thymus.

Discussion

It is quite clear that small cell carcinomas arise in various organ systems. They are probably biologically different from most other tumors originating from the given anatomical sites, perhaps because of their unique cellular origin. Many small cell cancers have been shown to have morphological and physiological similiarities to cells of the APUD series described by Pearse.[62,63] Chapter 6 of this monograph outlines the unitarian concept of lung cancer, in which small cell carcinoma represents a form with differentiation to cells with APUD characteristics. It is of interest that carcinoid tumors, which also share many characteristics of APUD cells, have a much more indolent clinical course, in contrast to the rapidly disseminating, aggressive pattern seen with SCC. This suggests that there may be subtle differences in their cells of origin, or that different characteristics may be acquired by the tumor cells during their neoplastic transformation. Most of the extrapulmonary small cell carcinomas in this review had a tendency for early systemic spread, and, in some patients, therapeutic trials with cytotoxic agents yielded gratifying results. However, this was not uniformly true, and it is possible that some of these tumors may represent biologic patterns forming a spectrum between the typical, indolent carcinoid tumors and highly malignant small cell anaplastic cancers. It is also likely that some of the patients who are considered to have SCC may, in fact, have carcinoid tumors or other poorly differentiated cancers with small cell size. While this type of misinterpretation can lead to an overdiagnosis of small cell carcinoma, it is equally likely that many small cell cancers presenting without a primary lung tumor are missed because of the lack of widespread recognition that these tumors may arise in unusual locations. Furthermore, since the subclassification of SCC, it is now established that the "intermediate cell" subtype is seen with equal frequency as the more typical "oat cell" subtype and is equally responsive to chemotherapy and radiotherapy.[64,65] The intermediate subtype consists of larger cells with more cytoplasm and is often confused with poorly differentiated tumors of other histologic varieties.[66] If a similar histologic variant exists in the extrapulmonary sites, it would certainly be susceptible to misinterpretation. Therefore, the true incidence of extrapulmonary small cell cancer is unknown at the present time.

Tumor markers have been frequently associated with small cell cancers, irrespective of their primary site, and may offer valuable tools in diagnosis and follow-up. Ectopic production of ACTH has been the most common humoral syndrome that has been reported in association with small cell cancers of nonpulmonary origin, particularly with those arising in the esophagus, uterine cervix, and prostate. Tumor markers, including polypeptide hormones, and clinical syndromes that result from their excess production should be specifically sought in suspected cases of small cell carcinomas presenting in unusual locations.

Although the natural history of extrapulmonary small cell neoplasms needs to be explored further, our experience indicates that many of these tumors are responsive to chemotherapy and radiotherapy. Subsets of patients and prognostic indicators may be determined as more patients are studied. Electron microscopy, tumor product and marker identification, and further follow-up on a greater number of patients will provide a firmer understanding of these neoplasms. It would appear that combination chemotherapy is indicated for patients presenting with extrapulmonary small cell carcinoma. Radiotherapy, in conjunction with chemotherapy, is a reasonable alternative to surgery for treating tumor bulk.

More optimal effects may be achieved as management of these relatively uncommon neoplasms is refined as further experience becomes available.

References

1. Cohen MH, Ihde DC, Bunn PA, et al: Cyclic alternating combination chemotherapy for small cell bronchogenic carcinoma. Cancer Treat Rep 63:163–170, 1979

2. Greco FA, Oldham RK: Small cell lung cancer. N Engl J Med 301:355–358, 1979

3. Greco FA, Richardson RL, Snell JD, et al: Small cell lung cancer: Complete remission and improved survival. Am J Med 66:625–630, 1979

4. Olofsson J, Van Nostrand AWP: Anaplastic small cell carcinoma of the larynx. Ann Otol Rhinol Laryngol 81:284–287, 1972

5. Koss LG, Spiro RH, Hajdu S: Small cell (oat cell) carcinoma of minor salivary gland origin. Cancer 30:737–741, 1972

6. Ferlito A: Oat cell carcinoma of the larynx. Ann Otol Rhinol Laryngol 83:254–256, 1974

7. Gelot R, Rhee TR, Lapidot A: Primary oat-cell carcinoma of head and neck. Ann Otol Rhinol Laryngol 84:238–244, 1975

8. Benisch BM, Tawfik B, Breitenbach, EE: Primary oat cell carcinoma of the larynx: An ultrastructural study. Cancer 36:145–148, 1975

9. Kyriakos M, Berlin BP, DeSchryver-Keeskemeti K: Oat-cell carcinoma of the larynx. Arch Otolaryngol 104:168–176, 1978

10. Mullins JD, Newman RK, Coltman CA: Primary oat cell carcinoma of the larynx. A case report and review of the literature. Cancer 43:711–717, 1979

11. Myerowitz RL, Barnes EL, Myers E: Small cell anaplastic (oat cell) carcinoma of the larynx: Report of a case and review of the literature. Laryngoscope 88:1697–1702, 1978

12. Bitran JD, Toledo-Pereyra LH, Matz G: Oat cell carcinoma of the larynx. Response to combined modality therapy. Cancer 42:85–87, 1978

13. Eusebi V, Betts CM, Giangaspero F: Primary oat-cell carcinoma of the larynx. Virchows Arch Pathol Anat Histol 380:349–354, 1978

14. Ferlito A: Primary oat-cell carcinoma of the larynx following supraglottic laryngectomy for squamous-cell carcinoma. J Am Geriatr Soc 26:278–283, 1978

15. Bone RC, Deer D: Oat cell carcinoma of the larynx. The Laryngoscope 88:1190–1195, 1978

16. Lorenz SA, Arena S: Primary oat cell carcinoma of the larynx. Pa Med 82:41–42, 1979

17. Pantridge JF: Primary carcinoma of the trachea. Br J Surg 37:48–49, 1949

18. Zarowitz H, Hoffman JB: Primary carcinoma of the trachea. Arch Int Med 89:454–462, 1952

19. Darch GH: Tracheal neoplasms presenting with mediastinal emphysema. Br J Dis Chest 56:212–213, 1962

20. Wengraf C: Oat cell carcinoma of the trachea. J Laryngol Otol 84:267–274, 1970

21. Jash DK: Oat cell carcinoma of the trachea. J Laryngol Otol 87:681–684, 1973

22. Deckert RE, Burgher LW: Serial flow-volume loops as an aid to management of primary oat cell carcinoma of the trachea. Chest 73:560–561, 1978

23. Soorae, AS, Gibbons JRP: Primary oat cell carcinoma of the trachea. Thorax 34:130–131, 1979

24. Raychowdhuri RN: Oat-cell carcinoma and paranasal sinuses. J Laryngol Otol 79:253–255, 1965

25. Koss LG, Spiro RH, Hajdu S: Small cell (oat cell) carcinoma of minor salivary gland origin. Cancer 30:737–741, 1972

26. Spiro RH, Koss LG, Hajdu, SI, et al: Tumors of minor salivary origin. A clinicopathologic study of 492 cases. Cancer 31:117–129, 1973

27. Wirman JA, Battifora HA: Small cell undifferentiated carcinoma of salivary gland origin. An ultrastructural study. Cancer 37:1840–1848, 1976

28. McKeown F: Oat cell carcinoma of the esophagus. J Pathol Bacteriol 64:889–891, 1952

29. Turnbull AD, Rosen P, Goodner JT, et al: Primary malignant tumors of the esophagus other than typical epidermoid carcinoma. Ann Thorac Surg 15:463–473, 1973

30. Taniguchi K, Iwanaga T, Kosaki G, et al: Oat-cell carcinoma of the esophagus producing ACTH. Report of two cases. (Japanese) Saishin Igaku 28:1834–1837, 1973

31. Rosen Y, Moon S, Kim B: Small cell epidermoid carcinoma of the esophagus. Cancer 36:1042–1049, 1975

32. Matsusaka, T, Watanabe H, Enjoji M: Anaplastic carcinoma of the esophagus. Report of three cases and their histogenetic consideration. Cancer 37:1352–1358, 1976

33. Cook MG, Eusebi V, Betts CM: Oat-cell carcinoma of the oesopha-

gus: a recently recognized entity. J Clin Pathol 29:1068–1073, 1976

34. Tateishi R, Taniguchi K, Horai T, et al: Argyrophil cell carcinoma (apudoma) of the esophagus. A histopathologic entity. Virchows Arch Pathol Anat Histol 371:283–294, 1976

35. Horai T, Kobayashi A, Tateishi R, et al: A cytologic study on small cell carcinoma of the esophagus. Cancer 41:1890–1896, 1978

36. Imai T, Sannohe Y, Okano H: Oat cell carcinoma (apudoma) of the esophagus. A case report. Cancer 41:358–364, 1978

37. Matsusaka T, Watanabe H, Enjoji M: Oat-cell carcinoma of the stomach. Fukuoka Acta Med 67:65–73, 1976

38. Chejfec G, Gould VE: Malignant gastric neuroendocrinomas. Hum. Pathol 8:433–440, 1977

39. Toker C: Oat cell tumor of the small bowel. Am J Gastoenterol 61:481–483, 1974

40. Gould VE, Chejfec G: Neuroendocrine carcinomas of the colon. Ultrastructural and biochemical evidence of their secretory function. Am J Surg Pathol 2:31–38, 1978

41. Cubilla AL, Fitzgerald PJ: Classification of pancreatic cancer (nonendocrine). Mayo Clic Proc 54:449–458, 1979

42. Corrin B, Gilby ED, Jones NF, et al: Oat cell carcinoma of the pancreas with ectopic ACTH secretion. Cancer 31:1523–1527, 1973

43. Wentz WB, Reagan JB: Survival in cervical cancer with respect to cell type. Cancer 12:384–388, 1959

44. Field CA, Dockerty M, Symmonds RE: Small cell cancer of the cervix. Am J Obstet Gynecol 88:447–451, 1964

45. Wentz WB, Lewis GC: Correlation of histologic morphology and survival in cervical cancer following radiation therapy. Obstet Gynecol 26:228–232, 1965

46. Van Nagell JR, Donaldson, ES, Wood EG, et al: Small cell cancer of the uterine cervix. Cancer 40:2243–2249, 1977

47. Tateishi R, Wada A, Hayadawa K, et al: Argyrophil cell carcinomas (Apudomas) of the uterine cervix. Virchows Arch Anat Pathol Anat Histol 366:257–274, 1975

48. Jones HW, Plymate S, Gluck FB, et al: Small cell non-keratinizing carcinoma of the cervix associated with ectopic ACTH production. Cancer 38:1629–1635, 1976

49. MacKay B, Osborne BM, Wharton JT: Small cell tumor of cervix with neuroepithelial features. Cancer 43:1138–1145, 1979

50. Lojek M, Fer MF, Kasselberg AG, et al: Cushings syndrome with small cell carcinoma of the uterine cervix. Am J Med 69:140, 1980

51. Wenk RE, Bhagavan BS, Levy R, et al: Ectopic ACTH, prostatic oat cell carcinoma, and marked hypernatremia. Cancer 40:773–778, 1977

52. Meissner WA, Warren S: Tumors of the thyroid gland. Atlas of tumor pathology (ser 2, fascicle 4). Washington, D.C., Armed Forces Institute of Pathology, 1969

53. Cameron RG, Seemayer TA, Wan N, et al: Small cell malignant tumors of the thyroid. Hum Pathol 6:731–740, 1975

54. Saito R, Sharma K: Fine structure of a diffuse undifferentiated small cell carcinoma of the thyroid. Am J Clin Pathol 65:623–630, 1976

55. Goncalves Y, Sousa-Le F, Magalhaes MP, et al: Ultrastructure of two small-cell carcinomas of the thyroid gland. J Submicrosc Cytol 10:457–463, 1978

56. Hayashi Y, Tokuoka S: Anaplastic carcinoma of the thyroid gland. An ultrastructural study on four cases. Acta Pathol (Jpn) 29:119–133, 1979

57. Heimann R, Vannineuse A, De Cloover C, et al: Malignant lymphomas and undifferentiated small cell carcinoma of the thyroid: A clinicopathological review in the light of the Kiel classification for malignant lymphomas. Histopathology 2:201–213, 1978

58. Soto-Velasco JM, Smith M, Albores-Saaredra J: Evidencia ultraestructural de la naturaleza linfoide del illamado "tipo diffuso de carcinoma indiferenciado de celulas pequenas del tiroides. Estudio de dos casos. Patologia 10:59–68, 1972

59. Rayfiled EJ, Nishiyama RH, Sisson JC: Small cell tumors of the thyroid. A clinicopathologic study. Cancer 28:1023–1030, 1971

60. Rossi R, Cady B, Meissner WA, et al: Prognosis of undifferentiated carcinoma and lymphoma of the thyroid. Am J Surg 135:589–596, 1978

61. Rosai J, Levine G, Weber R, et al: Carcinoid Tumors and Oat Cell Carcinomas of the Thymus. Pathology Annual. New York, Appleton-Century-Crofts, (vol 11), 1976, pp 201–226

62. Pearse AGE: The cytochemistry and ultrastructure of polypeptide hormone-producing cells of the APUD series and the embryologic, physiologic and pathologic implications of the concept. J Histochem Cytochem 17:303–313, 1969

63. Pearse AGE: The diffuse neuroendocrine system and the APUD concept: Related "endocrine" peptides in brain, intestine, pituitary and anuran cutaneous glands. Med Biol 55:115–125, 1977

64. Matthews MJ: Morphology of lung cancer. Sem Oncol 1:175–182, 1974

65. Cohen MH, Matthews MJ: Small cell bronchogenic carcinoma: A distinct clinicopathologic entity. Sem Oncol 5:234–243, 1978

66. Fer MF, Rogers LW, Richardson RL, et al: The intermediate subtype of small cell lung cancer: A frequently unrecognized neoplasm. Clin Res 384A, 1979 (Abst)

14

IMMUNOBIOLOGY OF SMALL CELL CARCINOMA

James T. Forbes
F. Anthony Greco
Robert K. Oldham

A basic tenet of tumor immunology is that neoplastic cells express antigenic determinants that are capable of eliciting an immune response in their host.[1] One possible outcome of this immunologic interaction is rejection of the tumor, and that is the goal to which immunotherapy is directed. Other aspects of these immunologic reactions may be used for diagnosis, may relate to prognosis, or may result in secondary pathology of clinical importance.

Introduction of an immunogenic substance such as tumor antigen into a mammalian host usually results in a demonstrable immune response that is composed of both humoral and cellular elements.[2] This response is the end result of recognition of the antigenic ligand by specific receptors on the surfaces of thymus-derived lymphocytes. This antigen–receptor interaction stimulates clonal expansion of these cells. Some of these thymus-derived lymphocytes (T cells) are capable of interacting with bone-marrow–derived lymphocytes (B cells) in such a manner that the B cells begin to produce antibody specific for the antigenic determinant. The antibody produced by B cells has the same specificity as the original antigenic receptor on the T cell.[3,4] Continued expansion and maturation of the

This work was supported in part by Grant NCI-CB-64007-31 from the National Cancer Institute.

primarily stimulated T cell subpopulation ultimately gives rise to clones of regulatory lymphocytes, cytotoxic lymphocytes, and memory lymphocytes. The actions of all these lymphoid elements, as well as their interactions with other, nonlymphoid reticuloendothelial elements (i.e., macrophages), comprise what we recognize as tumor immunity. The precise role each of these elements plays in the immune response has only been partially elucidated.

Antigens of Human Lung Cancer

Central to any discussion of the immunology of human tumors is demonstration of tumor-associated antigens (TAA) on the cancer cell surface. Many of the attempts to identify TAA in lung cancer have followed the same general protocol; injection of human lung cancer into rabbits, followed by absorption of the sera with normal lung and other normal tissues and demonstration of specific antibody in the absorbed sera by positive reactions with tumor that do not occur with normal tissue. This scheme has been followed by a number of investigators with varying degrees of success.[5,12] Most of these investigations have demonstrated two or three TAAs on human lung tumor tissue. These antigens have shown little or no histologic specificity, being found on all histologic types of human lung cancer and, in some cases, on tumors and tissues of other origin.

One of the most thoroughly studied antigens associated with human lung tumors is carcinoembryonic antigen (CEA).[13-19] Elevated serum levels of CEA have been associated with lung cancer of all histologic types, as well as with many neoplasms of nonpulmonary origin. Because of the presence of CEA in normal individuals and in patients with noncancerous conditions, this assay has little specificity. The majority of lung cancer patients with localized disease and 20 percent of patients with metastatic disease have normal CEA levels.[17] Preoperative values of CEA have shown some correlation with the extent of disease, and elevated values have been associated with poor prognosis.[15] A rising CEA may be associated with clinical recurrence, but serial measurements are of limited value in assessing responses to chemotherapy or radiotherapy. CEA values have not proved useful in the staging of lung cancer.

McIntire et al, [5,6,13] recently reported the isolation and characterization of human-lung-tumor–associated antigen (HuLTAA). This HuLTAA has been identified by antisera obtained from rabbits injected with perchloric acid extracts of pooled human lung tumors. The antisera were absorbed with normal human plasma, normal lung tissue, and ABO erythrocytes, and gave a single line in precipitation reactions with extracts of lung tumor tissue on Ouchterlony double-diffusion assay. There was no reaction with extracts of normal lung, but the antisera reacted with 85 percent of human lung tumors tested, regardless of histologic type. The same antisera also reacted with 20 percent of sarcomas tested. Physiochemical analysis of this antigen has suggested that it exists as an 80,000-dalton molecular species in its native state, and, when reduced and dissociated, it yields only a single species of 42,000 daltons. A radioimmunoassay has been developed for this antigen and is currently undergoing testing.

Several interesting lung TAA have been isolated from small cell carcinoma of the lung (SCC).[20-23] Bell[21] immunized rabbits with adenocarcinoma of the lung. Sera from these rabbits recognized an antigen that was present at high concentrations in normal adult and fetal lungs when assayed in radioimmunodiffusion. The antigen was detected at low concentrations in epidermoid carcinoma and in only trace amounts in oat cell carcinoma, thus suggesting some degree of histologic specificity. Bell et al.[22] reported that rabbits and monkeys immunized with plasma membranes of SCC produced an antiserum that, after absorption with normal lung, liver, colon, and peripheral nerve, failed to react with any normal adult tissue. These antisera reacted with 7 SCCs, but they failed to react with any of 7 lung adenocarcinomas, 6 epidermoid carcinomas of the lung, 7 colon adenocarcinomas, 8 breast carcinomas, 4 kidney carcinomas, and 1 pancreatic carcinoma. The expression of this tumor-specific antigen has been correlated with the presence of cytoplasmic neurosecretory granules in 6 of 6 cases studied.[24] In this same study, 4 of 4 antigen-negative tumors were also negative for neurosecretory granules. All of these tumors were histologically diagnosed as SCCs. These data support the concept that SCCs have unique antigenic specificity among lung cancers.

Further immunologic characterization of antigens from SCC has identified two other specificities.[22,23] One antigen was characteristic of certain normal endodermally derived epithelial cells of the digestive system, including those of colonic mucosa, hepatic ducts, pancreatic ducts and acini, and islets of Langerhans. The other antigen was characteristic of a variety of cells: some normal neural-crest–derived cells of the peripheral nervous system, including cells in the peripheral nerve, dorsal root ganglion, and other anterior roots of the spinal cord; parasympathetic ganglion cells in the colon; and small nerves and nerve processes in the lung, colon, and skin. Further characterization of this latter specificity has suggested that this antigen is identical to a differentiation antigen on Schwann cells. Studies by Bell[25] have further demonstrated the expression of differentiation antigens of both endodermal and neural-crest origin. Expression of neural-crest differentiation antigens was confined to SCC (6 positive of 6 tested) and adenocarcinoma of the lung (1 of 2 positive), while being absent in epidermoid carcinoma of the lung (2 tested) and adenocarcinoma (2 tested). By contrast, all of these tumors except 1 epidermoid carcinoma were demonstrated to exhibit differentiation antigens of endodermal origin. Luger et al.[26] have raised heteroantisera in rabbits to cultured human neuroblastoma cells and have found that such sera also reacts with human SCC. This reactivity can be removed by absorption with brain or adrenal homogenates, thus demonstrating a neural differentiation antigen that is also found on several types of malignant tissue (SCC, neuroblastoma, Wilms's tumor, and several sarcomas).

These observations have supported the classification of SCC with other cells, believed to be of endodermal and neural ectodermal origin, that are grouped under the acryonym APUD, for amine precursor uptake and decarboxylation.[27] In keeping with their expression of a differentiation antigen similar to that found on gut endocrine structures, SCCs have been shown to produce several endocrine secretions, including ACTH, ADH, calcitonin, glucagon, insulin, growth hormone, prolactin, and vasopressin. These data concerning ectopic production of hormones by SCC should be interpreted with care, in the light of observations by Haverman et al.,[28] who found immune complexes composed of IgG and "big" ACTH in 4 of 7 patients tested, only 1 of which displayed Cushing's syndrome. This complexing indicates that, in these patients, the "big" ACTH molecule is sufficiently different antigenically to become an autoimmunogen. Such molecules may thereby be more difficult to identify by radioimmunoassay, either because they are antigenically different from the normal molecule or because they exist in immune complexes. It is believed that SCC arises from pulmonary Kulchitsky-type cells that are closely related to the intestinal argentaffin (Kulchitsky) cell.[29] The demonstration of an antigen on the surface of SCC cells that cross-reacts with an antigen of Schwann cells is of interest, not only with reference to the histogenesis and biology of SCC but also in regard to certain clinical features of this disease and especially the neuromyopathy occasionally seen with SCC.

Immunobiology of Lung Cancer

Immunologic Assays

Any discussion of the immunobiology of the tumor–host relationship must consider not only the effect of the immunologic response by the host on the tumor but also the effect of the tumor-bearing state on the immunologic apparatus of the host. Oldham et al.[30] demonstrated that lung cancer

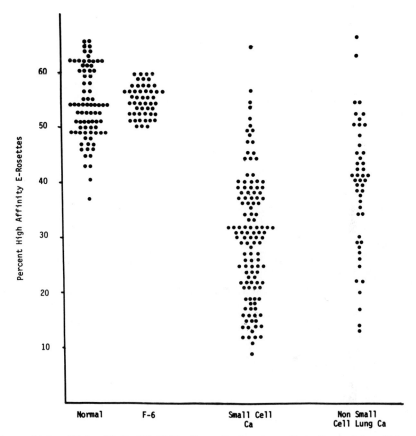

Figure 14-1. *High-affinity (29 C) T cell rosette-forming cells in the peripheral blood of normal individuals as compared with those having SCC or resectable non–small cell carcinoma of the lung. Cryopreserved normal standards (F-6) are run as technical controls.*

can result in varying degrees of immunosuppression. The proportion of peripheral blood T cells that form spontaneous rosettes with sheep erythrocytes at 29°C (high-affinity rosettes) is lower in lung cancer patients than in normal controls. As is shown in Figure 14-1, the levels of high-affinity T cell rosettes are lower in SCC patients than in non–small cell lung cancer. These data are also compared to cryopreserved standards (F-6) from a single donor as a technical control. The level of depression is correlated with the prognosis, extremely low levels being associated with poorer prognosis (T cell levels also fall prior to clinical recurrence). Lymphocyte transformation by the mitogens PHA and Con A is also depressed in patients

Forbes et al.

Table 14-1
Lymphocyte Stimulation Tests in Patients With
Bronchogenic Carcinoma

	Cell Type			
Stimulant	Epidermoid	Adenocarcinoma	Anaplastic	Small Cell
Phytohemagglutinin	55*	75	86	80
Con A	45	42	100	50
Pokeweed mitogen	40	65	100	75
Mixed lymphocyte culture	32	53	100	80

Adapted from Oldham et al.[30]
*Results expressed as percentage of patients with depressed blastogenesis.

with lung cancer[30] (Table 14-1). Those patients anergic to challenge with recall skin test antigens such as PPD, SK-SD, mumps, or candidin tend to have poorer prognoses than do patients with normal responses.[30]

For a variety of technical reasons, relatively few studies of specific tumor immunity have been carried out in patients with lung cancer. One technique of studying specific immunity to lung cancer antigens is to test for delayed hypersensitivity to either crude or partially purified lung tumor antigens. Stewart[31] found that 4 of 9 lung cancer patients had positive skin reactions to crude autologous lung extracts. Hollingshead et al.[32] reported similar results with partially purified extracts, in studies that included control skin tests with similarly treated extracts of normal tissues. Weese et al.[33] examined the specificity of delayed cutaneous hypersensitivity to crude and partially purified extracts of several human tumors, including lung cancer (Table 14-2). These studies reported wide variation in degrees of reactivity and disease-related specificity among extracts from tumors of different histologic types. Some extracts showed high degrees of disease-related discrimination, whereas others, such as lung tumor extracts, demonstrated little discrimination between lung tumor patients and controls. These studies illustrate the need for extensive testing and standardization of putative tumor-specific extracts, as well as the need for highly purified tumor extracts. The data from these and other studies[34] suggest that carefully purified tumor antigen preparations might exhibit higher degrees of specificity and utility.

Two other assays of specific immunity in lung cancer have been studied extensively. Lymphocyte-mediated cytotoxicity reactions specific for various types of cancer have been reported,[35,36] but recent studies of Oldham et al.[37,38] have emphasized the difficulty of interpreting the specificities of these cytotoxicity reactions. Dean et al.[39,40] reported lymphocyte stimulation by autologous extracts of lung cancer (Table 14-3). Most of the

Table 14-2
Delayed Hypersensitivity to Lung Tumor Extracts

Source of Extracts	Percentage Positive Reactions in Patients with Lung Cancer							
	Stages I and II	Stage III	Stage IV	Epidermoid	Adeno-carcinoma	Large Cell Undifferentiated	Small Cell	Control Patients*
Primary tumors	58	49	43	47	50	37	54	69
Pleural effusion	14	33	0	25	25	20	0	17
Liver metastases	50	46	44	40	50	60	40	58

Adapted from Weese et al.[33]
*Patients with cancer other than lung cancer.

Table 14-3
Lymphoproliferative Responses to
Autologous Lung Cancer Cells and to
Membrane Extracts of Tumor Cells

Stimulant	Percentage of Patients Positive
Intact autologous tumor cells	62
Membrane extracts (autologous)	
Cancer lung	48
Normal lung	6

Data from Dean et al.[40]

positive reactions were from patients with localized disease. Some of the negative reactions were attributed to the presence of suppressor cells, since reactivity was restored following surgical resection of the tumor.[40]

Leukocyte migration inhibition (LMI) is an in vitro assay of tumor-specific immunity that has wide application in the study of human tumor immunobiology.[41] In this assay the positive interaction of antigen with sensitized lymphoid cells results in production of a soluble factor (MIF/LIF) that inhibits leukocyte migration in vitro. Figure 14-2 demonstrates the specificity of the LMI assay using lung cancer extract 7661 in tests with lung cancer patients versus normal controls. Less specificity is seen in other cancer patients as compared with controls. Tables 14-4 and 14-5 present examples of LMI assays used with lung cancer patients. Table 14-4 shows the specificity of 7661 lung cancer extract as compared with control extracts, but there was lack of histologic specificity for the different types of lung carcinomas.[30] Table 14-5 demonstrates that the specificity of these reactions in lung cancer patients for lung cancer extracts is still open to question.[42] Boddie et al.[43] and Vose et al.[44] have reported similar results. In certain of these tests, the reaction with nonhomologous pairing of lymphocytes and antigen (i.e., lung cancer patient's lymphocytes and breast antigen and Ewing's sarcoma) is stronger than with homologous pairing (i.e., lung tumor patient's lymphocytes and lung tumor antigens). In paired experiments, McCoy found that, when lung cancer patients were tested simultaneously with 7661, MCF-7, and 5838TC, the homologous reactivity was greater (by ranking analysis) to the lung cancer extracts than to the controls.[42] These findings may result from the presence of TAA associated with many types of neoplasms (i.e., embryonic antigens), regardless of histologic type, from nonspecific factors capable of affecting the immune response, or from a combination of both these elements. It is possible that further purification of the antigenic determinants used to

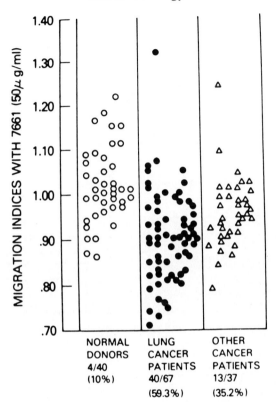

Figure 14-2. *Inhibition of migration of leukocytes from normal donors, lung cancer patients, and patients with other cancers by extracts of 7661.*

elicit these responses will eliminate those reactions that make interpretation of the results difficult.[42]

Recent results with the indirect agarose migration inhibition assay have demonstrated that approximately 50 percent of lung cancer patients versus 7 percent or less of normals reacted to the 7661 lung cancer antigen.[45] These same investigators have reported an increased reactivity to this antigen among normals "exposed" to lung cancer patients, suggesting some transmission of reactivity.[46]

Natural cell-mediated cytotoxicity (NCMC) was originally described as a complicating factor in the in vitro demonstration of tumor-specific cytolysis.[37,47-49] NCMC involves the ability of lymphocytes from normal individuals to effect lysis of tumor cells in vitro. The correlation of this

Table 14-4
LMI in Lung Cancer Patients to Lung Cancer Extracts
and Controls

Histologic Cell Type	Percentage Positive LMI*		
	Extracts of 7661	Other Lung Cancer Extracts	Other Cancer and Normal Tissue Extracts
Epidermoid	73	29	5
Adenocarcinoma	55	36	20
Large cell anaplastic	50	39	10
Small cell	89	9	0
Total	75	30	11

Data from Oldham et al.[30]
*7661 is a 3-M KC extract of fresh pleural effusion from a patient with pulmonary adenocarcinoma.

phenomenon to the clinical course of cancer patients is especially interesting in light of the demonstrations of beneficial antitumor effects of NCMC in animal tumor models.[50-53]

Since NCMC can be reproduced on a day-to-day basis, baselines for NCMC in normal populations may be established in advance. These data, which are reported elsewhere[54,55] and summarized here in Table 14-6, represent a total sample of over 250 normal nonpregnant individuals. The data (Table 14-6) serve as the baseline values with which the NCMC of cancer patients may be compared.

Studies were also designed for evaluating the NCMC of peripheral blood lymphocytes from patients being treated for SCC. This disease has been demonstrated to be remarkably responsive to chemotherapy[56] and,

Table 14-5
LMI Reactivity of Cancer Patients with 3-M KC1 Extracts
of 7661, MCF-7, and 5838TC

Patient Category	Percentage Positive LMI		
	7661*	MCF-7[†]	5838TC[‡]
Lung carcinoma	60	17	56
Breast carcinoma	29	76	60
Ewing's sarcoma	18	20	76

Adapted from McCoy et al.[42]
*Fresh pleural effusion cells from patient with pulmonary adenocarcinoma.
[†]Tissue culture cell line from pleural effusion of breast carcinoma.
[‡]Tissue culture cell line from pleural effusion of Ewing's sarcoma.

Table 14-6
NCMC Values in the Normal Population

Age Group	No. Tested	NCMC*
11–20	29	31.50 ± 2.31
21–30	89	21.10 ± 1.93
31–40	35	24.94 ± 2.86
41–50	38	23.19 ± 1.73
51–60	23	24.99 ± 2.94
>60	49	27.08 ± 2.30

*Mean percent ± S.E. at effector: target, 50:1.

as such, represents a good model for assessing NCMC in relationship to tumor burden. Patients with this disease may be initially classified according to the extent of their disease as either limited or extensive. The values for NCMC from patients with either limited- or extensive-stage SCC are shown in Figure 14-3. These data demonstrate that, among those patients with limited disease, the NCMC values are not significantly different from normal (Table 14-6) prior to chemotherapy but fall during and after chemotherapy. Those patients with extensive-stage SCC show a similar low NCMC when on chemotherapy ($p < 0.05$). There are currently too few pretherapy values for analysis of change with treatment.

Initial examination of these data would suggest that the decrease in levels of NCMC found in patients being treated for SCC is attributable to the chemotherapy and radiotherapy, as described by Greco et al.[56] for limited-stage disease. Those patients in complete remission at this time were randomized to treatment with methotrexate alone or with *Corynebacterium parvum* for 7 mo. Almost all (90 percent) of these patients initially showed a complete clinical response to this treatment. The NCMC of patients during and after such therapy is shown in Figure 14-4. These data are divided according to those patients who are receiving chemotherapy and those patients who are disease free and not receiving chemotherapy. The data indicate that both groups are below normal, but that the group receiving chemotherapy is the lowest. Those patients receiving induction therapy (cyclophosphamide, adriamycin, and vincristine) are only slightly less reactive in NCMC (Figure 14-5) than those receiving consolidation or maintainence therapy. These data suggest that perhaps the chemotherapy regimen can affect levels of NCMC. The differences between these groups is not statistically significant ($p > 0.1$).

That chemotherapy is not solely responsible for the decrease in NCMC in these patients is supported by the data in Figure 14-6. These data are NCMC values of blood from patients with extensive SCC. These

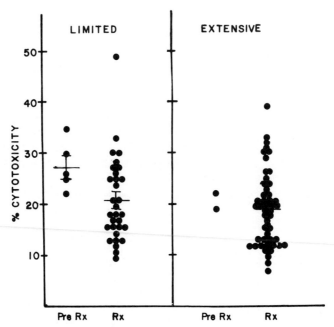

Figure 14-3. *NCMC from patients with limited or extensive SCC, tested prior to and during therapy.*

patients were all being treated with chemotherapy (cyclophosphamide, adriamycin, vincristine, and methotrexate) and prophylactic radiation (10 × 300 rads) to the brain. Those patients not in remission are generally sicker and more protein depleted and have a lower performance status than those whose disease is in remission. As seen in Figure 14-6, those patients in remission have lower NCMC than those patients in relapse. These data would suggest that NCMC levels are related to tumor burden and that, when the tumor burden is high, the NCMC is elevated; This value then decreases as the tumor burden is decreased. Reexamination of the data in Figures 14-3 to 14-5 also supports this hypothesis, as tumor burden would be highest in the pretreatment population and would be lowest in those patients undergoing intensive treatment (Figure 14-5).

This interpretation of these data is further supported by comparing serial values for NCMC from each of 3 selected individuals with the clinical history of each of those patients (Figure 14-7). All 3 of these patients (C.S., W.H., and R.C.) had limited-stage SCC and demonstrated complete responses to treatments, with complete disappearance of all clinical signs and symptoms of disease. Two of these patients (C.S. and W.H.) were

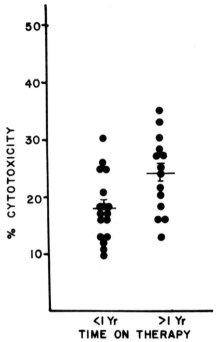

Figure 14-4. *NCMC for patients with limited-stage SCC re-ceiving chemotherapy (< 1 yr) and those having finished che-motherapy (> 1 yr).*

tested for NCMC against K-562 prior to the initiation of therapy, and this value was the highest obtained for these patients. Values obtained subse-quently, when the tumor burden of these patients was greatly reduced, were also reduced. Patient R.C., who had demonstrated a complete re-sponse and clinical remission following therapy, suffered a recurrence of disease at 16 mo after beginning treatment. This clinical recurrence was predated and accompanied by an increase in the level of NCMC against K-562. These data are preliminary, and no attempt has yet been made to assess the accuracy of the serial measurement of NCMC for predicting tumor burden.

In Vivo Phenomena

Some of the in vivo manifestations of immunity to SCC are worthy of note. One of the hallmarks of an antitumor immune response is the pres-ence of an inflammatory infiltrate at the tumor site.[57] This cellular infiltrate

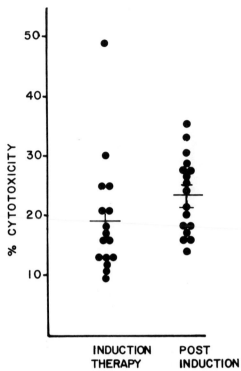

Figure 14-5. *NCMC for patients with limited stage SCC during induction therapy and following induction therapy.*

is most pronounced in squamous cell carcinomas and least pronounced or nonexistent in SCC.[58]

   It is possible that the antitumor response may in some way contribute to the pathological manifestations of SCC. The carcinomatous neuro-myopathies are the paraneoplastic syndromes most frequently associated with bronchogenic carcinoma. This group of secondary diseases is associated particularly with SCC; 56 percent of lung cancer patients exhibiting carcinomatous neuromyopathy have SCC.[56] The broad range of diseases classified as carcinomatous neuromyopathy are listed in Table 14-7. It has been suggested that these diseases may have an autoimmune basis.[60,61] This suggestion is largely based on the similarity of these syndromes to diseases such as myasthenia gravis or multiple sclerosis, in which autoimmunity is highly suspect, and to experimental disease models such as allergic encephalomyelitis, which has been proved to have an autoimmune cause.[61,62] The proposition is especially intriguing in light of the evidence

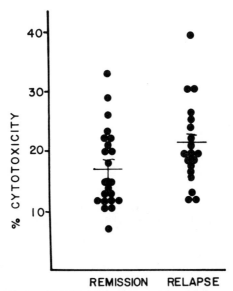

Figure 14-6. *NCMC for patients with extensive-stage SCC either in clinical remission or in relapse.*

(vide supra) that the cells of small cell carcinoma have antigens on their surfaces that share determinants with antigens on the surfaces of normal Schwann cells. There is evidence that the antigens on the surfaces of Schwann cells in the peripheral nervous system are shared by glial cells in the central nervous system.[69-71] Whether or not these glial cell antigens cross-react with antigens of SCC is not known at present.

It is interesting to speculate on the mechanisms involved in the causes of the neuromyopathies of SCC. A schematic representation of one possible mechanism is presented in Figure 14-8. In this proposed mechanism, both tumor antigens and those antigens that share determinants with Schwann cells would be present on the surfaces of cells of SCC. These antigens would be capable of eliciting an immune response in the host to both antigens on the surfaces of tumor cells. Such an immune response would consist of both cellular and humoral elements that would be capable of reacting with tumor cells, with circulating antigen shed from tumor cells, and with nervous system elements expressing the appropriate antigens. It is this last reaction that has been postulated to lead to carcinomatous neuromyopathy.

Some of the diseases listed in Table 14-7 are associated with mononuclear inflammatory infiltrate, whereas others are not. It has been sug-

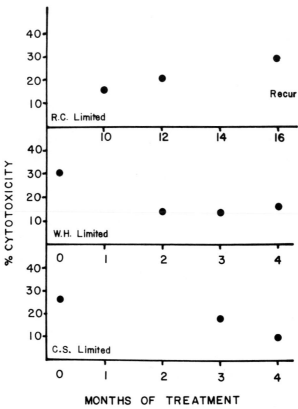

Figure 14-7. *NCMC serial values for 3 patients with limited-stage SCC.*

Table 14-7
Carcinomatous Neuromyopathies

Neuromyopathies	Reference No.
Neuropathies	
Peripheral neuropathy	62
Subacute cerebellar degeneration	63
Carcinomatous amytrophic lateral sclerosis	64
Myopathies	
Eaton-Lambert myasthenic syndrome	59, 65, 66
Polymyositis	59, 67, 68
Dermatomyositis	59, 67, 68

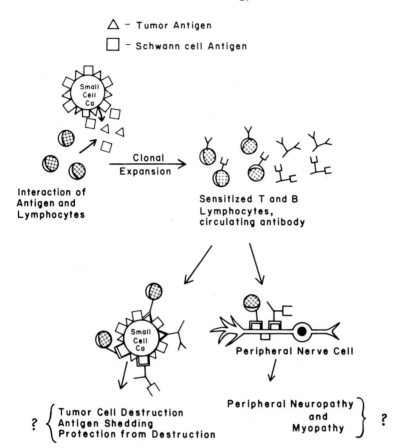

Figure 14-8. *Schematic representation of proposed causes of neuromyopathies associ- ated with SCC.*

gested that the lack of such infiltrate is evidence against an autoimmune cause. However, noninflammatory demyelinating lesions have been pro- duced in the dorsal roots of experimental animals by immunization with Schwann cells.[71,72] Demyelination of Schwann cells and glial cells in vitro has been produced by antibodies.[73] Thus, these lesions could be caused by elements of the host immune response to the tumor, and, as such, would be classified as autoimmune disease. Alternative causes have been suggested for the carcinomatous neuromyopathies, but they will not be discussed here.

Immunotherapy of SCC

The major approaches to immunotherapy in cancer are outlined in Table 14-8. Although many immunotherapy studies have included patients with SCC, those patients have been studied exclusively in only a few studies.[72] Israel[75] reported on 60 patients with SCC who were treated with chemotherapy, 30 of whom also received weekly treatments with *Corynebacterium parvum*. The *C. parvum* group had a statistically significant longer survival, which the authors felt was attributable to increased resistance to viral and bacterial infections. These patients were not prospectively randomized nor were they staged as to limited versus extensive disease. The latter omission could be responsible for the differences in survival noted. Another study by Israel[76] and one by Tenezynski[77] utilized *C. parvum* in treating SCC, but neither study was well designed to test its effectiveness.

Immunotherapy of SCC using BCG has been tested in several studies. McCracken,[78] using BCG in combination with chemotherapy, noted a higher, but not statistically significant, response rate in the BCG arm. Aisner[79] tested MER-BCG in combination with chemotherapy versus chemotherapy alone and found no difference. Holoye[80] tested BCG in conjunction with chemotherapy, and reported improved survival. This study was compared to historical controls, which limits any conclusion that may be drawn. Einhorn[81] treated 58 patients with chemotherapy plus BCG in a nonrandomized study where all the patients received BCG. He later dropped the BCG, and could not determine from the study if it had any effect.[82]

Cohen,[84] in a randomized trial, treated 61 patients (42 extensive and 19 limited stage) with chemotherapy followed by thymosin fraction V in 31 patients. In this study thymosin did not increase the response rate but did increase survival ($p < 0.05$) in the patients receiving the higher dose of thymosin. The lower dose had no effect. This study, which utilized a small number of patients, is ready to be confirmed in a larger trial.

In the Vanderbilt study of combined modality therapy of limited-stage SCC, we have studied the effect of *Corynebacterium parvum* in a controlled, prospective manner. Patients were given induction chemotherapy with cyclophosphamide, Adriamycin, and vincristine concommittently with thoracic irradiation followed by consolidation chemotherapy with VP-16 and hexamethylmelamine as previously described.[56] Patients in complete remission after extensive restaging[56] were randomized to methotrexate (75 mg/m² i.v. q-3-wk) or methotrexate plus *C. parvum* (2.5 mg/m² s.c. on day 1 and 14 q-3-wk). The methotrexate was given for 9 cycles and

Table 14-8
Approaches to Immunotherapy of Cancer

Active Immunization
    Specific
    Nonspecific

Transfer of immune cells, sera, or immune cell products
    Adoptive transfer with cells
    Passive transfer of antisera
    Transfer factor
    RNA from immune lymphocytes

Removal of inactivation of tumor-promoting factors

the *C. parvum* for 12 cycles. The results of this still ongoing trial are summarized in Table 14-9. No significant difference between the two groups is apparent up to now. Approximately 25 patients will be on each arm at the completion of this study, and, given the current results, it is unlikely *C. parvum* will have any impact on disease remission or survival over the first 2 yr from the beginning of treatment for limited-stage SCC.

Thus, of the immunotherapeutic agents studied, only thymosin has given preliminary evidence of effect in a controlled trial. Increased knowledge of the mechanism of action of each of these agents and the immunologic defects of the patient may lead to improved immunotherapy trials. Isolation and characterization of tumor-specific antigens or the use of monoclonal antibody, or both, may also eventually make specific immunotherapy more successful.

Conclusion

The natural history of the tumor–host relationship in SCC is of interest for several reasons. First, the changes this tumor causes in the host immune system could have some diagnostic and prognostic value. Sec-

Table 14-9
C. parvum Immunotherapy in SCC

	Methotrexate	Methotrexate–*C. parvum*
Number of patients	18	14
Median survival (range)	18 mo (9–40+)	18 mo (9–32+)
Number alive at 1 yr	16	10
Number alive at 2 yr	4	5

ond, the antigenic nature of this tumor may lead, via an autoimmune mechanism, to the expression of the neuromyopathic changes in this disease. Third, an increased knowledge of the immunobiology of this tumor may offer increased hope for immunodiagnosis and immunotherapy.

References

1. Prehn RT, Main JM: Immunity to methylcholanthrene induced sarcomas. J Natl Cancer Inst 18:769–778, 1957
2. Smith RT: Possibilities and problems of the immunologic intervention in cancer. N Engl J Med 287:439–450, 1972
3. Krammer PH: Alloantigen receptors on activated T-cells in mice. I. Binding of alloantigens and anti-idiotypic antibodies to the same receptor. J Exp Med 147:25–36, 1978
4. Binz H, Wigzell H: Induction of specific immune unresponsiveness with purified mixed leukocyte culture-activated T lymphoblasts as an autoimmunogen. III. Proof for the existence of autoanti-idiotype killer T-cells and transfer of suppression to normal syngeneic recipients by T or B lymphocytes. J Exp Med 147:63–76, 1978
5. McIntire KR, Adams WP, Braatz JA, et al: Identification of antigen associated with lung cancer suitable for diagnosis and monitoring, in Muggia FM (ed): Proceedings of the Second Conference on Lung Cancer Treatment. Virginia, Arlie House, 1977, p 27
6. McIntire KR, Sizaret PP: Human lung tumor antigens, in Bucalossi P, Veronesi U, Cassenelli N (eds): Proceedings of the XIth International Cancer Congress (vol. 1). Amsterdam, Excerpta Medica, 1974 pp 295–299
7. Sega E. Natali PG, Ricci C, et al: Lung cancer tumor associated antigen isolated by gel filtration and characterized by immunodiffusion. J Int Res Communic Med Sci 2:1278, 1974
8. Schlipkoter HW, Idei H, Barsoum AL, et al: Antigens characteristic for tumors in bronchial carcinoma. Zentralbl Bakteriol (Orig B) 158:109–124,1973
9. Veltri RW, Mergoli HF, Maxim PE, et al: Isolation and identification of human lung tumor associated antigens. Cancer Res 37:1313–1322, 1977
10. Yachi A, Matsura Y, Carpenter CM, et al: Immunochemical studies on human lung cancer antigens soluble in 50 % saturated ammonium sulfate. J Natl Cancer Inst 40:663–682, 1968
11. Frost MJ, Rogers GT, Bagsharve KD: Extraction and preliminary

characterization of a human bronchogenic carcinoma antigen. Br J Cancer 31:379–380, 1975

12. Gold P, Freedman SO: Demonstration of tumor-specific antigen in human colonic carcinomata by immunologic tolerance and absorption techniques. J Exp Med 121:439–462, 1965

13. Herberman RB, McIntire KR, Braatz J, et al: Antigen markers associated with lung cancer, in Proceedings Symposium on Clinical Application of Carcinoembryonic Antigen and Other Antigenic Markers Assays. Amsterdam, Excerpta Medica, 1974, pp 295–299

14. LoGerffo LP, Herter FP, Braun J, et al: Tumor associated antigen with pulmonary neoplasms. Ann Surg 175:495–500, 1972

15. Laurence DJR, Stevens U, Bettilheim R, et al: Role of plasma carcinoembryonic antigen in diagnosis of gastrointestinal, mammary and bronchial carcinoma. Br Med J 3:605–609, 1972

16. Vincent RG, Chu TM: Carcinoembryonic antigen in patients with carcinoma of the lung. J Thorac Cardiovasc Surg 66:320–328, 1973

17. Concannon JP, Dalbow MH, Liebler GH, et al: The carcinoembryonic antigen assay in bronchogenic carcinoma. Cancer 34:184–192, 1974

18. Stevens DP, Mackay IR: Increased carcinoembryonic antigen in heavy cigarette smokers. Lancet 2:1238–1239, 1973

19. Pauwels R, Van Der Straeten M: Plasma levels of carcinoembryonic antigen in bronchial carcinoma and chronic bronchitis. Thorax 30:560–562, 1975

20. Bell CE, Seetharam S: A plasma membrane antigen highly associated with oat-cell carcinoma of the lung and undetectable in normal adult tissue. Int J Cancer 18:605–611, 1976

21. Bell CE: A normal adult and fetal lung antigen present at different quantitative levels in different histologic types of lung cancer. Cancer 37:705–713, 1976

22. Bell CE, Seetharam S, McDaniel RC: Endodermally-derived and neural crest-derived differentiation antigens expressed by a human lung tumor. J Immunol 116:1236–1243, 1976

23. Bell CE, Seetharam S: Identification of the Schwann cell on a peripheral nervous system cell possessing a differentiation antigen expressed by a human lung tumor. J Immunol 118:826–831, 1977

24. De Schryver-Kecskemeti K, Kyriakos M, Bell CE, et al: Pulmonary oat cell carcinomas. Expression of plasma membrane antigen correlated with presence of cytoplasmic neurosecretory granules. Lab Invest 41:432–436, 1979

25. Bell CE, Seetharam S: Expression of endodunially derived differentiation antigens by human lung and colon tumors. Cancer 44:13–18, 1979

26. Seeger RC, Zeltzer PM, Rayner SA: Onco-neural antigen: A new neural differentiation antigen expressed by neuroblastoma, oat cell carcinoma, Wilms' tumor and sarcoma cells. J Immunol 122:1548–1555, 1979

27. Tischler AS, Dichter MA, Bialer B, et al.: Neuroendocrine neoplasms and their cells of origin. N Engl J Med 296:919–925, 1977

28. Havemann K, Gropp C, Scheuer A, et al: ACTH-like activity in immune complexes of patients with oat-cell carcinoma of the lung. Br J Cancer 39:43–50, 1979

29. Bonikor DS, Bensch KG: Endocrine cells of bronchial and bronchiolar epithelium. Am J Med 63:765–771, 1977

30. Oldham RK, Weese JL, Herberman RB, et al: Immunoembryonic monitoring and immunotherapy in carcinoma of the lung. Int J Cancer 18:739–749, 1976

31. Stewart THM: The presence of delayed hypersensitivity reactions in patients toward cellular extracts of their malignant tumors. 2. A corretation between the histologic picture of lymphocyte infiltration of the tumor stroma and the presence of such a reaction and a discussion of the significance of this phenomenon. Cancer 23:1368–1379, 1969

32. Hollingshead AC, Stewart THM, Herberman RB: Delayed hypersensitivity reactions to soluble membrane antigens of human malignant lung cells. J Natl Cancer Inst 52:327–338, 1974

33. Weese JL, Herberman RB, Hollingshead AC, et al: Specificity of delayed cutaneous hypersensitivity reactions to extracts of human tumor cells. J Natl Cancer Inst 60:255–263, 1978

34. Stewart THM, Hollingshead AC, Harris JE, et al: Immunochemotherapy of lung cancer. Ann NY Acad Sci 277:436–466, 1976

35. Hellström I, Hellström KE, Sjögren HO, et al: Demonstration of cell mediated immunity to human neoplasms of various histological types. Int J Cancer 7:1–16, 1971

36. Oldham RK, Djeu JY, Cannon GB, et al: Cellular microcytotoxicity in human tumor systems: Analysis of results. J Natl Cancer Inst 55:1305–1318, 1975

37. Oldham RK, Sivarski D, McCoy JL, et al: Evaluation of a cell-mediated cytotoxicity assay utilizing ^{125}Iododeoxy-uridine-labeled tissue-culture target cells. Natl Cancer Inst Monogr 37:49–58, 1973

38. Herberman RB, Oldham RK: Problems associated with study of cell-mediated immunity to human tumors by microcytoxicity assays. J Natl Cancer Inst 55:749–753, 1975

39. Dean JH, McCoy JL, Cannon GB, et al: Cell-mediated immune re-

sponses of breast cancer patients to autologous tumor-associated antigens. J Natl Cancer Inst 58:549–555, 1977

40. Dean JH, McCoy JL, Cannon GB, et al: Lymphocyte proliferation responses of patients with carcinoma of the breast and lung to mitogens, alloantigens and tumor-associated antigens, in Proceedings of the Symposium on Detection and Prevention of Cancer. (in press)

41. McCoy JL: Clinical applications of assays of leukocyte migration inhibition, in Herberman RB, McIntire KR (eds): Immunodiagnosis of Cancer. New York, Marcel Dekker, 1979, pp 979–998

42. McCoy JL, Jerome LF, Cannon GB, et al: Reactivity of lung cancer patients in leukocyte migration inhibition assays to 3M potassium chloride extracts of fresh tumor and tissue-cultured cells derived from lung cancer. J Natl Cancer Inst 59:1413–1418, 1978

43. Boddie AW, Urist MM, Chee DO, et al: Detection of human tumor-associated antigens by the leukocyte migration in agarose assay. Int J Cancer 18:161–167, 1976

44. Vose BM, Kimber I, Moore M: Leukocyte migration inhibition in human pulmonary neoplasm. J Natl Cancer Inst 58:483–488, 1977

45. Suslov I, McCoy JL, Herberman RB: Indirect leukocyte migration inhibition reactions to lung tumor-associated antigens by lung cancer patients. J Natl Cancer Inst (in press)

46. Suslov I, McCoy JL, Cannon GB, et al: High incidence of migration inhibition reactivity to lung tumor-associated antigen by normal donors in close contact with lung cancer. J Natl Cancer Inst 65:708–713, 1980

47. Takasuzi M, Mickey MR, Terasaki PI: Reactivity of lymphocytes from normal persons on cultured tumor cells. Cancer Res 33:2898–2902, 1973

48. Herberman RB, Nunn M, Lavrin DH, et al: Effect of antibody to theta antigen on cell-mediated immunity induced in syngeneic mice by nurine sarcoma virus. J Natl Cancer Inst 51:1509–1512, 1973

49. Rosenberg EB, McCoy JL, Green SS, et al: Destruction of human lymphoid tissue culture cell lines by human peripheral lymphocytes in ^{51}Cr-release cellular cytotoxicity assays. J Natl Cancer Inst 52:345–352, 1974

50. Shov CB, Holland JM, Perkins EH: Development of fewer tumor colonies in lungs of athymic nude mice after intravenous injection of tumor cells. J Natl Cancer Inst 56:193–195, 1976

51. Fidler IJ, Caines S, Dolan Z: Survival of hematogenously disseminated allogenic tumor cells in athymic nude mice. Transplantation 22:208–212, 1976

52. Gillette RW, Fox A: The effect of T-lymphocyte deficiency on tumor induction and growth. Cell Immunol 19:328–335, 1975

53. Bonmassar E, Canupanile F, Houchens D, et al: Impaired growth of a radiation induced lymphoma in intact or lethally irradiated allogenic athymic (nude) mice. Transplantation 20:343–346, 1975.

54. Forbes JT, Oldham RK: Natural cytotoxicity of human lymphocytes: population distribution. Fed Proc 37:1591, 1978

55. Forbes JT, Niblack GD, Fuchs R, et al: Human natural cell-mediated cytotoxicity. I. Distribution in normal populations. Cancer Immunol Immunotherapy (in press).

56. Greco FA, Richardson RL, Snell JA: Small cell lung cancer. Complete remission and improved survival. Amer J Med 66:625–630, 1979

57. Fisher ER, Fisher B: Local lymphoid response as an index of tumor immunity. Arch Pathol 94:137–146, 1972

58. Ioachim HL, Dorsett BH, Paluck E: The immune response at the tumor site in lung carcinoma. Cancer 38:2296–2307, 1976

59. Morton DL, Itabashi HH, Grimer DF: Nonmetastatic neurological complications of bronchogenic carcinoma: The carcinomatous myopathies. J Thorac Cardiovasc Surg 51:14–29, 1966

60. Prehn RT: Immune responses in cancer, in Brain WT, Norris FH (eds): The Remote Effects of Cancer on the Nervous System. New York, Grune & Stratton, 1965, p 185

61. Alvord EC: Brain antigens and antibodies: The possible relationship between carcinomatous and experimental allergic neuro-encephalomyelitides, in Brain WT, Norris FH (eds): The Remote Effects of Cancer on the Nervous System. New York, Grune & Stratton, 1965, p 188

62. Richardson EP: Progressive multifocal leukoencephalopathy, in Brain WT, Norris FH (eds): The Remote Effects of Cancer on the Nervous System. New York, Grune & Stratton, 1965, p 6

63. Brain WT, Wilkinson M: Subacute cerebellar degeneration in patients with carcinoma, in Brain WT, Norris FH (eds): The Remote Effects of Cancer on the Nervous System. New York, Grune & Stratton, 1965, p 17

64. Norris FH, Engel WK: Carcinomatous amyotrophyic lateral sclerosis, in Brain WT, Norris FH (eds): The Remote Effects of Cancer on the Nervous System. New York, Grune & Stratton, 1965, p 24

65. Kennedy WR, Jimenez-Paton E: The myasthenic syndrome associated with small cell carcinoma of the lung (Eaton-Lambert syndrome). Neurology (Minneap) 18:757–766, 1968

66. Norris FH, Izzo AJ, Garvey PH: Tumor site and Lambert-Eaton syn-

drome, in Brain WT, Norris FH (eds): The Remote Effects of Cancer on the Nervous System. New York, Grune & Stratton, 1965, p 81

67. Rowland LP, Schotland DL: Neoplasms and muscle disease, in Brain WT, Norris FH (eds): The Remote Effects of Cancer on the Nervous System. New York, Grune & Stratton, 1965, p 83

68. Bohan A, Peter JB, Bowman RL, et al: A computer associated analysis of 153 patients with polymyositis and dermatomyositis. Medicine 56:255–286, 1977

69. Waksman BH, Adams RD: A comparative study of experimental allergic neuritis in the rabbit, guinea pig and mouse. J Neuropathol Exp Neurol 15:293–314, 1956

70. Kies MW, Alvord EC (eds): Allergic Encephalomyelitis. Springfield, Illinois, Charles C Thomas, 1959

71. Palacios O, Pette E: Zur Frage der Erzengung einer allergischen Polyneuritis in Kanimchen mit Schwannscehm Zellgewebekultur-Antigen. Z Imm Allerg 126:122–124, 1964

72. Pette E, Mannweiler K, Palacios O, et al: Phenomena of the cell membrane and their possible significance for the pathogenesis of so-called autoimmune diseases of the nervous system. Ann NY Acad Sci 122:417–428, 1965

73. Bornstein MB, Appel SH: Tissue culture studies of demyelination diseases. Ann NY Acad Sci 122:280–286, 1965

74. Mikulski SM, McGuire WP, Louie AL, et al: Immunotherapy of lung cancer II. Review of clinical trials in small cell carcinoma. Cancer Treat Rep 6:125–130, 1979

75. Israel L: Nonspecific immune stimulation with Corynebacteria in lung cancer, in Israel L, Chahinian P (eds): Lung Cancer: Natural History, Prognosis and Therapy. New York, Academic Press, 1976, p 273

76. Israel L, Depierre A, Choffel C, et al: Immunochemotherapy in 34 cases of oat cell carcinoma of the lung with 19 complete responses. Cancer Treat Rep 61:343–347, 1977

77. Tenczynski TF, Valdivieso M, Hersh EM, et al: Chemoimmunotherapy (CI) of small cell bronchogenic carcinoma (SCBC). Proc Am Soc Clin Oncol 19:376, 1978

78. McCracken J, White J, Reed R, et al: Combination chemotherapy, radiotherapy, and immunotherapy for oat cell carcinoma of the lung. Proc Am Soc Clin Oncol 19:395, 1978

79. Aisner J, Esterkay RJ, Wiernik PH: Chemotherapy versus chemoimmunotherapy for small cell carcinoma of the lung. Proc Am Assoc Cancer Res 18:310, 1977

80. Holye PY: Chemoimmunotherapy of small cell bronchogenic carcinoma. Proc Am Soc Clin Oncol 18:278, 1977

81. Einhorn LH, Hornback NB, Bond WH: Combination chemotherapy, radiotherapy, and immunotherapy in small cell undifferentiated lung cancer. Proc Am Soc Clin Oncol 18:267, 1977

82. Einhorn LH, Bond WH, Hornback N, et al: Long-term results in combined modality treatment of small cell carcinoma of the lung. Sem Oncol 5:309–313, 1978

83. Cohen MH, Ihde DC, Fossieck BE, et al: Cyclic alternating combination chemotherapy of small cell bronchogenic carcinoma (SCBC). Proc Am Soc Clin Oncol 19:359, 1978

84. Cohen MH, Chretien PB, Ihde DC, et al: Thymosis fraction V and intensive combination chemotherapy. Prolonging the survival of patients with small cell lung cancer. JAMA 241:1813–1815, 1979

15

CLINICAL MANAGEMENT OF PATIENTS WITH SMALL CELL LUNG CANCER

F. Anthony Greco
Robert K. Oldham

The management of patients with small cell lung cancer (SCC) is undergoing evolution and refinement.[1] Although current therapy is more effective than ever, therapeutic toxicity and the high relapse rate remain major problems. While working to develop a rational therapy comparable in effectiveness to the antibiotics used for many infectious diseases, we are faced with the reality of caring for many thousands of patients yearly with this neoplastic disorder.

Although the most rational method for improving therapy is first to gain a better understanding of the etiology and pathogenesis of the disease, improvements in therapy do not necessarily depend on such understanding. Progress thus far in the management of patients with several neoplastic diseases has hinged upon semiempirical therapy developed by clinical investigators. Like many other neoplasms that are sensitive to various chemotherapeutic agents and radiotherapy, SCC has partially yielded to therapy.

Unfortunately, the number of patients with SCC is expected to increase during the next decade. Unless cigarette smoking decreases dra-

This work was supported in part by Grants CA 19429, CA 23909-01, and 1 R01 CA 27333-01 from the National Cancer Institute and by Grant JFCF 394A from the American Cancer Society.

matically, lung cancer will reach even greater epidemic proportions. Small cell lung cancer accounts for 20–25 percent of all lung cancer and will be diagnosed in approximately 30,000 patients in the United States in 1980. Although relatively rare in women in the past, the incidence is steadily increasing in parallel with the accelerated level of cigarette smoking among women.

We would be remiss to ignore the primary prevention of a disease that is very difficult to treat after it develops. In nonsmokers or in those who have stopped smoking for at least 10 yr, small cell lung cancer is extremely rare.[2] There is a latent period from the beginning of cigarette-smoking to the clinical appearance of the neoplasm. Total cessation of cigarette smoking by a large segment of the population would not be expected to diminish the disease substantially for 10–15 yr. Nonetheless, it remains the responsibility of medicine and the medical community to support antismoking programs in order to prevent the many diseases linked to cigarette smoking.

Once clinically diagnosed, the management of the SCC patient becomes the primary problem. Current therapy offers the patient the opportunity to obtain effective palliation and prolongation of useful life. This chapter deals primarily with the spectrum of the illness and some general management concepts. Unfortunately, therapy has not yet reached a point where toxicity is trivial and the disease easily curable. Therefore absolutely safe and effective therapy is not available. It is in the best interest of each patient to be seen and managed by an oncologist. Ideally, each patient should also have the opportunity of receiving a potentially improved therapy as a part of an ongoing clinical investigative program.

Spectrum of the Illness

Symptomatic male cigarette smokers between the ages of 40 and 70 represent the majority of patients who present with this illness. Recently the incidence in women has been escalating, subsequent to increased cigarette smoking by teenage girls and young women.

In keeping with its origin and growth characteristics, SCC produces a variety of clinical manifestations related to rapid local growth, visceral metastases, ectopic hormone or peptide production, and poorly understood nonmetastatic or remote effects. At presentation, most patients have respiratory symptoms related to the primary tumor (cough, chest pain, dyspnea, wheezing, or hemoptysis). Less frequently presenting problems are related to regional spread (superior vena cava syndrome, hoarseness, dysphagia, pericardial effusion, pleural effusion), visceral metastases (bone pain, hepatomegaly, liver dysfunction, neurologic deficits), ectopic hormone production (Cushing's syndrome, the syndrome of inappropriate secretion of antidiuretic hormone), or remote effects (anorexia, weight loss, Eaton-Lambert myasthenic syndrome, neuromyopathies). During the course of the illness a composite of some of these clinical problems is the rule, although any one may dominate.

Several important and some unique clinical associations have been identified. Greater than 80 percent of patients have symptoms for less than 3 mo prior to diagnosis, as a consequence of rapid growth and metastases. Mediastinal tumor produces superior vena cava syndrome and hoarseness more often than any other pulmonary neoplasm.[3] Chest radiographs typically show a central tumor mass, often with hilar and mediastinal involvement reminiscent of a lymphoma. Metastases are a formidable problem occurring in nearly every patient prior to diagnosis, and, in the absence of effective therapy, they soon become clinically apparent. Symptomatic metastases in the central nervous system, liver, bone or bone marrow from an occult primary tumor is not an unexpected finding. Symptomatic central nervous system involvement is present in 10 percent of patients initially and at least 30 percent during the untreated course of the disease.[4] Cerebral symptoms and signs or the spinal cord compression syndrome may dominate the clinical picture. Although bone involvement is frequent and often extensive, hypercalcemia is only rarely seen.[5] Anemia, thrombocytopenia, or a leukoerythroblastic blood reaction may result from bone marrow involvement. However, bone marrow involvement is usually clinically silent even though demonstrable by bone marrow examination in 25 percent of all patients.[6] Bone marrow aspiration and biopsy may be diagnostic in patients with lesions in otherwise poorly accessible areas such as the brain, retroperitoneum, kidney, or mediastinum. Constitutional manifestations such as anorexia, weight loss, anemia, and weakness are extremely common. These manifestations are often not adequately explained by the clinical location or volume of the tumor and are best viewed as remote effects of the tumor.

Current Therapy

Chemotherapy for SCC has evolved largely over the past decade. As is illustrated in Table 15-1, early studies administered placebo or no therapy to some patients. These results, a reflection of the natural history of the neoplasm, showed a median survival of 10 wk, with approximately 95

Table 15-1
Evolution of More Successful Therapy for SCC in the
Past 15 Years

Therapy	No. of Patients	Complete Response (%)	Median Survival (weeks)	Survival at 1 yr (%)
Placebo[7,8]	55	0	10	5
Surgery[9,†]	187	25	20	20
Radiotherapy[45–48,†]	235	—	24	20
Single drugs[10]	831	1.8	22	16
Combination chemotherapy[10,‡]	452	23	36	40
Combination chemotherapy plus radiotherapy[10,‡]	984	31	44	47

*Represents the mean 1-yr survival of all series.
†Primarily limited-stage patients.
‡Review of multiple series with therapy of varying efficacy.

percent of the patients dead within the first year. Patients rarely survived longer than 35 wk with limited-stage (median 14 wk) and 20 wk with extensive stage-disease (median 7 wk).[7,8] Local therapy, in the form of surgery or radiotherapy, improved the short-term survival only slightly and primarily for a small subset of patients with limited-stage disease. However, the overwhelming majority of patients were not benefited, and 80 percent of the patients died within 1 yr.

Single chemotherapeutic agents have been evaluated during the last decade. Initially, these drugs were tested in previously untreated patients. Since more effective therapy has been developed, new drugs are now evaluated in heavily pretreated patients. Several single drugs have produced impressive, but transient, clinical responses and a statistically significant increase in survival. Unfortunately, the overwhelming majority of patients were not benefited to any extent. The combined use of active single drugs has been a major therapeutic advance and has increased the complete response rate, the median survival, and the 1-yr survival significantly.[10] The data outlined in Table 15-1 are from a large, heterogeneous group of patients, some with limited and some with extensive disease, of mixed ages and performance status, who received a large number of drug combinations, each having a different efficacy. Nonetheless, the complete response rate and survival have increased substantially.

Table 15-2
Survival in Selected Series of Extensive-Stage SCC

Therapy*,†	Number of Patients	Complete Response (%)	Median Survival (weeks)	Relapse-free at 2 yr (%)
CTX, DOX, VCR, MTX, RT[49]	250	14	28	2
CTX, DOXO, VCR, RT[50]	35	40	40	—
CTX, DOXO, VCR, RT, CCNU, MTX, BCG[51]	39	22	36	—
CTX, DOXO, VCR, RT, HEXA, VP-16, MTX[52]	20	15	44	5
CTX, DOXO, CCNU, MTX, VCR, BLEO, Emetine, *C. parvum*[53]	16	62	52	—
CTX, MTX, CCNU, DOXO, VCR, PROCAR[54]	42	42	40	—
CTX, DOXO, VP-16, VCR[11]	21	24	62	—
Various Intensive regimens (Vanderbilt)[52,55–57]	98	21	51	4
Various Intensive regimens (National Cancer Institute)[58]	95	—	—	4

*CTX, cyclophosphamide; DOXO, doxorubicin; MTX, methotrexate; RT, radiotherapy; VCR, vincristine; HEXA, hexamethylmelamine; BLEO, bleomycin; BCG, bacillus calmette Guérin; *C. parvum, Corynebacterium parvum*; PROCAR, procarbazine.

Therapy of Extensive-Stage Disease

A more specific look at recent therapy for patients with extensive-stage disease is illustrated in Table 15-2. The complete response rate in these patients ranges from 14 to 62 percent but more commonly is 15–25 percent. The median survival of all patients ranges from 28 to 62 wk. Approximately 40 percent are alive at 1 yr. Patients attaining a complete response usually survive beyond the median. Increasing numbers of patients have been treated and followed for a period of 2 to 3 yr. However, few data have been published at this time regarding long-term survival. From our series and a few others it appears that 1–5 percent of these patients will be relapse free at 2 yr following the initiation of therapy (Table 15-2). A critical look at patients in complete remission who have been aggressively restaged suggests that these patients may have a prognosis similar to complete responders with limited-stage disease.[11]

Therapy of Limited-Stage Disease

For those unusual patients who present with a solitary peripheral nodule or a small bronchial lesion, surgical resection may be the treatment of choice.[12] These patients should receive postoperative combination chemotherapy. No large series of resected patients treated subsequently with effective chemotherapy has been reported. Studies in these patients are in progress. Logically, chemotherapy should be very effective in this setting, since the majority of patients do have micrometastases, regardless of the size of the primary lesion. Unfortunately, patients rarely present with resectable lesions, and even more rarely are these lesions the only areas of disease.

Survival in selected series of patients with limited-stage disease is illustrated in Table 15-3. A majority of these therapies also include chest radiotherapy but there is no definitive evidence that this is necessary to produce these results. Preliminary results from studies using sequential chest radiotherapy and chemotherapy have shown no advantage for radiotherapy.[13-14] However, simultaneously administered radiotherapy and chemotherapy may be superior to chemotherapy alone.[15] Complete response rates after various treatment regimens ranges from 33 to 100 percent. The 1-yr survival ranges from 50 to 80 percent and the relapse-free survival at 2 yr from 11 to 40 percent. Overall, approximately 25 percent of patients with limited-stage disease are relapse free at 2 yr following a variety of the effective combination chemotherapies, often, but not necessarily, combined with thoracic radiotherapy. Prophylactic whole brain radiotherapy is required in all patients to prevent the growth of brain metastases.[4]

Detailed results obtained in one illustrative series of patients with limited-stage disease will now be presented. Between January 1976 and January 1979, 51 patients with limited-stage disease were treated with combined radiotherapy and combination chemotherapy at Vanderbilt University Medical Center. The rationale for the regimen was based on several factors. Radiotherapy alone could eradicate the primary tumor in a minority of patients,[16] and the primary tumor was a frequent site of relapse in those treated with chemotherapy alone.[10] Each drug selected for combination chemotherapy (cyclophosphamide, doxorubicin, and vincristine) was active as a single agent. Furthermore, therapeutic synergism between doxorubicin and cyclophosphamide had been demonstrated,[17] and vincristine could be added without increasing the myelotoxicity. In addition, a few patients had at that time experienced improved survival following combinations of cyclophosphamide and vincristine plus chest

Table 15-3
Survival in Selected Series of Limited-Stage SCC

Therapy[*],[†]	Number of Patients	Complete Response (%)	1-yr Survival (%)	Relapse-free at 2 yr (%)
CTX, VCR, RT[59]	16	50	50	19
CTX, DOXO, VCR, RT[49]	108	41	50	15
CTX, DOXO, VCR, RT, CCNU, MTX, BCG[61]	19	89	80	26
CTX, DOXO, CCNU, MTX, VCR, BLEO, Emetine, C. parvum[53]	20	70	—	25
CTX, DOXO, VCR, CCNU, MTX, RT[†]	12	—	—	17
CTX, CCNU, MTX, VCR, RT[†]	110	—	—	11
CTX, DOXO, VCR, RT[†]	10	100	—	40
CTX, DOXO, VCR, MTX, RT[†]	12	100	—	17
CTX, VP-16, RT[60]	12	40	—	25
DOXO, VP-16, RT[60]	9	33	—	11
CTX, MTX, CCN, DOXO, VCR, PROCAR[54]	19	74	—	16
CTX, VCR, CCNU, DOXO, HEXA, RT[61]	36	64	—	22
CTX, DOXO, VCR, HEXA, RT, VP-16, MTX ± C. parvum (this chapter)	51	80	72	25

*CTX, cyclophosphamide; DOXO, doxorubicin; MTX, methotrexate; RT, radiotherapy; VCR, vincristine; HEXA, hexamethylmelamine; BLEO, bleomycin; BCG, bacillus calmette Guérin; C. parvum, Corynebacterium parvum; PROCAR, procarbazine.
†As reported from Greco et al.[10]

radiotherapy.[18] The simultaneous administration of radiotherapy and cyclophosphamide, doxorubicin, and vincristine produced an enhanced effect on normal tissues and probably against the tumor.[19] Therefore, we felt the schedule and dose of radiotherapy and drug administration was an important issue. Our goal was to begin combination chemotherapy and chest radiotherapy simultaneously and to give full doses of drugs unless severe clinical toxicity was present. The radiosensitizing potential of the drugs, particularly doxorubicin, when given simultaneously with radiotherapy was felt to represent a potential therapeutic advantage.

Supervoltage radiotherapy was given to the area of the primary tumor and mediastinum, to a total dose of 3000 rads in 10 300-rad daily fractions. The first 12 patients in this program were not given prophylactic whole brain radiotherapy, but the remaining patients received prophylactic whole brain radiotherapy in the same schedule as the chest radiotherapy. Each patient received cyclophosphamide 1000 mg/m^2, doxorubicin 40 mg/m^2, and vincristine 1 mg/m^2 intravenously simultaneously with the beginning of radiotherapy and thereafter once every 3 wk for a total of 6 cycles. Following this induction phase, a non-cross-resistant combination of the epipodophyllotoxin VP-16 (200 mg/m^2 intravenously on days 1 and 8 of each month) and hexamethylmelamine (8 mg/kg orally on days 1–14 of each month) was administered for 3 monthly cycles. Patients were then randomly assigned to receive continued therapy during remission with either cyclic methotrexate (75 mg/m^2) intramuscularly every 3 wk or the same dose and schedule of methotrexate plus *Corynebacterium parvum* (2.5 mg/m^2 subcutaneously) on days 1 and 14 for 7 mo. Following this period all treatment was stopped. Doses were attenuated as necessary based upon severe bone marrow depression, particularly if accompanied by infection.

The patients were evaluated for response to therapy after the course of radiotherapy and at least 3 cycles of chemotherapy (10–12 wk). Complete response was defined as disappearance of all clinical evidence of disease as judged by physical examination, chest radiographs, and fiberoptic bronchoscopy with biopsy, brushings, and washings.

It is well known that radiation changes such as fibrosis in the lung may mimic residual or progressive tumor and make it very difficult to evaluate response to therapy. This is certainly true several months after the initiation of radiotherapy. The radiographic changes produced by radiotherapy or the combination of radiotherapy and chemotherapy do not usually begin to occur until 3 mo. Therefore, if the patient is evaluated for response between 7 and 12 wk after the initiation of treatment, a clearer definition of response as judged by the radiograph can be made. This is illustrated in Figures 15-1 and 15-2. Fiberoptic bronchoscopy is also useful. The area of the previous intrabronchial lesion can be visualized, biopsied, brushed, and washed for pathologic examination.

All 51 patients were evaluated for response. Forty-two of these patients had a complete re-staging evaluation, while 9 patients did not have

Figure 15-1. *(A) Chest radiograph showing a left hilar mass before therapy. (B) The appearance 10 wk after the start of therapy. There is a complete radiographic resolution of the mass, and no changes in the lung from the radiotherapy are apparent.*

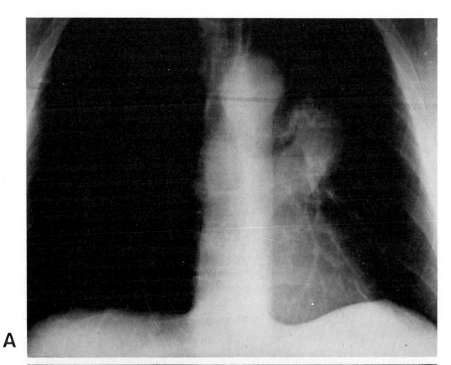

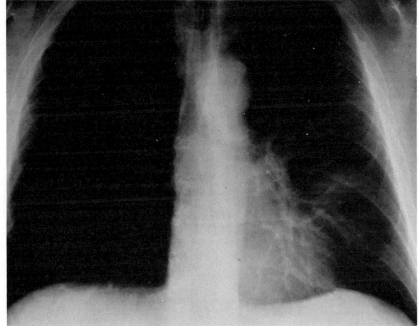

361

a repeat bronchoscopy. Complete responses occurred in 36 of the 42 patients (85 percent) as judged by both chest radiographs and bronchoscopy, and in 5 of the remaining 9 patients as judged by chest radiographs alone. Therefore, 41 of the 51 (80 percent) patients had a complete response to therapy and 10 of 51 (20 percent) had a partial response, for an overall response rate of 100 percent.

Every symptomatic patient in this series showed improvement following therapy. The majority of patients with chest pain had complete relief of their pain, usually within 1–3 wk, whereas all other patients had a decrease in the quantity of chest pain. Cough and shortness of breath were usually greatly relieved. Twenty-three patients with hemoptysis had complete resolution of bleeding. Anorexia also substantially decreased between treatments, and 38 percent of the patients regained lost weight. Considering the universal, but transient, nausea and frequent vomiting associated with intermittent chemotherapy, the weight gain was impressive. The performance status or functional status of the patients also improved.

The median duration of partial response was 8 mo, while the median duration of complete response was 16 mo. Partial responses ranged from 3 to 17 mo, whereas complete responses have ranged from 3 to over 42 mo. Seventeen patients remained in complete response or relapse free from 11 to over 42 mo. Immunotherapy given late in remission had no effect on duration of response or survival (see Chapter 14, this monograph). The major emphasis will now focus on the survival of the 51 patients.

Sixteen patients were treated between January 1976 and January 1977. The minimum follow-up on any 1 patient has been 34 mo, with the longest surviving patient now having survived over 42 mo from the time of first therapy. The first 12 patients were not treated with prophylactic whole brain radiotherapy, and 3 of these patients died of isolated cranial metastases without clinical evidence of disease outside the brain at the time of relapse. Unfortunately, postmortem examinations were not obtained on these patients. One other patient died of a myocardial infarction while in complete remission 5 mo after beginning therapy. Three patients (19 percent) are alive and disease free at 34, 39 and 42 mo. Seven of the initial 16 patients were alive at 2 yr (44 percent), but only 4 were relapse free (25 percent). One of these 4 patients who was relapse free at 2 yr subsequently relapsed and died at 36 mo. Therefore, 3 of the 16 patients are currently disease free with a median follow-up in excess of 3 yr.

Figure 15-2. *(A) A large left hilar mass shown before therapy. (B) The radiographic appearance 12 wk following the start of therapy shows complete resolution of the lesion and no apparent radiation changes.*

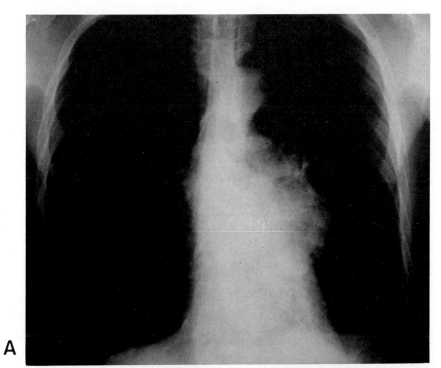

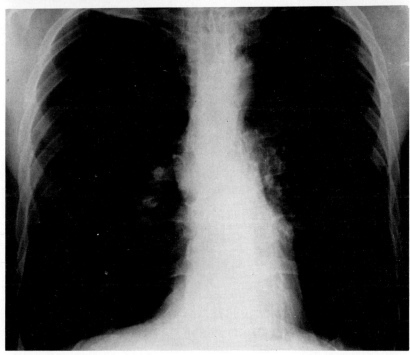

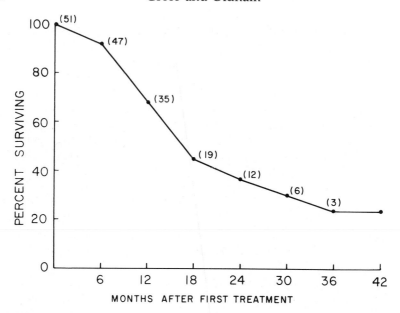

Figure 15-3. *Life-table analysis of survival for all 51 patients. Numbers in parentheses represent patients surviving at each time interval.*

There were also 16 patients entered on the study between January 1977 and January 1978. All 16 patients received prophylactic whole brain radiotherapy in addition to the therapy previously outlined. Five of these 16 patients (31 percent) have survived 2 yr, and all are clinically free of disease. Minimum follow-up is 26 mo. Three other patients in this group died of causes not clearly related to their cancer or the therapy. Two patients died of myocardial infarctions and 1 of encephalitis. One patient died from pneumonia that was treatment-related. Although he was clinically free of tumor, microscopic residual cancer was found at autopsy.

In summary, 8 of 32 patients (25 percent) treated with this program between January 1976 and January 1978 are alive and free of disease with a minimum follow-up in excess of 2 yr. Four patients who had had a complete response to therapy died of diseases other than cancer. These deaths were not clearly related to therapy. One patient died from pneumonia and sepsis directly related to therapy.

Twenty-one patients have been entered in the final year of this evaluation between January 1978 and January 1979, making a total of 51 patients. Median follow-up for this latter group is 15 months, and these patients do not substantially add to the information concerning 2-yr relapse-free survival. Nonetheless these patients appear to have relapse-

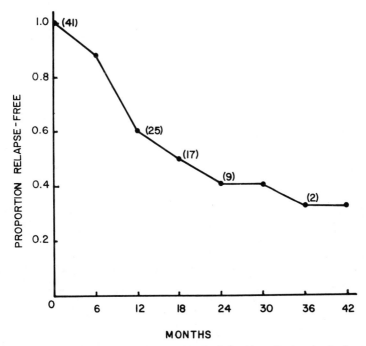

Figure 15-4. *Analysis of relapse-free survival of the 41 patients who had a complete response to therapy.*

free survival rates similar to the earlier groups in that 5 of the 8 (63 percent) at risk for 14 months are alive and relapse free.

Life-table analysis of all 51 patients is illustrated in Figure 15-3. The minimum follow-up is in excess of 1 yr, and the median follow-up for all patients is greater than 2 yr. The relapse-free or disease-free survival curve (Fig. 15-4) shows that approximately 40 percent of the patients who had complete responses will have no evidence of the disease 2 yr after the initiation of the therapy. The *actuarial* survival curve (Fig. 15-3) indicates that approximately 40 percent of all the patients will be alive 2 yr after beginning therapy. The *actual* survival of patients at risk for 2 yr or greater in this series of patients is 25 percent (8 of 32 patients at risk are alive and disease free). Only those patients achieving a complete response can be expected to reach the 2-yr period.

One of the 51 patients (2 percent) entered in this program between January 1976 and January 1978 died from a treatment-related cause. He had pneumonia and severe pulmonary insufficiency. Mild to moderate esophagitis has occurred in 50 percent of the patients but none developed an esophageal stricture. No patient had recurrent episodes of severe esophagitis following subsequent chemotherapy or "recall" esophagitis. Only an occasional patient required hospitalization for intravenous fluids during a period of moderate esophagitis. Nonhemotologic toxicity has not been a serious problem in these patients. None developed doxorubicin-related heart disease or radiation myelitis. One patient had a transient acute radiation–drug-induced pneumonia. Two patients had acute hemorrhagic cystitis from cyclophosphamide. Hematologic toxicity was the important toxicity. Most patients had a drop in their total white blood cell count during induction therapy to below 1000/mm³. The mean nadir was 725 mm³ with a range of 100–1750 mm³. Thrombocytopenia was not a major problem, and only 1 patient required a platelet transfusion. The mean platelet nadir was 75,000 mm³ with a range of 20,000–130,000 mm³. Nine patients required hospitalization a total of 12 times for fever and suspected infection during periods of leukopenia. Two had documented infections, and every patient except 1, who died with pneumonia, recovered.

Several other series of patients with limited disease have been reported as is shown in Table 15-3. A plateau of the survival curve is definitely present, and, unless there are late relapses in the majority of patients, therapy is curative for a portion of patients. More data on extensive-stage patients who attain a complete response are necessary to make conclusions concerning these patients. However, it is reasonable to speculate that patients who are re-staged aggressively and who are in complete remission will do as well as limited-stage patients who achieve a complete response.

General Concepts

The optimal management of patients with SCC is still evolving. As yet there is no therapy that can cure the majority of patients. Nevertheless, the natural history of this disease has been impressively modified by combination chemotherapy. Today patients are surviving as a group much longer than before. Those with limited-stage disease have a median survival of approximately 1.5 yr, whereas those with extensive-stage disease approach a median survival of about 1 yr. Because most patients die of their disease within 2 yr, it is not surprising that the median survival figures have not changed dramatically. There has been a major improvement for a subset of surviving patients reflected as a plateau in the survival curve. Most of these patients will probably not relapse.

A less dramatic, although important, result has been the successful palliation of most patients with current therapy. The protean clinical manifestations of SCC can often be completely ameliorated for variable periods.

Since local therapy had no meaningful impact on the quality of life or survival for the majority of patients, chemotherapy developed in a fashion similar to that for other previously successfully treated metastatic cancers also characterized by rapid growth rates, such as Burkitt's lymphoma, testicular carcinoma, diffuse histiocytic lymphoma, and Ewing's sarcoma. Several active drugs have been identified to date and include nitrogen mustard, cyclophosphamide, methotrexate, doxorubicin, vincristine, CCNU, procarbazine, hexamethylmelamine, and the epipodophyllotoxin (VP-16-213).

Combination chemotherapy is superior to single drugs in producing a complete response.[10] A complete response to treatment is the first step in providing symptomatic relief for the patient and for increasing useful survival. The optimal type and duration of therapy for SCC have not yet been determined. The most frequently administered combination regimens have consisted of cyclophosphamide given with either doxorubicin and vincristine, methotrexate and vincristine, or methotrexate and CCNU. Combination chemotherapy has usually been given rather intensively and intermittently. More intensive induction therapy, including higher doses administered more frequently, is more effective in increasing complete response rate and survival, but it is also associated with greater toxicity.[10]

There are factors that make it quite difficult to give intensive therapy to some patients. Often these patients are elderly chronic cigarette smokers with other major medical problems, including chronic obstructive pulmonary disease, arteriosclerotic cardiovascular disease, and alcoholism. Frequently they are malnourished because of these underlying diseases or because of their neoplasm and are less able to withstand intensive induction chemotherapy. Therefore, clinical judgment is necessary in selecting patients for more intensive approaches. Elderly patients and those with poor performance status or with other major medical illnesses are not good candidates for trials of more intensive chemotherapy. Most of these patients can be palliated with moderate doses of any of the available combination programs. Patients who are malnourished but otherwise reasonable candidates for intensive treatment should be considered for enteral or parenteral hyperalimentation before and during the course of therapy. Nutritional counseling is extremely important for all patients, particularly during the induction phase of therapy, when gastrointestinal side effects may produce further nutritional deterioration and compromise an otherwise good response to therapy.

Although radiotherapy produces more dramatic responses in SCC than in the other histological varieties of lung cancer, there is still considerable controversy about the exact role of radiotherapy in the management of patients.[20] Radiotherapy is a necessary adjuvant to chemotherapy in patients with cerebral metastases and spinal cord compression, and irradiation is also often helpful for painful bone lesions. Preliminary studies suggested that radiotherapy to the primary lesion in patients with limited-stage disease did not add to adequate combination chemotherapy when the radiotherapy and chemotherapy were given in a sequential fashion. However, the simultaneous use of chest radiotherapy and effective combination chemotherapy may be superior to chemotherapy alone in limited-stage patients.[15] Primary tumor relapse has been a persistent problem, even following combined modality therapy. The doses and timing of radiation and chemotherapy appear to be important issues and await further evaluation. Several large cooperative groups in the United States are comparing the combined use of radiotherapy and combination chemotherapy with that of combination chemotherapy alone in patients with limited-stage disease. Better control of the primary tumor is a necessity, and various new approaches are currently under study. The use of "prophylactic" or preventative whole brain radiotherapy definitely prevents symptomatic cerebral metastases from developing but has not significantly prolonged overall survival.[4] It is not surprising that survival was not prolonged, since the tumor outside the brain was not adequately controlled by chemotherapy. It is anticipated that whole brain radiotherapy will prolong survival in limited-stage patients who remain disease free for 2 yr or longer. Because chemotherapy has become more effective and patient survival significantly prolonged, there has been an increased incidence of leptomeningeal involvement analogous to that observed previously with acute lymphoblastic leukemia.

The use of the staging system designating limited and extensive stages is simple and has clinical utility. However, the system is artificial, since a complete response to therapy, regardless of stage, is the major prognostic determinent. Therefore, accurate documentation of the sites of metastases and estimation of the volume of involvement may eventually lead to the recognition of various subsets of patients with different prognoses. Subcatergorization is already beginning, with the demonstration that patients with ipsilateral pleural effusion, even though classically considered extensive stage, have a prognosis similar to that for patients with limited disease.[21] Similarly, those with contralateral supraclavicular node involvement, classically considered extensive stage, appear to have a prognosis similar to patients with limited-stage disease.[22] Further refinements in staging are likely to continue, and a modification of the tumor–node–metastases (TNM) system may be more suitable for patients with this disease in the future. Patients should be thoroughly staged before therapy is begun. Those patients with documented extensive-stage disease achieve a complete response less often, and therefore generally do worse than do limited-stage patients. Many believe that, before therapy is discontinued, thorough restaging must be repeated to document the absence of detectable disease. Bronchoscopy can detect otherwise occult tumor and should be a part of the restaging. There is controversy regarding the routine use of peritoneoscopy to visualize and biopsy the liver, but peritoneoscopy may also detect otherwise occult disease.

A reliable tumor marker or tumor-associated product that can be measured in the blood has not yet been recognized for this neoplasm. The biology and probable histogenesis of this neoplasm from embryologic neuroendocrine cells[23] has stimulated the search for a tumor marker. There are preliminary reports of elevated plasma calcitonin,[24] antidiuretic hormone,[25] and neurophysin[26] measurements as reasonably reliable tumor markers. This is particularly true in patients who manifest the syndrome of inappropriate antidiuretic hormone secretion, in whom the plasma levels of antidiuretic hormone often correlate with the volume of tumor present.[25] These preliminary observations were made on only a few patients, however, and the magnitude of false-positive and false-negative values are not known at this time. Therefore, for all practical purposes, there is no reliable biologic marker generally available. Because SCC produces several tumor-associated products, there is reasonable hope that, in the near future, a marker or group of markers will be found that will be useful in monitoring the effect of therapy and in determining remission status. Such markers may be critical for the detection of disease before micrometastases develop, for staging patients prior to therapy, for determining when to stop therapy, and for follow-up of the patients after stopping therapy.

Following intensive combination chemotherapy of SCC, variable histopathologic patterns have recently been observed[27-29] (see also Chapter 10, this monograph). A group of intensively treated patients have relapsed with mixed cell types, or with completely different cell types, as determined either by repeated biopsy or at autopsy. The reasons for these new pathologic observations made in intensively treated patients are not clear. The early studies of Abeloff et al.[29,30] have shown not only histologic changes but also biochemical changes following intensive therapy of SCC. In 5 of 40 autopsied patients only non-small carcinomas were found. However, at the original diagnosis, each of these patients had SCC (1 oat cell subtype, and 4 intermediate cell subtype). Furthermore, 4 of the 5 tumors initially had elevated dopa-decarboxylase, as measured by radioimmunoassay, and intracellular histaminase, as demonstrated by immunoperoxidase methods. Following intensive therapy and at autopsy none of these tumors contained these substances, and, histologically, 3 squamous cell carcinomas, 1 adenocarcinoma, and 1 large cell carcinoma were found. There are several possible explanations for these phenomena: (1) the initial biopsy was not originally classified correctly; (2) sampling errors were made in the initial biopsy; (3) mixed tumor was initially present and small cell components were selectively "cured" or eradicated; (4) a second tumor developed after "cure" of small cell tumor and (5) an alteration occurred in the histologic appearance and biochemical characteristics of the tumor. The most likely explanation appears to be a true alteration of the biochemical and histologic features following intensive therapy. A similar phenomenon has been observed following intensive therapy for testicular and ovarian germinal neoplasms, where "benign" teratomas are all that remains of a previously documented germinal neoplasm.[31] Both histological and biochemical (human chorionic gonadotropin, α-fetoprotein) changes following therapy have been demonstrated in these neoplasms as well. Similarly, neuroblastoma may spontaneously "convert" to benign ganglioneuroma.[32] There are several possible implications of the alterations of histology and biochemistry in SCC following intensive therapy. It may provide further evidence that SCC is but one part of a spectrum of lung cancers,[33] and that the other histologic types may, indeed, arise from SCC. Increased knowledge of this possible histologic and biochemical conversion may provide insight into a way of therapeutically changing this tumor to a "more benign" histology. Does this alteration mean that some patients may be "cured" of their small cell tumor only to have squamous, adenocarcinoma, or large cell tumors with which to deal? The possibility of a change in histologic type and, therefore, the clinical behavior of the tumor should be kept in mind when managing a patient whose tumor does not appear to behave like SCC. For example, a patient who relapses with a slowly growing tumor or with hypercalemia would be unusual for typical SCC and would suggest another cell type. A biopsy of the tumor is indicated for determining whether a "change" in histology has occurred. If mixed tumors are more common than generally believed, then the role of the adjuvant surgical resection of the primary tumor needs further consideration.

The intermediate subtype is not as easily recognized as the oat cell subtype of SCC.[34] Therefore, patients with unrecognized intermediate cell subtype may not receive appropriate therapy. This distinction between

SCC and the other varieties of lung cancer is now very important. Large cell carcinomas and the intermediate subtype of SCC are at times difficult to distinguish by light microscopy from each other or from poorly differentiated adenocarcinoma or squamous cell carcinomas. Added to these problems are the rare patients who have mixed varieties of lung cancer which contain small cell and large cell components, small cell and squamous cell components, or small cell and adenocarcinoma components. The recognition of the intermediate subtype of SCC is often a matter of subjective interpretation relating to (1) the amount of tissue available and the adequacy of fixation; (2) a knowledge of the therapeutic importance of recognizing lung cancer types; (3) the expertise of the pathologist in lung cancer pathology; and (4) the inherent difficulty of classifying poorly differentiated lung cancer utilizing standard light microscopy. Pathologists whose primary interest is lung cancer are probably better able to identify the different morphologic subtypes of lung cancer and particularly the intermediate cell subtype. Even such experienced pathologists recognize their shortcomings.[35] For example, when slides submitted from a large cooperative cancer therapy group in the United States were reviewed, it was observed that the majority of SCC submitted were of the oat cell subtype (lymphocytelike subtype).[36] However, within the overall incidence of SCC, it appears that approximately 50 percent of the patients have the oat cell subtype and 50 percent the intermediate cell subtype.[37] That the majority of the slides submitted by the cooperative group were of the oat cell subtype may relate either to the lack of recognition of the intermediate cell subtype or to the belief that these patients do not have a biologically equivalent neoplasm.

Data from our series at Vanderbilt University Medical Center substantiates this.[38] Of the first 40 patients referred for management to our center for SCC between January 1976 and October 1976, 38 had the classic oat cell subtype and only 2 had the intermediate cell subtype. Therefore, we initiated a retrospective study to evaluate the magnitude of this problem at our medical center. One hundred slides were pulled from our pathology files with the diagnosis of "poorly differentiated carcinoma" from tissue obtained from the lung by thorocotomy, bronchoscopy, or needle biopsy between 1969 and 1974. Of these 100 specimens, 52 were found to be either large cell undifferentiated carcinoma or metastatic tumors, as determined by chart review. We decided to exclude large cell carcinomas, since they may be confused less often with the intermediate subtype than the other poorly differentiated carcinomas. The remaining 48 slides were reviewed by a pathologist, along with 8 cases of the intermediate subtype which were added as "positive controls." Seven of the 8 controls were correctly identified. In addition, 12 of the 48 study slides were the intermediate cell subtype of SCC. They had been initially diagnosed as either poorly differentiated carcinoma, poorly differentiated squamous carcinoma, or poorly differentiated adenocarcinoma. Review of the records showed that these patients had a median survival of 14 wk. They were treated with surgery or radiotherapy alone, and no patient survived more than 2 yr. This is certainly consistent with the clinical biology of this neoplasm. Analysis of 19 other intermediate subtype patients subsequently seen between 1976 and 1978 revealed that 7 were initially diagnosed as poorly differentiated carcinoma, leading to a median delay of 8 wk before appropriate therapy was initiated. Nonetheless, 16 of these 19 patients responded to chemotherapy plus radiotherapy (8 complete responses). We believe that, when many physicians who refer patients to our medical center receive a diagnosis of poorly differentiated carcinoma, poorly differentiated adenocarcinoma, poorly differentiated squamous cell carcinoma, or large cell carcinoma from their pathologist, they do not refer these patients with unresectable cancer because the patients are not considered to have "treatable neoplasms." Since the therapy of SCC has improved, all lung cancer histology should be carefully scrutinized. During the past 2 yr, SCC diagnosed at Vanderbilt University Medical Center has been about equally divided between the oat cell subtype and the intermediate cell subtype. The problems and limitations of the morphologic diagnosis of lung cancer, particularly of poorly differentiated tumors, remains an important issue. Electron microscopy may be useful in selected cases, but further research of other methods may be necessary to improve our understanding and recognition of these tumors.

Combination chemotherapy has been developed to such a point that it is now relatively effective in providing palliation of the majority of tumor-associated clinical problems, and in a minority of patients is curative. Chest pain, cough, or hemoptysis are often completely relieved for variable periods. The anorexia, weight loss, and general weakness are often reversed, except for the brief periods of gastrointestinal side effects related to the administration of therapy. Symptoms related to metastatic disease are also frequently palliated for variable periods. Painful hepatomegaly, jaundice, liver function abnormalities, or pain in various portions of the body related to metastatic disease are usually adequately controlled. The additional judicial use of radiotherapy for specific problems such as bone pain and the spinal cord compression syndrome is indicated.

The therapy of patients presenting with superior vena cava syndrome is controversial.[39,40] Small cell lung carcinoma is now the most frequent cause of superior vena cava syndrome. Although radiotherapy is very effective in treating superior vena cava syndrome, the primary therapy of patients with SCC involves the use of combination chemotherapy whether or not radiotherapy is added. Many physicians choose to give radiotherapy for superior vena cava syndrome, followed by combination chemotherapy. Others believe combination chemotherapy alone is adequate for most patients, even for those with superior vena cava syndrome. There are fewer published data on the use of chemotherapy alone for this complication. However, there appear to be sufficient data to support the view that effective combination chemotherapy alone is certainly adequate therapy. In two separate reports,[41,42] a total of 29 patients were treated with one of the effective drug combinations (cyclophosphamide, methotrexate, and CCNU). Every patient had a partial disappearance of superior vena cava syndrome after a median period of 7 days. Twenty-eight of the 29 patients had complete disappearance of the obstruction after a median of 14 days. We have seen similar results in several patients treated with another effective drug combination (cyclophosphamide, doxorubicin, vincristine, and methotrexate). There have been no randomized comparisons of radiotherapy alone versus chemotherapy alone for patients with the superior vena cava syndrome. Because radiotherapy alone is inadequate therapy, this study should never be done. However, the question remains whether chest radiotherapy given with effective combination chemotherapy improves the remission rate or the survival of patients with limited-stage disease. There is reasonable evidence that radiotherapy does not add to the current combination chemotherapy for patients with extensive disease. However, the use of combination chemotherapy and radiotherapy for superior vena cava syndrome in limited-stage patients is a reasonable approach.

Several of the paraneoplastic syndromes associated with SCC may also respond favorably to combination chemotherapy. These include the ectopic ACTH syndrome, the Eaton Lambert myasthenic syndrome and other carcinomatous neuromyopathies, and the syndrome of inappropriate antidiuretic hormone secretion. The syndrome of inappropriate antidiuretic hormone secretion is a common paraneoplastic syndrome. It rarely occurs with other types of lung cancer. Approximately 5–10 percent of all patients with SCC will present or develop this complication.[43] Considerable controversy and confusion about the appropriate management of these patients exists. For example, a major question has been whether demeclocycline or lithium is more effective "treatment."[44] Since the overwhelming majority of these patients have SCC, neither of these drugs should be considered primary therapy in this setting. Indeed, they should be used initially only as adjuvants to the more effective treatment of the underlying disorder with combination chemotherapy. A review of our patients with the syndrome of inappropriate antidiuretic hormone secretion will illustrate this point.[25] From March 1976 to August 1979, we evaluated and treated 195 patients for SCC, and 13 (6.5 percent) presented with the syndrome of inappropriate secretion of antidiuretic hormone. Sodium values in these patients ranged from 106 to 126 mEq/liter. All patients had relative urinary hypertonicity, normal renal and adrenal function, and no signs of intravascular volume depletion. Two patients had limited-stage disease and 11 had extensive-stage disease. All patients received intensive combination chemotherapy. The drug combination was usually cyclophosphamide, doxorubicin, and vincristine. Restaging after induction therapy documented objective responses in all patients. After 3–6 wk of therapy, serum sodium returned to normal (greater than 135 ml/liter), despite unrestricted fluid intake in 12 of 13 patients. One patient had persistent hyponatremia, despite having a documented partial remission. Plasma antidiuretic hormone levels were measured by radioimmunoassay in the last 4 patients. Initial antidiuretic hormone levels were 16.1, 20.0, 25.7, and 250 pg/ml (normal 1–6 pg/ml). In 3 of 4 patients, antidiuretic hormone values became normal coincident with the resolution of the clinical syndrome. The fourth patient with persistent clinical syndrome showed a persistently elevated antidiuretic hormone (30.1 pg/ml). Effective chemotherapy controls the syndrome of inappropriate antidiuretic hormone secretion in most patients by reducing the tumor cell population and, thereby, the production of antidiuretic hormone. Chronic fluid restriction and demeclocycline or lithium administration are indirect therapies which are useful before chemotherapy produces a response or when tumors are resistent to chemotherapy.

Combination chemotherapy is not effective for lesions in the central nervous system, which represents a pharmacologic santuary site for most effective drugs.[4] Two major clinical problems are cerebral metastases at presentation and carcinomatous leptomeningitis occurring during the course of the illness. Intensive radiotherapy to documented lesions in the brain can be effective in producing marked palliation and, rarely, eradication of the metastases. Treatment of carcinomatous leptomeningitis is more difficult.[4] Although cranial–spinal irradiation can be used, it produces extensive bone marrow damage and severely limits subsequent chemotherapy. Intrathecal methotrexate and cytosine arabinoside may provide some palliation. Because carcinomatous leptomeningitis has increased as patients survive longer, the prevention of this complication may become a major challenge, as it is in acute lymphoblastic leukemia.

Prophylactic whole brain radiotherapy can prevent the progression of most brain metastases. Studies are in progress regarding the efficacy of high-dose methotrexate or intrathecal methotrexate in preventing lepto-meningitis.

References

1. Greco FA, Oldham RK: Small cell lung cancer. New Engl J Med 301:355–358, 1979
2. Wynder EL, Berg JW: Cancer of the lung among non-smokers: Special reference to histologic patterns. Cancer 20:1161–1172, 1967.
3. Polackwich RJ, Straus MJ: Superior vena caval syndrome, in Straus (ed): Lung Cancer: Clinical Diagnosis and Treatment. New York, Grune & Stratton, 1977, pp 249–260
4. Bunn PA, Nugent JL, Matthews MJ: Central nervous system metastasis in small cell bronchogenic carcinoma. Sem Oncol 5:314–322, 1978
5. Bender RA, Hansen HH: Hypercalcemia in bronchogenic carcinoma: A prospective study of 200 patients. Ann Intern Med 80:205–208, 1974
6. Hansen HH, Dombernowsky P, Hirsch FR: Staging procedures and prognostic features in small cell anaplastic bronchogenic carcinoma. Sem Oncol 5:280–288, 1978
7. Green RA, Humphrey E, Close H, et al.: Alkylating agents in bronchogenic carcinoma. Am J Med 46:516–525, 1969
8. Wolff J, Patno ME, Roswit B, et al.: Controlled study of survival of patients with clinically inoperable lung cancer treated with radiation therapy. Am J Med 40:360–367, 1966
9. Mountain CF: Clinical biology of small cell carcinoma: Relationship to surgical therapy. Sem Oncol 5:272–279, 1978
10. Greco FA, Einhorn LH, Richardson RL. Oldham RK: Small cell lung cancer: Progress and perspective. Sem Oncol 5:323–335, 1978
11. Minna JD, Ihde DC, Bunn PA, et al.: Extensive stage small cell carcinoma of the lung: effect of increasing intensity of induction chemotherapy. Proc Am Soc Clin Oncol 21:448, 1980
12. Meyer JA, Comis RL, Ginsberg SJ, et al.: Selective surgical resection in small cell carcinoma of the lung. Thorac Cardiovasc Surg 77:243–248, 1979
13. Stevens E, Einhorn LH, Rohn R: Treatment of limited small cell lung cancer. Proc Am Assoc Can Res 20:435, 1979

14. Hansen HH, Dombernowsky P, Rorth M: Chemotherapy versus chemotherapy plus radiotherapy in regional small cell carcinoma of the lung—A randomized trial. Proc Am Assoc Can Res 20:277, 1979

15. Cohen MH, Lichter AS, Bunn PA, et al: Chemotherapy–radiation therapy versus chemotherapy in limited small cell lung cancer. Proc Am Soc Clin Oncol 21:448, 1980

16. Rissanen PM, Tikka U, Holsti LR: Autopsy findings in lung cancer treated with megavoltage radiotherapy. Acta Radiol Therap (Stockh) 7:433–438, 1968

17. Tobias JS, Parker LM, Tattersall MHN: Adriamycin–cyclophosphamide chemotherapy in advanced L1210 leukemia. Br J Cancer 32:199–207, 1975

18. Holoye PY, Samuels ML: Cyclophosphamide, vincristine and sequential split-course radiotherapy in the treatment of small cell lung cancer. Chest 67:675–679, 1975

19. Greco FA, Brereton HD, Kent H, et al.: Adriamycin and enhanced radiation reaction in normal esophagus and skin. Ann Int Med 85:294–298, 1976

20. Seydel HG, Creech RH, Mietlowski W, et al.: Radiation therapy in small cell lung cancer. Sem Oncol 5:288–298, 1978

21. Livingston RB: Personal communication.

22. Maurer LH, Tulloh M, Weiss RB, et al.: A randomized combined modality trial in small cell carcinoma of the lung. Cancer 45:30–39, 1980

23. Tischler AS: Small cell carcinoma of the lung: cellular origin and relationship to other neoplasms. Sem Oncol 5:244–252, 1978

24. Wallach SR, Royston I, Taetler R, et al.: Plasma calcitonin as a marker of disease activity in patients with small cell carcinoma of the lung during chemotherapy. Clin Res 28:56A, 1980

25. Hainsworth J, Oldham RK, Sismani AR, et al.: Treatment of the syndrome of inappropriate secretion of antidiuretic hormone in small cell lung cancer. Proc Am Assoc Can Res 21:157, 1980

26. North WG, LaRochelle FT, Melton J, et al.: Human neurophysins as potential tumor markers for small cell carcinoma. Clin Res 26:536A, 1978

27. Brereton HD, Matthews MM, Costa J, et al.: Mixed anaplastic small cell and squamous cell carcinoma of the lung. Ann Intern Med 88:805–806, 1978

28. Matthews MJ: Effects of therapy on the morphology and behavior of small cell carcinoma of the lung—A clinicopathologic study, in Mug-

gia F, Rozencweig M (eds): Lung Cancer: Progress in Therapeutic Research. New York, Raven Press, 1979, pp 155–165

29. Abeloff MD, Eggleston JC, Mendelsohn G, et al.: Changes in morphologic and biochemical characteristics of small cell carcinoma of the lung. Am J Med 66:757–764, 1979

30. Baylin SB, Weisburger WR, Eggleston JC, et al.: Variable content of histaminase, L-dopa decarboxylase and calcitonin in small cell carcinoma of the lung. N Engl J Med 299:105–110, 1978

31. Hajdu SI: Pathology of germ cell tumors of the testis. Sem Oncol 6:14–25, 1979

32. Aterman K, Schueller EF: Maturation of neuroblastoma to ganglioneuroma. Am J Dis Child 120:217–222, 1970

33. Yesner R: Pathologic diagnosis of lung cancer: overview, in Muggia F, Rozencweig M (eds): Lung Cancer: Progress in Therapeutic Research. New York, Raven Press, 1979, pp 79–82

34. Cohen MH, Matthews MJ: Small cell bronchogenic carcinoma: A distinct clinicopathologic entity. Sem Oncol 5:234–243, 1978

35. Yesner R, Von Hoff DD: Pathologic diagnosis of lung cancer: reappraisal and prospects, in Muggia F and Rozencweig M (eds): Lung Cancer: Progress in Therapeutic Research. New York, Raven Press, 1979, pp 175–178

36. Matthews MJ: Personal communication

37. Matthews MJ: Personal communication

38. Fer MF, Rogers LW, Richardson RL, et al.: The intermediate subtype of small cell lung cancer: a frequently unrecognized neoplasm. Clin Res 27:384A, 1979

39. Mittal BB: Treatment of SVC syndrome. N Engl J Med 302:61, 1980

40. Greco FA, Oldham RK: SVC syndrome in small cell carcinoma. N Engl J Med 302:61, 1980

41. Kane RC, Cohen MH, Broder LE, et al.: Superior vena caval obstruction due to small cell anaplastic lung carcinoma: Response to chemotherapy. JAMA 235:1717–1718, 1976

42. Dombernowsky P, Hansen HH: Combination chemotherapy in the management of superior vena caval obstruction in small cell anaplastic carcinoma of the lung. Acta Med Scand 204:513–516, 1978

43. Richardson RL, Greco FA, Oldham RK, et al.: Tumor products and potential markers in small cell lung cancer. Sem Oncol 5:253–263, 1978

44. Forrest JN, Cox M, Hong C, et al.: Demeclocycline versus lithium for

inappropriate secretion of antidiuretic hormone. N Engl J Med 298:173–177, 1978

45. Bergsagel D, Jenkin R, Pringle J, et al.: Lung cancer: clinical trial of radiotherapy alone versus radiotherapy plus cyclophosphamide. Cancer 30:621–627, 1972

46. Fox W, Scadding AG: Medical research council comparative trials, surgery and radiotherapy for primary treatment of small cell or oat cell carcinoma of the bronchus: 10-year followup. Lancet 2:63–65, 1973

47. Laing AH, Berry RJ, Newman CR: Treatment of small cell carcinoma of the bronchus. Lancet 1:129–132, 1975

48. Lee RE, Carr DT, Childs DS: Comparison of split-course radiation therapy and continuous radiation therapy for unresectable bronchogenic carcinoma: five year results. Am J Roentgenol Radium Ther Nucl Med 126:116–122, 1976

49. Livingston RB, Moore TN, Heilburn L, et al: Small cell carcinoma of the lung: combined chemotherapy and radiation. Ann Intern Med 88:194–199, 1978

50. Johnson RE, Brereton HD, Kent CH.: "Total" therapy for small carcinoma of the lung. Ann Thor Surg 25:510–515, 1978

51. Einhorn LH, Bond WH, Hornback N, et al.: Long term results in combined modality treatment of small cell carcinoma of the lung. Sem Oncol 5:309–313, 1978

52. Greco FA, Richardson RL, Schulman SF, et al.: Therapy of oat cell carcinoma of the lung: complete remissions, acceptable complications and improved survival. Br Med J 2:10–11, 1978

53. Israel L, DePierre A, Choffel C.: Immunochemotherapy in 34 cases of oat cell carcinoma of the lung with 19 complete responses. Cancer Treat Rep 61:343–347, 1977

54. Cohen MH, Ihde DC, Fossieck BE, et al.: Cyclic alternating combination chemotherapy of small cell carcinoma. Proc Am Soc Clin Oncol 19:359, 1978

55. Greco FA, Hande KR, Richardson RL, et al.: High-dose methotrexate in combination chemotherapy in small cell lung cancer, in Mathe G, Muggia F (eds): Recent Results in Cancer Research, in press

56. Fer MF, Greco FA, Richardson RL, et al.: Alternating non–cross resistant combination chemotherapy for small cell lung cancer. Clin Res 28:414A, 1980

57. Greco FA, Oldham RK: Unpublished data

58. Minna J, Lichter A, Brereton H, et al.: Small cell lung cancer: Long

term potentially cured survivors in National Cancer Institute trials. Clin Res 28:419A, 1980

59. Holoye PY, Samuels ML, Lanzotti VJ, et al.: Combination chemotherapy and radiation therapy for small cell carcinoma. JAMA 237:1221–1224, 1977

60. Eagan RT, Carr DT, Lee RE, et al.: Phase II studies of polychemotherapy regimens in small cell lung cancer. Cancer Treat Rep 61:93–95, 1977

61. Ginsberg SJ, Comis RL, Gottlieb AJ, et al.: Long term survivorship in small cell anaplastic lung carcinoma. Cancer Treat Rep 63:1347–1349, 1979

16

COMPLICATIONS OF TREATMENT AND OF IMPROVED SURVIVAL IN PATIENTS WITH SMALL CELL CARCINOMA OF THE LUNG

Joseph Aisner
Peter H. Wiernik

Small cell bronchogenic carcinoma is now considered a distinct clinical and histopathological entity.[1] This tumor has a high growth fraction and a short doubling time, which are seen clinically as a short symptomatic period and early dissemination.[2-4] The median duration of survival in untreated patients is short, 6–8 wk, and palliative therapy such as radiation alone results in only moderate prolongation of life.[3-6] Without systemic therapy there have been virtually no long-term survivors.[6-8] Some patients may present with complications of rapidly advancing disease, such as superior vena cava syndrome, brain or adrenal metastases, or paraneoplastic endocrine syndromes,[3,4,9,10] but, in the past, few patients survived sufficiently long to develop complications of the disease or its treatment.

Recently, small cell carcinoma (SCC) has been shown to be a highly treatable disease. Many recent studies have demonstrated a high response rate and significant prolongation of survival.[11-20] More importantly, however, those studies are also showing a small, but real, percentage of long-term disease-free survivors.[11-19] These data suggest that current treatment has the potential of curing this disease. With this improvement in survival, however, certain complications, both of the natural history of the disease and of its treatment, are becoming evident. These complications will need to be considered in planning future treatment trials, if the percentage of long term survivors is to increase. The purpose of this chapter is to review the recognized complications of the disease, as well as the potential complications yet to be seen but predictable on the basis of experience in the long-term follow-up of other diseases.

Classification of the Complications

Any division of complications must be arbitrary, since treatments and their toxicities overlap. Thus, complications are not necessarily caused by one treatment modality or another, and, similarly, long-term complications may be caused by treatments, natural history of the disease, or treatment-induced changes in the biologic behavior of the disease. For the purposes of discussion, however, the complications are divided here according to acute and chronic periods, according to treatment modalities (chemotherapy or chemotherapy with radiotherapy—so-called combined modality therapy), and according to late complications in the evolution of the disease (Tables 16-1 to 16-3).

Acute Complications

Many of the acute toxicities of both chemotherapy and radiotherapy (Table 16-1) are generally known by both professional and lay personnel. Nausea, vomiting, and blood count suppression are toxicities common to both treatment modalities and may be augmented by the simultaneous application of both modalities. Nausea and vomiting, although unpleasant, are generally transient and should not guide dose or drug modification. Similarly alopecia, frequently seen in most treatment regimens from drugs or cranial irradiation, is not a serious problem and does not provide a rationale for dosage modification.

Myelosuppression

Blood count suppression is, however, a more serious problem. Most combination chemotherapy programs utilize cyclophosphamide along with two or more other drugs, such as doxorubicin, vincristine, methotrexate, VP16-213, or CCNU.[9] When such drugs are given in maximal doses, the predominant myelosuppression is leukopenia,[11-16] which increases the risk of infectious complications. Patients who develop febrile

Table 16-1
Acute Complications of Treatment

Toxicities shared by chemotherapy alone and
     combined modality therapy
  Nausea and vomiting
  Alopecia
  Myelosuppression
    Leukopenia
    Febrile episodes
    Serious infections
  Neuropathies

Additional toxicities observed in combined
     modality therapy
  Esophagitis
  Pneumonitis `
  Central nervous system toxicity

episodes during periods of granulocytopenia are treated with parenteral broad-spectrum antibiotics on an empirical basis,[23] and this treatment practice results in variable periods of hospitalization in 10–25 percent of patients. Serious infections such as pneumonia or bacteremia are documented in a small fraction of the patients, ranging from 1 percent to 13 percent, and infectious deaths occur in 0–5 percent of patients treated with combination therapy.[11–16] In our own studies, we have observed an infection rate of 10–15 percent, with 4–5 percent infectious deaths.[11,12] These serious infections tend to originate as pneumonias, usually behind partially occluded bronchi, and tend to occur early on in therapy, before dosage modifications are made.[12] They also usually occur in the patients who are partially debilitated by their disease (poor performance status).[11,12] Therefore, careful attention to prevention of infection is indicated, and preliminary data suggest that suppression of colonizing aerobic microbial flora by agents such as trimethoprim/sulfamethoxazole may be useful in reducing infection incidence.[24]

Thrombocytopenia and anemia are far less important problems, partly because of the availability of replacement therapy and partly because the drugs are less likely to cause serious suppression of the platelet count and hematocrit than suppression of the granulocyte count.

Other Drug-Related Acute Toxicities

Other drug-related toxicities are drug specific. Thus, when neurotoxic drugs such as vincristine, hexamethylmelamine, or procarbazine are used, one might see neuropathies in the form of parasthesias, muscle weakness, or foot drop; myalgias, lethargy, or confusion; obstipation or osthostatic hypotension.[25] Cis-platinum may produce nephrotoxicity, neurotoxicity, or hearing loss.[26] Some agents such as methotrexate or bleomycin can cause skin toxicity, pulmonary fibrosis, or mucositis.[27-29] Many of these toxicities may be augmented by radiation.[28,29] The inclusion of these various agents in combination chemotherapy should therefore be based on evidence of single-agent activity. For example, the rationale for including bleomycin is weak, since there is little data to suggest that this agent possesses any activity in SCC as a single agent.

Acute Toxicities from Combined Modality Therapy

In addition to those toxicities that are shared with combination chemotherapy alone, such as nausea and vomiting, there are a number of acute toxicities associated specifically with the addition of adjuvant radiotherapy (Table 16-1). The majority of these reactions are probably caused by drug augmentation of the tissue reaction to the irradiation.

Skin Toxicity

Mild skin changes are frequently seen with irradiation. However, with the addition of certain agents, unusually severe skin reactions can occur. Doxorubicin given in combination concurrently with irradiation has been associated with unusually severe skin reactions, requiring modification of both the radiation and chemotherapy doses.[30] Such reactions can produce moist epithelitis, skin necrosis, and desquamation,[14,15,30-32] all with prolonged healing times. These could be particularly important complications if they were to delay systemic therapy. Furthermore, doxorubicin may produce recall reactions in previously irradiated ports. Bleomycin alone may produce skin toxicity, and the combination of bleomycin as well as certain other agents and irradiation is known to induce enhanced skin toxicity.[33] Fortunately, the incidence of severe skin toxicity in SCC therapy trials has generally been low (5 percent).[14,15,31] In two studies in which bleomycin was used, however, skin toxicity occurred in 21 percent of patients[32] and 10 percent of patients,[34] respectively.

Pulmonary Toxicity

Combined modality therapy can result in pneumonitis or fibrosis that are more severe than expected from either modality alone. Combined modality studies including doxorubicin, methotrexate, or bleomycin are especially likely to yield such toxicity.[13-15,28,31,32,34] It is well established that these agents will increase the pulmonary response to radiation therapy.[28,35-37] The incidence of pneumonitis varies among reports, ranging from only a small incidence to roentgoenographic changes in all patients.[13,15,31,32,34-36] More importantly, however, severe pneumonitis, which may sometimes be severe enough to cause pulmonary insufficiency and death, occurs in 2–30 percent (generally 2–5 percent) of the treated patients, depending on such variables as drugs, radiation dose, and timing of treatment modalities.

Esophageal Toxicity

Another worrisome acute toxicity of combined modality therapy is the occurrence of esophagitis. Mild transient esophagitis, manifested by burning and dysphagia, is frequent with mediastinal irradiation, resolves spontaneously, and does not constitute a major problem.[38]

Severe esophagitis, however, can be a very bothersome clinical problem and has been seen in most combined modality studies.[13-15,31,36,39] The incidence of severe esophagitis is probably 5–10 percent.[13-15,31,36,39] Severe esophagitis has produced significant morbidity, necessitating tube feeding. Esophageal strictures and death by inanition have occurred in some studies.[14,36,39] The severity is generally related to volume and time of irradiation, but, with the addition of chemotherapy, the likelihood of this toxicity is probably enhanced.[38] In virtually all series reporting severe esophagitis, doxorubicin-containing combination chemotherapy was used. Recently, however, severe esophagitis was also noted in combined modality therapy without doxorubicin.[40] Furthermore, timing of irradiation and chemotherapy appear important, since concurrent chemotherapy and irradiation result in higher rates of severe esophagitis[13,14,31,36,39] than does serial scheduling of the modalities.

As in the case of pulmonary toxicity, the frequency and severity of esophagitis warrant extreme care in the use of adjuvant radiotherapy. The planning of treatment ports to exclude the esophagus, especially when drug combinations containing doxorubicin are to be used, should be considered.

Neurological Toxicity

Mediastinal irradiation for lung cancer has occasionally produced transverse myelitis,[38] although with appropriate port planning and dose sequencing, this complication occurs with an incidence of 1 percent or less. It is thus not surprising that transverse myelitis has been seen as well in combined modality therapy for SCC.[15] The incidence of this complication increases with increasing ret dose, so that more aggressive radiation treatment programs are likely to produce a higher incidence.[38] There is currently no information about the effect of chemotherapy on this reaction, and there does not appear to be an excess incidence of this complication in combined modality therapy.

Another neurological complication of combined modality therapy is a syndrome consisting of poor attention span, memory loss, intention tremor with occasional myoclonus, and slurred speech.[36] This self-limited syndrome became clinically evident after 4 mo of treatment. So far, this syndrome remains unexplained. Loss of consciousness soon after methotrexate administration was also seen in one study utilizing combined modality therapy,[34] thereby raising the question of drug–radiation interaction in the central nervous system.

Chronic Toxicities

Until recently, chronic toxicities were essentially nonexistent, owing to the lack of long-term survival. Long-term toxicities are thus just beginning to be observed. Therefore, it is necessary to look to other diseases that have been successfully treated with either combination chemotherapy alone or combined modality therapy in order to predict what chronic toxicities may be expected as the therapy for SCC becomes more effective.

As in the case of acute toxicities, the chronic drug-associated toxicities are shared by both treatments with chemotherapy alone and combined modality therapy. Distinctions made according to treatment modality are, therefore, both difficult and artificial (Table 16-2).

Chronic Drug-Related Toxicities

Myelosuppression

The prolonged administration of myelotoxic agents can be expected to produce chronic depletion of bone marrow reserve, resulting in progressively greater hypocellularity of the marrow. Thus, one might anticipate the emergence of aplastic anemia, particularly with prolonged drug administration. In point of fact, this complication is only rarely reported.[18,40] We have seen one such case among more than 150 patients treated with aggressive combination chemotherapy for up to 2 yr. This infrequency would suggest that this will be a rare complication of therapy, although additional follow-up is still needed.

Table 16-2
Complications of Therapy—Chronic
Toxicities from Treatment

Toxicities common to both chemotherapy alone
    and combined modality therapy
  Marrow hypoplasia—aplasia
  Second malignancies
    Acute leukemia
    Others
  Cardiomyopathies

Toxicities related to combined modality therapy
  Second malignancies
  Esophageal fibrosis and stricture
  Pulmonary fibrosis and insufficiency
  Cardiac disease
    Pericarditis
    Coronary artery disease

Second Malignancies

Another difficulty with chronic myelo- and immunosuppressive drug treatment is the potential for the emergence of second malignancies. Many of the chemotherapeutic agents are themselves carcinogenic. Long-term cytotoxic chemotherapy, particularly with alkylating agents, has been associated with acute leukemia.[40–44] Risk estimates have been generally calculated from 1 to 4 percent, ranging to as high as 7 percent in some calculations. These cases of "secondary" acute leukemia are frequently heralded by bone marrow aspirates showing ring sideroblasts and chromosomal aberrations.[43,44] The precise mechanism for the evolution of this secondary process is currently unknown, but the low incidence of acute leukemia does not constitute a justification for withholding effective therapy. At present only 10–15 percent of the overall population with SCC will be long-term survivors, so that the risk of acute leukemia is still far less than 1 percent. As more effective therapy is established, the duration of therapy may become a more critical issue in view of this potential complication.

Lymphomas, particularly "histiocytic" lymphomas, have been seen with chronic immunosuppressive therapy, particularly in renal transplants,[44] but, so far, there has not been any evidence of an increased risk of lymphoma in patients treated with cytotoxic agents for cancer and particularly SCC.

Other second malignancies, such as other lung cancers or bladder cancer (see below) may occur, but it would be difficult to evaluate the relative risk factors, since the patients affected have generally been exposed to certain common carcinogens, such as cigarette smoke.

Cardiac Toxicity

Many combination therapy programs include doxorubicin. Thus, there is the potential for doxorubicin cardiomyopathy. Severe, progressive congestive heart failure secondary to doxorubicin-induced cardiomyopathy is seen as a complication of prolonged administration, generally at cumulative doses exceeding 540 mg/m^2.[46] Thus, it is necessary to limit the dose of doxorubicin, and, in most treatment programs using 30–45 mg/m^2 per course, this means about 10–14 mo of chemotherapy before doxorubicin must be stopped.

Chronic Radiation-Related Toxicity

Chronic toxicities in combined modality therapy, like acute toxicities, are related to the interacting effects of both modalities on tissue, and the assignment of the toxicities or complications to irradiation is arbitrary. For example, acute leukemia secondary to cytotoxic therapy occurs in combined modality therapy and may even be more frequent in this group than among patients who receive chemotherapy alone.[42-44]

Long-Term Effects of Acute Toxicities

As has been previously noted, acute severe esophagitis can lead to strictures requiring bougienage and long term tube feedings.[14,36,39] Similarly, acute radiation pneumonitis can lead to interstitial fibrosis, with subsequent respiratory insufficiency and its sequelae.[31,32,34] Thus, the acute toxicities seen from combined modality can potentially become severely incapacitating chronic problems. Currently, these problems are relatively infrequent, as only about 20–30 percent of the limited-disease population (the group likely to receive combined modality therapy) will achieve long-term survival. However, when a greater percentage of patients achieve this status, the long-term complications are likely to present considerably more important management problems.

Radiation-Related Cardiac Diseases

As has been discussed, the interaction of doxorubicin and irradiation can produce enhanced toxicity.[30,31,36,39] Thus, it is conceivable that the combination of doxorubicin and irradiation would enhance the doxorubicin-associated cardiotoxicity. Animal and histopathology series suggest that the combination of radiation and doxorubicin can produce enhanced cardiac toxicity,[47,48] and clinical evidence of enhanced toxicity is now reported.[49] Such enhanced toxicity may further restrict the amount of doxorubicin that can be administered if further follow-up of the patients treated with combined modality therapy discloses enhanced cardiotoxicity.

Among patients treated for Hodgkin's disease with mediastinal irradiation, a significant proportion will develop clinical or roentgoenographic evidence of pericarditis or pericardial effusion, or both.[38,50] Among various reports this incidence varies from 2 to 30 percent.[38,50] Symptoms generally appear within 1 yr, and cardiac-tamponade may require surgical intervention. Doxorubicin, and possibly other agents, can potentiate these complications, so that we may expect to find this complication in a small fraction of patients surviving after combined modality therapy.

It is also known that radiation injury may cause arterial intimal proliferation,[51] possibly leading to coronary artery occlusion. Occasionally, young patients with Hodgkin's disease undergoing mediastinal irradiation have been noted to have narrowing of all coronary arteries, leading to myocardial infarction.[52] We have also observed such patients. Because most patients with SCC are older and are heavy smokers, this complication can be expected to occur as well among long-term survivors with SCC who receive combined modality therapy. Eagen et al.[53] recently reported three deaths from myocardial infarction or pericarditis among 61 patients treated with such therapy.

Because the precise risk of these cardiac complications is unknown, they should not, by themselves, be an impediment to therapy if combined modality therapy proves to be superior to chemotherapy alone (see below).

Evolution of the Natural History of the Disease

Another aspect of improving survival is the appearance of new or previously unusual manifestations of the disease process (Table 16-3). In view of the relatively small percentage of long-term survivors, this area has not yet been fully defined. However, certain problems are already emerging.

Table 16-3
Late Complications in the
Natural History of SCC

CNS diseases
  Brain metastases
  Leptomeningeal metastases
Subsequent histological changes

Central Nervous System Disease

Brain Metastases

Brain metastases are seen frequently in patients with SCC. They occur at presentation in more than 12 percent of patients and are diagnosed clinically in more than 30 percent of patients during the course of their disease.[3,5,10,54-56] Necropsy series suggest that brain metastases occur in an even larger percentage of the patients.[55,56] Hansen[54] predicted that some form of treatment to the brain would be necessary when response and survival improved. This is now undoubtedly true. Because most patients still relapse systemically, however, central nervous system prophylaxis does not yet make an impact on survival in the disease. Nevertheless, most centers now perform "prophylactic" whole brain irradiation in order to treat the micrometastases in this pharmacologic sanctuary.[3,13-15,55-60] In our program we have now seen nonirradiated patients who relapsed only in the central nervous system and who had only central nervous system metastases at necropsy.[12] Thus, "prophylactic" whole brain irradiation is necessary to prevent or delay the morbidity of brain metastases, particularly when the patient is doing well and is in systemic remission. Furthermore, this treatment is likely to become more important with further improvement in survival.

Leptomeningeal Metastases

Leptomeningeal carcinomatosis was unusual in the past, and reports involved individual observations. With improving survival, this complication has become a more common finding.[56,61-64] Diagnosis on the basis of cerebrospinal fluid cytology, myelograms, or necropsy have shown that such metastases occurred in 9–12 percent of patients in several recent series.[56,61-64] In our study, we have noted 18 cases among 147 patients, with greater than 25 patients still at risk.[64] Prophylactic whole brain irradiation apparently did not prevent this complication,[56,62] which presented with diverse clinical signs and symptoms, ranging from confusion, limb weakness, or incontinence to diplopia and neck pain.[64] Cerebrospinal fluid when examined was generally diagnostic in our series.[63] Therapy for leptomeningeal metastases has, so far, been unrewarding, and survival from the time of diagnosis of this complication was short, despite treatment with combinations of intrathecal drugs, whole brain irradiation, and spinal irradiation.[64] Pathologic examination disclosed thick tumor deposits along leptomeninges, invading deep into neurosubstance and distally along nerve roots, a finding which suggests an anatomic explanation for failure.[64]

Leptomeningeal carcinomatosis was generally associated with extensive disease and systemic relapse. However, in 5 of our 18 cases, this was the first evidence of relapse, and, in one of the 5, leptomeningeal metastases were the only evidence of disease at necropsy.[64] Because of the current lack of effective therapy for this complication and the possibility that the complication may be a barrier to cure, there may be a need for prophylactic therapy analogous to the need existing in pediatric acute lymphoblastic leukemia. However, only a fraction of SCC patients achieve long-term survival at present, and most long-term survivors present with limited disease. Thus, the number of patients with this complication as a major barrier to cure remains small. Methods of prophylaxis that might impair ability to deliver systemic chemotherapy are not warranted at this time. If, however, there is an improvement in survival, particularly among patients with extensive disease, then it is likely that methods of prevention will need to be considered.

Subsequent Tumors

It has been suggested, on the basis of ultrastructure and immunologic assessment of endocrine precursor molecules that the various subtypes of bronchogenic carcinoma may be related.[65] Support for this thesis comes from the observation that occasionally these tumors will be of mixed histologic type (e.g., mixed epidermoid–small cell).[66–68] In general, these tumors are found after therapy (e.g., an epidermoid carcinoma may be found within a radiation treatment portal, such as the lung[66–68]), raising the possibility that the small cell tumor matured into another histology. This is certainly an interesting concept and raises questions about our classification system for bronchogenic carcinoma and particularly about possible subtypes of SCC which might actually not be "oat cell."

Others have described patients who present with multiple mixed or bilateral primary lung cancers,[69-71] raising questions about the possibility of separate diseases arising concomitantly in similar carcinogenic settings.

Regardless of the explanation, patients who develop subsequent histologies present an unusual opportunity for study and reopen the question regarding the role of surgery in the management of SCC. Firstly, surgical intervention would occasionally be necessary for confirming the histology of a new mass. Secondly, if the subsequent histology is truly localized, it might still be resected for long-term survival benefit. Finally, if some tumors will "mature" or evolve into other histologies, surgical removal following chemical or irradiation debulking should, perhaps, be considered. Further study in this area will likely lead to a better understanding of the basic disease and its sequelae.

Therapeutic Alternatives in View of Acute and Chronic Toxicities

There can be little question today that systemic combination chemotherapy, administered in maximally tolerated doses, is the main treatment for SCC. Radiotherapy, once considered the standard, is now an adjuvant therapy, added for the purpose of achieving local control in limited disease. Recent, prospectively randomized trails have suggested that irradiation of the chest primary does not affect response or survival,[60,72,73] but these are preliminary reports and leave considerable question about the appropriate timing of drugs and radiotherapy (sandwich technique versus concurrent administration).[14,15] The question of the role of radiotherapy is of considerable interest, since its addition adds both acute and chronic toxicities. It must be remembered, however, that toxicities, particularly chronic toxicities, are complications that are seen or only potentially seen in a group of patients who might otherwise not survive. Thus, if careful study shows that one or all of the treatment modalities improve survival, then it will be necessary to deal with these complications and to assess the potential gains from therapy relative to the complication rate.

References

1. Cohen MH, Matthews MJ: Small cell bronchogenic carcinoma: A distinct clinicopathologic entity. Sem Oncol 5:234–243, 1978
2. Muggia FM, Krezoski SK, Hansen HH: Cell kinetic studies in pa-

tients with small cell carcinoma of the lung. Cancer 34:1683–1690, 1974

3. Bunn PA, Cohen MH, Ihde DC, Fossieck BE, Matthews MJ, Minna JD: Advances in small cell bronchogenic carcinoma. Cancer Treat Rep 61:333–342, 1977

4. Cohen MH: Signs and symptoms of bronchogenic carcinoma. Sem Oncol 1:183–189, 1974

5. Kato Y, Fergusson TB, Bennett DE, Burford TH: Oat cell carcinoma of the lung. A review of 138 cases. Cancer 23:517–524, 1969

6. Roswit B, Panto ME, Rapp R, Veinbergs A, Feder B, Stuhbarg J, Reid CB: The survival of patients with inoperable lung cancer: a large scale randomized study of radiation therapy vs. placebo. Radiology 90:688–697, 1968

7. Mountain CF: Clinical biology of small cell carcinoma: Relationship to surgical therapy. Sem Oncol 5:272–279, 1978

8. Fox W, Scadding JG: Medical research council comparative trial of surgery and radiotherapy for primary treatment of small celled or oat-celled carcinoma of the bronchus. Lancet 2:63–65, 1973

9. Esterhay RJ Jr: Current concepts in the management of small cell carcinoma of the lung. Am J Med Sci 274:232–246, 1977

10. Hansen HH, Dombernowsky P, Hirsch FR: Staging procedures and prognostic features in small cell anaplastic bronchogenic carcinoma. Sem Oncol 5:280–287, 1978

11. Aisner J, Wiernik PH: Chemotherapy vs. chemoimmunotherapy for small cell undifferentiated carcinoma of the lung. Cancer 46:2543–2549, 1980

12. Aisner J, Whitacre M, Van Echo DA, Esterhay RJ Jr, Wiernik PH: Alternating non-cross resistant combination chemotherapy for small cell carcinoma of the lung (SSCL). Proc ASCO/AACR 21:453, 1980

13. Livingston RB, Moore TN, Heilbrun L, Bottomley R, Lehane D, Rivkin SE, Thigpen T: Small cell carcinoma of the lung: Combined chemotherapy and radiation. Ann Intern Med 88:194–199, 1978

14. Brereton HD, Kent CH, Johnson RE: Chemotherapy and radiation therapy for small cell carcinoma of the lung: A remedy for post therapeutic failure in lung cancer, in: Muggia FM, Rozencweig M (eds): Progress in Therapeutic Research. New York, Raven Press, 1979, pp 575–586

15. Greco FA, Richardson RL, Snell JN, Stroup SL, Oldham RK: Small cell lung cancer. Complete remission and improved survival. Am J Med 66:625–630, 1979

16. Cohen MH, Ihde DC, Bunn PA Jr, Fossieck BE Jr, Matthews MJ,

Shackney SE, Early AJ, Makuch R, Minna JD: Cyclic alternating combination chemotherapy for small cell bronchogenic carcinoma. Cancer Treat Rep 63:163–170, 1979

17. Ginsberg SJ, Comis RL, Gottlieb AJ, King GB, Goldberg J, Zamkoff A, Meyer JA: Long term survivorship in small cell anaplastic lung carcinoma. Cancer Treat Rep 63:1347–1349, 1979

18. Einhorn LH, Bond WH, Hornbach M, Beng-Teh J: Long term results in combined modality treatment of small cell carcinoma of the lung. Sem Oncol 5:309–313, 1978

19. Holoye PY, Samuels ML, Smith T, Sinkovics JG: Chemoimmunotherapy of small cell bronchogenic carcinoma. Cancer 42:34–40, 1978

20. Greco FA, Oldham RK: Current concepts in cancer: Small cell lung cancer. N Engl J Med 301:355–358, 1979

21. Broder LE, Cohen MH, Selawry OS: Treatment of bronchogenic carcinoma II small cell. Cancer Treat Rep 4:219–260, 1977

22. Cohen MH, Fossieck BE Jr, Ihde DC, Bunn PA Jr, Matthews MJ, Shackney SE, Minna JD: Chemotherapy of small cell carcinoma of the lung: Results and concepts, in F. Muggia, M. Rozencweig (eds): *Lung Cancer in Therapeutic Research*. New York, Raven Press, 1979, pp 559–566

23. Schimpff SC, Aisner J: Empiric antibiotic therapy. Cancer Treat Rep 62:673–680, 1978

24. Wade J, Schimpff SC, Hargadon M, Bender J, Aisner J, Young V, Wiernik PH: Trimethoprim/sulfamethoxazole: Infection prophylaxis during granulocytopenia. Proc AACR/ASCO 20:350, 1979

25. Weiss HD, Walker MD, Wiernik PH: Neurotoxicity of commonly used antineoplastic agents. N Engl J Med 291:75–81, 127–133, 1974

26. Von Hoff DD, Schilsky R, Reichert CM, Reddick RL, Rozencweig M, Young RC, Muggia FM: Toxic effects of cis-Dichlorodiammine-platinum (II) in man. Cancer Treat Rep 63:1527–1531, 1979

27. Bennett JM, Reich SD: Bleomycin: Diagnosis and treatment. Ann Int Med 90:945–948, 1979

28. Weiss RB, Muggia FM: Cytotoxic drug induced pulmonary diseases: Update, 1980. Am J Med 68:259–266, 1980.

29. Spittle MF: Methotrexate and radiation. Int J Radiat Oncol Biol Phys 4:103–107, 1978

30. Aristizabal SA, Miller RC, Schlichtemeier AL, Jones SE, Boone MLM: Adriamycin-irradiation cutaneous complications. Int J Rad Oncol Biol Phys 2:325–331, 1977

31. Moore TN, Livingston R, Heilbrun L, Durrance FY, Tesh D, Hickman B, Bogardus C: An acceptable rate of complications in combined doxorubicin-irradiation for small cell carcinoma of the Lung: A Southwest Oncology Group Study. Int J Rad Oncol Biol Phys 4:675–680, 1978

32. Van Houtte P. Tancini G, De Jager R, Lustman-Marechal J, Milani F, Bonadonna G, Kenis Y: Small cell carcinoma of the lung: a combined modality treatment. Eur J Cancer 15:1159–1165, 1979

33. Levantine A, Almeyda J: Cutaneous reactions to cytostatic agents. Br J Dermatol 90:239–242, 1974

34. Livingston RB, Mira J, Haas C, Heilbrun L: Unexpected toxicity of combined modality therapy for small cell carcinoma of the lung. Int J Rad Oncol Biol Phys 5:1637–1641, 1979

35. Einhorn L, Krause M, Hornback N, Furnas B: Enhanced pulmonary toxicity with bleomycin and radiotherapy in oat cell lung cancer. Cancer 37:2414–2416, 1976.

36. Kent CH, Brereton HD, Johnson RE: "Total" therapy for oat cell carcinoma of the lung. Int J Rad Oncol Biol Phys 2:427–432, 1977

37. Mayer EG, Poulter CA, Aristizabal SA: Complications of irradiation related to apparent drug potentiation by adriamycin. In J Radiat Oncol Biol Phys 1:1179–1188, 1976.

38. Seydel HG, Creech RH, Mietlowski W, Perez C: Radiation therapy in small cell lung cancer. Sem Oncol 5:288–298, 1978

39. Chabora BM, Hopfan S, Wittes R: Esophageal complications in the treatment of oat cell carcinoma with combined irradiation and chemotherapy. Radiology 123:185–187, 1977.

40. Cohen MH, Lichter AS, Bunn PA Jr, Glatstein EJ, Ihde DC, Fossieck BE jr, Matthews MJ, Minna JD: Chemotherapy-radiation therapy versus chemotherapy in limited small cell lung cancer. Proc Am Soc Clin Oncol 21:448, 1980

41. Bradley E, Matthews MJ, Cohen M, Fossieck B, Bunn P, Ihde D, Minna J: Erythroleukemia, pancytopenia, and peripheral blood aneuploidy as complications of therapy in long term survivors of small cell carcinoma of the lung (SSCL). Proc Am Soc Clin Oncol 21:321, 1980

42. Reimer RR, Hoover R, Fraumeni J Jr, Young RC: Acute leukemia after alkylating-agent therapy of ovarian cancer. N Engl J Med 297:177–181, 1977

43. Casciato DA, Scott JL: Acute leukemia following prolonged cytotoxic agent therapy. Medicine (Baltimore) 58:32–47, 1979.

44. Rosner F, Grunwald HW, Zarrabi MH: Acute leukemia as a complication of cytotoxic chemotherapy. Int J Rad Oncol Biol Phys 5:1705–1707, 1979

45. Hoover R, Fraumeni JF: Risk of cancer in renal-transplant recipients. Lancet 2:55–57, 1973

46. Lefrak EA, Pitha J, Rosenheim S, Gottlieb JA: A clinicopathologic analysis of adriamycin cardiotoxicity. Cancer 32:302–314, 1973

47. Fajardo LF, Eltringham JR, Stewart JR: Combined cardiotoxicity of adriamycin and x-radiation. Lab Invest 34:86–96, 1976

48. Billingham ME: Endomyocardial changes in anthracycline treated patients with and without irradiation. Front Radiat Therap Oncol 13:67–81, 1979

49. Kinsella TJ: Ahman DL: Guiliani ER, Lie JT: Adriamycin cardiotoxicity in stage IV breast cancer: Possible enhancement with prior left chest radiation. Inter J Radiat Oncol Biol Phys 5:1997–2002, 1979

50. Ruckdeschel JC, Chang P, Martin RG, Byhardt RW, O'Connell MJ, Sutherland JC, Wiernik PH: Radiation-relation pericardial effusions in patients with Hodgkin's disease. Medicine 54:245–259, 1975

51. Warren S: The Pathology of Ionizing Radiation. Springfield, Illinois, Charles C Thomas, 1961

52. McReynolds RA, Gold GL, Roberts WC: Coronary heart disease after mediastinal irradiation for Hodgkin's disease. Am J Med 60:39–45, 1976

53. Eagen RT, Lee RE, Frytak S, Ingle JN, Creagen ET: Combination chemotherapy with and without cis-Diammine Dichloride Platinum (II) plus thoracic radiation therapy for limited small cell lung cancer. Proc Am Assoc Cancer Res 21:131, 1980

54. Hansen HH: Should initial treatment of small cell carcinoma include systemic chemotherapy and brain irradiation? Cancer Chemother Rep Part II 4:239–241, 1973

55. Bunn PA, Nugent JL, Matthews MJ: Central nervous system metastases in small cell bronchogenic carcinoma. Sem Oncol 5:314–322, 1978

56. Nugent JL, Bunn PA Jr, Matthews MJ, Ihde DC, Cohen MH, Gazdar A, Minna JD: CNS metastases in small cell bronchogenic carcinoma: Increasing frequency and changing patterns with lengthening survival. Cancer 44:1885–1893, 1979

57. Jackson DV, Richards F II, Cooper R, Ferree C, Muss HB, White DR, Spurr C: Prophylactic cranial irradiation in small cell carcinoma of the lung: A randomized study. JAMA 237:2730–2733, 1977

58. Tulloh M, Mourer L, Forcier RT: A randomized trial of prophylactic whole brain irradiation in small cell carcinoma of the lung. Proc Am Soc Clin Oncol 18:268, 1977

59. Moore TN, Livingston R, Heilbrun L, Eltringham J, Skinner O, White J, Tesh D: The effectiveness of prophylactic brain irradiation in small cell carcinoma of the lung. Cancer 41:2149–2153, 1978

60. Williams C, Alexander M, Glatstein EJ, Daniels JR: Role of radiation therapy in combination with chemotherapy in extensive oat cell cancer of the lung: A randomized study. Cancer Treat Rep 61:1427–1431, 1977

61. Greco FA, Fer MF: Oat cell carcinoma of the lung with carcinomatosis meningitis. N Engl J Med 298:1146, 1978

62. Brereton HD, O'Donnell JF, Kent CH, Matthews MJ, Dunnich NR, Johnson RE: Spinal meningeal carcinomatosis in small cell carcinoma of the lung. Ann Int Med 88:517–519, 1978

63. Aisner J, Aisner SC, Ostrow S, Govindan S, Mummert K, Wiernik PH: Meningeal carcinomatosis from small cell carcinoma of the lung: Consequence of improved survival. Acta Cytol (Baltimore) 23:292–296, 1979

64. Aisner J, Govindan S. Wiernik PH, Gallagher RE: Meningeal carcinomatosis with small cell carcinoma of the lung: A clinicopathologic correlation. Medical Pediatric Oncology (in press)

65. Yesner R: A unified concept of lung cancer histopathology. Proc Am Soc Clin Oncol 18:271, 1977

66. Brereton HD, Mathews MM, Costa J, Kent H, Johnson RE: Mixed anaplastic small cell and squamous cell carcinoma of the lung. Ann Intern Med 88:805–806, 1970

67. Abeloff MD, Eggleston JC, Mendelsohn G, Ettinger DS, Baylin SB: Changes in morphological and biochemical characteristics of small cell carcinoma of the lung: A clinicopathologic study. Am J Med 66:757–764, 1979

68. Matthews MJ: Effects of therapy on the morphology and behavior of small cell carcinoma of the lung—A clinicopathologic study, in: F. Muggia, M. Rozencweig (eds): Lung Cancer: Progress in Therapeutic Research. New York, Raven Press, 1979

69. Hanbury WJ: Two histologically different carcinomas in the same lung. J Pathol Bacteriol 81:540–541, 1961

70. Mobley DF, Martinez J: Two histologically different primary carcinomas of the lung. Cancer 22:287–292, 1968

71. Chaudhuri MR: Independent bilateral primary bronchial carcinomas. Thorax 26:476–480, 1971

72. Stevens E, Einhorn L, Rohn R: Treatment of limited small cell lung cancer. Proc Am Assoc Clin Oncol 20:435, 1979
73. Hansen HH, Dombernowsky P, Hansen HS, Rorth M: Chemotherapy vs. chemotherapy plus radiotherapy in regional small-cell carcinoma of the lung. A randomized trial. Proc Am Assoc Cancer Research 20:277, 1979

17

INVESTIGATIONAL NEW DRUGS IN THE TREATMENT OF SMALL CELL BRONCHOGENIC CARCINOMA

John Y. Killen, Jr.
John S. Macdonald

The responsiveness of small cell bronchogenic carcinoma (SCC) to a large number of chemotherapeutic agents and the dramatic increments in patient survival which have resulted from the use of multimodality therapy have been extensively reviewed in other chapters of this monograph. The optimism generated by these exciting developments must be tempered by the fact that very few patients are cured. It is therefore imperative that new drugs be continuously screened for activity, in the hope that, like VP-16, they may be included in future treatment and further improve upon the results achieved thus far.

One of the ironies of success in the treatment of malignant disease is that the identification of promising leads from among the many available investigational new drugs becomes less and less likely. This phenomenon is seen in leukemias, lymphomas, and breast cancer, for example, and is multifactorial. Patients who become candidates for single-agent phase II trials have almost always failed one or, more likely, several multiagent regimens, thereby decreasing the chance of response to new drugs that may have similar mechanisms of action. A closely related problem is the unwillingness of many physicians to treat first-relapse patients with investigational single agents, in spite of the poor performance of "pick-up" regimens for these cases. Finally, patients relapsing a second or third time invariably present with severely compromised performance status, limiting the number of cases acceptable for entry into a study.

Interpretation of the available data is also complicated by the fact that each reported trial may be composed of a patient population that is heterogeneous with respect to amounts and types of prior therapy. This information is often not given in detail. Furthermore, there are very few single-institution or cooperative-group trials that include more than 10–20 patients with SCC.

Within the framework of these limitations, we will review the available data on investigational agents (excluding VP-16 and hexamethylmelamine) in the treatment of SCC, concentrating on single-agent trials. Unless otherwise stated, conventional and generally accepted criteria for partial (PR) and complete (CR) response apply, PR being a 50 percent or greater decrease in the product of perpendicular diameters of a clearly measurable tumor and CR being a complete disappearance of all tumor and tumor-related morbidity.

Cisplatin

Cis-diamminedichloroplatinum (CDDP), a coordination complex that has alkylating-agent properties, has been evaluated by a number of investigators. From the standpoint of incorporation into combination chemotherapy regimens, this drug has the advantage of being relatively non-myelosuppressive. Greco et al.[1] reported 3 partial responses among 17 patients (17 percent) who had failed a combination regimen of cyclophosphamide, adriamycin, vincristine, VP-16, and hexamethylmelamine. Mean Karnofsky performance status was 50, and the dose schedule was 80 mg/m^2 every 2–3 wk. Mean response duration was only 3.5 mo, however. Dombernowsky et al.[2] reported the results of a trial in which 28 patients were treated with doses ranging from 30 to 100 mg/m^2 every 3 wk. All had received prior chemotherapy, and some had received irradiation; performance-status data are not included. Partial responses were seen in 3 of the 28 evaluable patients, 2 of whom were among the 17 who had received at least 60 mg/m^2 (see Table 17-1). Cavalli et al.[3] treated 11 patients with CDDP at 80 mg/m^2 every 3 wk. ECOG performance status was 0–1 in 4 patients and 2–3 in 7; 6 patients had been previously treated with 1 combination chemotherapy regimen, and 5 with 2 or more; and 5 patients had extensive and 6 had limited disease at the start of the CDDP therapy. Partial responses were seen in 4 patients, 2 of whom had subsequent irradia-

Table 17-1
Single-Agent Cisplatin Trials in SCC

No. Evaluable Patients	Prior Therapy	Performance Status	Stage	CDDP Dose	No. of Responses			Reference No.
					CR	PR	MR	
17	CAVH*	50 (20–90)	NA	80 mg/m² Q 2–3 wk	0	3 (17%)	—	1
7	Variable*	NA	NA	30 mg/m² Q 3 wk	0	0	—	
4	Variable	NA	NA	45 mg/m² Q 3 wk	0	1	—	
9	Variable	NA	NA	60 mg/m² Q 3 wk	0	2 } (12%)	—	
3	Variable	NA	NA	90 mg/m² Q 3 wk	0	0	—	2
5	Variable	NA	NA	100 mg/m² Q 3 wk	0	0	—	
28					0	3 (12%)		
11	1 Prior Comb. (n = 6)* ≥2 Prior Comb. (n = 5)*	0–1 (n = 4) 2–3 (n = 7)	L (n = 6) E (n = 5)	80/m² Q 3 wk	0	4 (36%)	2 (18%)	3
10	POCC-VAM*	≥70	NA	100/m² Q 3 wk	1 (10%)	2 (20%)	5 (50%)	4
18	Variable*	0–1 (n = 7) 2–3 (n = 11)	L (n = 6) E (n = 5)	100/m² Q 3 wk	0	1 (6%)	2 (12%)	5
19	Variable*	NA	NA	75/m² Q 3 wk	0	0	0	6
103 Total					1 (1%)	13 (13%)	—	

*See text for further explanation.

tion during response; in the remaining 2 patients, the duration of response was 2.5 and over 2.5 mo. An additional 2 patients, classified as minor responders (MR), met criteria for partial response in pulmonary lesions, while showing stable hepatic metastases. Rosenfelt et al.,[4] from the Northern California Oncology Group, reported the results of a phase II trial of 10 patients who had failed a 7-drug combination of procarbazine, vincristine, cyclophosphamide, CCNU, VP-16, adriamycin, and methotrexate. All had Karnofsky performance status of 70 or better. The overall response rate was 30 percent (1 CR, 2 PR), with an additional 5 minor responses. Levenson et al.,[5] from the NCI–VA Medical Oncology Branch, observed 1 partial response and 2 minor responses in 18 patients treated with 100 mg/m² every 3 wk. The patient population was relatively unfavorable, with 12 having extensive disease and 11 having ECOG performance status of 2–3 at the initiation of CDDP. The Eastern Cooperative Oncology Group (ECOG)[6] recently completed a phase II trial in which patients were randomized between three treatments, one being CDDP at a dose of 75 mg/m². They were stratified on the basis of performance status (ECOG 0–1 or 2) and extent of disease at start of study, and all had failed prior treatment. No responses were seen in 19 evaluable patients. The results of all the above-mentioned studies are summarized in Table 17-1.

The response data for platinum cited above vary from study to study but indicate at least a modest degree of activity. The most important test will be to determine whether CDDP increases the effectiveness of existing first-line chemo- or multimodality therapies. Eagan et al.[7] reported on preliminary data from the Mayo Clinic, comparing the VOCA regimen (VP-16, 50 mg/m², days 1–3; vincristine, 1.4 mg/m² day 1; cyclophosphamide, 150 mg/m², days 1–3; and adriamycin, 15 mg/m², days 1–3; all IV) with VOCA plus *low-dose* CDDP at 40 mg/m² on day 1 (VOCAP). All patients had limited-stage disease, and all received a total of 4000 rads to the primary tumor and mediastinum, concurrent with cycles 3 and 4. The two groups were well balanced with respect to performance status, age, and sex. The overall response rates (CR + PR) prior to irradiation were 87 percent (30 percent CR) for VOCA and 81 percent (29 percent CR) for VOCAP. Following irradiation, the CR rate increased to 43 percent for VOCA and 39 percent for VOCAP. Median survival was virtually identical between the two groups (72 versus 73 wk). The authors concluded that no significant benefit could be found with the addition of low-dose CDDP. Whether higher doses of platinum can improve on the results of established combinations, without undesirable toxicity, in limited-stage disease, and whether any dose of platinum adds to the results thus far achieved in extensive-stage disease remain unanswered questions.

VM-26

The epipodophyllotoxin, VM-26, has received remarkably little attention, given the activity of the closely related compound VP-16: only two adequately recorded phase II trials have been reported, and the results are conflicting (Table 17-2). Samson et al.[8] from Wayne State University treated 14 patients at 30 mg/m² for 5 consecutive days; dose escalation was allowed in the absence of prohibitive toxicity. All patients had received prior chemotherapy and some had received prior irradiation. They saw no objective responses. Woods et al.[9] from Sydney, Australia, treated 25 patients: 5 at 100 mg/m² and 20 at 60 mg/m², both in daily doses for 5 consecutive days every 3 wk. Using the previously described criteria, they identified 7 objective responders (2 CR, 5 PR). Interestingly, 2 of 4 patients who had received no prior chemotherapy responded. Furthermore, there did not seem to be a dose–response effect over the range tested: 1 PR occurred in the group treated with 100 mg/m², and the remaining 6 responses (including 2 CR's in limited-disease patients) occurred in the 60 mg/m² group. The number of patients who had received prior VP-16 is not known for either trial. In summary, the usefulness of VM-26 in SCC, especially in view of the widespread use of VP-16, remains unsettled. Other studies of the drug's effectiveness are currently in progress or are about to be activated.

Streptozotocin and Chlorozotocin

Two investigational nitrosoureas, streptozotocin and chlorozotocin, have undergone phase II testing (Table 17-2). The former is of special interest, both because it is relatively nonmyelosuppressive and because it has proven activity against neoplasms generally regarded as being of neural crest origin—the amine precursor uptake and decarboxylation (APUD) tumors, such as islet cell carcinoma and malignant carcinoid. A similar site of origin has been postulated for SCC.[10] In three published phase II studies incorporating a total of 41 patients, no responses were seen.[11–13] It is important to note that virtually all of these patients had previously received up to 6 chemotherapeutic agents, and at least 29 had received CCNU.

Whereas streptozotocin is a water-soluble methyl nitrosourea derivative, chlorozotocin is a water-soluble chloroethyl nitrosourea. In the previously noted ECOG study, a total of 16 evaluable patients were treated with a dose of 120 mg/m² every 6 wk.[6] Again, no responses were seen; it is not

Table 17-2
Single-Agent Phase II Trials in SCC

Drug	Starting Dose	No. Evaluable Patients	No. of Responses		Duration PR	Reference No.
			CR	PR		
VM-26	30 mg/m² × 5 d	14	0	0	—	8
	100 mg/m² × 5 d	5	0	1	—	9
	60 mg/m² × 5 d	20	2 (10%)	3 (15%)	3–20+ wk	9
Streptozotocin	1 g/m² weekly	13	0	0	—	11
	1 g/m² weekly	13	0	0	—	12
	Variable	15	0	0	—	13
Chlorozotocin	120 mg/m² Q 6 wk	16	0	0	—	6
	NA	13	0	0	—	14
AMSA	90–100 mg/m² Q 3–4 wk or 30–40 mg/m²/d × 3 Q 3–4 wk	54	0	0	—	15
5-FU	600 mg/m² × 5 d	8	0	3 (38%)	42–45 d	16
	400 mg/m² × 5 d	15	0	0	—	16
Maytansine	1.5 g/m² Q 3 wk	18	0	0	—	6
Dibromodulcitol	NA	17	0	4 (24%)	NA	17

known how many of these patients had received prior nitrosourea therapy. An additional 13 patients, 11 from a single institution, are cited in the annual report to the FDA.[14] No details of the patient population are available. There were no objective responses.

AMSA

AMSA (4'-(9-acridinylamine)-methansulfon-m-ansidine) is an acridine dye derivative that appears to act by a mechanism similar to that of the anthracycline antibiotics. It has shown very promising activity in the treatment of acute leukemia in second and third relapse.[15] A compilation of several phase II trials, using either a single dose of 90–100 mg/m² or a 3-day schedule of 30–40 mg/m²/day every 3–4 wk, reveals no responses among 54 evaluable cases of SCC (Table 17-2).[15] These doses are substantially less than those employed in the successful acute leukemia regimens, but are consistent with those used in other solid-tumor studies.

5-Fluorouracil

In an interesting report by Hovsteen et al.,[16] 5-fluorouracil (5-FU) was evaluated for activity in 26 patients with advanced, previously treated SCC (Table 17-2). Ten patients received 600 mg/m² for 5 consecutive days, followed by 1000 mg/m² every other week. Three partial responses of 42, 45, and 45 days were reported, but myelosuppressive toxicity, including one fatal case, was unacceptable. No responses were seen in 15 evaluable patients subsequently treated at a lower dose of 400 mg/m² for 5 days, followed by the maintenance dose of 1000 mg/m² every other week. When 5-FU is administered by continuous infusion, myelosuppression can be significantly reduced and much larger doses delivered, as compared to the usual, bolus technique. The results seen in the higher dose regimen raise the possibility that infusional therapy may be worth phase II investigation.

Other Single Agents

The macrolide antibiotic, maytansine, has also been tested by the ECOG, employing a dose schedule of 1.5 mg/m² every 3 wk.[6] No responses were seen among the 18 evaluable patients treated.

Dibromodulcitol appears to act as a bifunctional alkylating agent. The only data available are from a study reported by the Central Oncology Group, describing 4 responses among 17 poorly characterized patients who were treated with an unspecified dose according to an unspecified schedule.[17] No further work has been reported for this agent.

Ifosphamide, an alkylating agent similar to cyclophosphamide, has been extensively tested in non–small cell bronchogenic carcinoma and has shown signs of activity.[18] There are virtually no data to support its efficacy in SCC, in spite of the fact that it has been incorporated into several combination chemotherapy/multimodality regimens under active study.

The results of the above studies are summarized in Table 17-2.

High Dose Methotrexate with Citrovorum Factor Rescue

High-dose methotrexate with citrovorum factor rescue (HDMTX) is of particular interest in the treatment of SCC for two reasons. First, it can be incorporated into combination chemotherapy regimens with essentially no additive myelosuppression. Second, this treatment approach results in tumoricidal drug levels in the central nervous system, suggesting a potential role in prophylactic central nervous system therapy by encompassing areas not included in conventional cranial irradiation portals, e.g., the spinal leptomeninges. Unfortunately, very few phase II single-agent data are available. Frei et al.[10] reported 6 "objective responses" among 15 evaluable patients (40 percent) treated with a weekly i.v. bolus dose of $3-7.5$ g/m², followed by citrovorum factor rescue.[10] These patients were previously untreated, and, at first evidence of response, conventional combination chemotherapy was added to the HDMTX; therefore, full degree and duration of response cannot be evaluated. Bunn et al.[20] treated 16 patients with at least 2.5 g/m² over a 30-hr period every 3 wk and observed no responses. All patients had been previously treated with regimens containing conventional-dose methotrexate.

HDMTX has been incorporated into combination regimens for first-line therapy in three published, uncontrolled trials.[21–23] All that can be said from these trials is that the available data on frequency of response, response duration, and percentage of long-term responders do not appear dramatically different from those obtained in other studies without HDMTX (see Table 17-3).

The role of HDMTX in central nervous system prophylaxis has been addressed in three studies, with conflicting results. Neijstrom et al.[24] reported on 31 patients *sequentially* assigned to receive either high-dose (500 mg/m²) or conventional-dose methotrexate in conjunction with vincristine, adriamycin, and cyclophosphamide. No prophylactic cranial irradiation was employed. Updated information indicates no difference between the two groups with respect to type or frequency of central nervous system relapse, tumor response, or duration of response or patient survival.[25] No information is available on cerebrospinal fluid levels to confirm that the dose of methotrexate employed actually resulted in tumoricidal drug concentrations.

Skarin et al.,[21] from the Sidney Farber Cancer Institute, included HDMTX (3 g/m² for a total of 14 doses) in a 6-drug combination regimen without other central nervous system prophylaxis. A preliminary report on 31 evaluable patients suggested that fewer central nervous system relapses were seen than had been expected. Data with longer follow-up are not available.

At the Vincent T. Lombardi Cancer Research Center, 43 patients were treated with a combination regimen of cyclophosphamide, adriamycin and VP-16.[26] After two cycles, HDMTX at 100 mg/kg was added for the next 6 cycles. Actuarial analysis at 15 mo of follow-up shows a 56 percent incidence of parenchymal brain and leptomeningeal relapse. It should be noted that the doses of cyclophosphamide, adriamycin, and VP-16 were somewhat less than those used in most current protocols.

Tattersal et al.[27] randomized 84 patients with limited-stage disease into two groups which received either high-dose or intrathecal methotrexate in conjunction with vincristine, adriamycin, and cyclophosphamide. There were no differences between the two groups with respect to number of central nervous system relapses, tumor response, duration of response, or patient survival.

Thus, there seems to be little role for HDMTX in the treatment of SCC. There is no evidence that its addition has improved upon current combination chemotherapy regimens, and there are no data indicating its superiority over the much simpler conventional dose. Likewise, its role in central nervous system prophylaxis does not seem promising. It is hoped that these questions will be answered definitively by the results of several ongoinng, randomized trials comparing standard- and high-dose methotrexate.

Conclusion

For the most part, the data reviewed are discouraging. The only agent that appears reasonably promising is cisplatin. Randomized trials evaluating its contribution to current therapy when used in full dose are clearly needed.

Table 17-3
Trials Incorporating HDMTX in the Treatment of SCC

Concurrent Therapy*	Dose MTX	No. of Patients†	Responses	Median Survival	Reference No.
None	3–7.5 g/m²	15	6 "obj. resp."†	NA	19
All previously treated All had received low dose MTX	2.5 g/m²/30 hr	16	0	NA	20
CYC, 400 mg/m² Q 3 wk ADR, 40 mg/m² Q 3 wk VP-16, 100 mg/m² d 1,3,5 Q 3 wk.	100 mg/kg	L = 32 E = 11 ——— 43	CR = 41% CR = 27% CR + PR = 74%	11.3+ mo 7.2+ mo.	
CYC, 700 mg/m² Q 3 wk ADR, 45 mg/m² Q 3 wk VCR, 1.0 mg/m² Q 3 wk MeCCNU + CYC maint.	3 g/m² d 7,14	L = 12 E = 19 ——— 31	CR = 58% CR = 37% CR + PR = 87%	CR pts: 15 mo PR, NR pts: 9 mo	21

ADR, 400 mg/m² Q 4 wk CYC, 750 mg/m² Q 4 wk VCR, 1.0 mg/m² Q 4 wk RT to Primary	500 mg/m² or 40 mg/m² (nonrandom)	31	CR 33% Groups identical	Overall 300 days Groups identical	24
VCR, 1 mg/m² 1 Q 3 wk CYC, 750 mg/m² 1 Q 3 wk ADR, 50 mg/m² 1 Q 3 wk ± chest R.T.	12 mg IT or 1g/m² IV (Randomized)	49 35 (All limited)	CR = 40% CR = 32%	63 wks 58 wks	27
CYC, 1g.m² ADR, 40 mg/m² VCR, 1.0 mg/m² Alternating with HEX, 8 mg/kg/d × 14 VCR, 1.0 mg/m² 2 VP-16, 180 mg/m²/d × 3	6 g/m²	21 (All extensive)	CR = 33% PR = 47% 80%	7+ mo	23

*CYC, cyclophosphamide; ADR, adriamycin; VCR, vincristine; MeCCNU, methyl-CCNU; HEX, hexamethylmelamine.
†L, limited disease; E, extensive disease.
‡See text for further explanation.

409

Investigations of a number of agents, including PALA, AMSA, VM-26, neocarzinostatin, MGBG, and AZQ are planned or are currently underway in various cooperative groups and institutions. It is encouraging that the protocols for many of these studies stipulate that patients must be in their first relapse to be eligible. This will help address some of the issues outlined in the introduction to this chapter.

Virtually unexplored in the treatment of SCC is the role of so-called "biochemical modulation." The report by Hovsteen et al., indicating some activity for high-dose 5-FU, raises this approach as another avenue for investigation in future studies, which may include 5-FU and thymidine, 5-FU and PALA, and sequenced methotrexate and 5-FU.

A final area "ripe" for development is the use of in vitro sensitivity assays, both in the design of individual patient therapy and, more importantly, in the screening of new agents for antitumor activity. Once their validity is definitively established, it is possible to imagine that systems such as that reported by Salmon et al.[28] might be adapted to serve the additional role of a screening resource for new agents. Drugs that appear promising in vitro could then be taken to conventional in vivo phase II testing in patients with minimal prior therapy. This potential development seems especially attractive for diseases like SCC, in which heavy pretreatment before phase II therapy is the rule.

References

1. Greco FA, Einhorn LH, Hande KR, et al: Phase II studies in resistant small cell lung cancer. Proc Am Assoc Cancer Res 20:28, 1979
2. Dombernowsky P, Sorenson S, Aisner J, et al: Cis-dichlorodiammineplatinum (II) in small cell anaplastic bronchogenic carcinoma: A phase II study. Cancer Treat Rep 63:543–545, 1979
3. Cavalli F, Jungi WF, Sonntag RW, et al: Phase II trial of cis-dichlorodiammineplatinum (II) in advanced malignant lymphoma and small cell lung cancer: Preliminary results. Cancer Treat Rep 63:1599–1603, 1979
4. Rosenfelt FP, Sikic BI, Daniels JR, et al: Phase II evaluation of cis-diammine-dichloroplatinum (DDP) in small cell carcinoma of lung (SCC). Proc Am Soc Clin Oncol 21:449, 1980
5. Levenson RM: Personal communication
6. Creech RH: Personal communication
7. Eagen RT, Lee RE, Frytak S, et al: Combination chemotherapy with and without cis-diamminedichloroplatinum (II) plus thoracic radia-

tion therapy for limited small cell lung cancer. Proc Am Assoc Cancer Res 21:131, 1980

8. Samson MK, Baker LH, Talloy RW, et al: VM-26 (NSC 122819): A clinical study in advanced cancer of the lung and ovary. Eur J Cancer 14:1395–1399, 1978

9. Woods RL, Fox RM, Tattersall MHN: Treatment of small cell bronchogenic carcinoma with VM-26. Cancer Treat Rep 63:2011–2013, 1979

10. Smith LH: Oat cell carcinoma as a malignant apudoma. J Thorac Cardiovasc Surg 70:147–151, 1975

11. Bunn PA, Ihde DC, Cohen MH, et al: Streptozotocin in advanced small cell bronchogenic carcinoma: An ineffective nonmyelosuppressive agent. Cancer Treat Rep 62:479–481, 1978

12. Kane RC, Bernath AM, Cashdollar MR: Phase II trial of streptozotocin for small cell anaplastic carcinoma of the lung. Cancer Treat Rep 62:477–478, 1978

13. Maurer LH, Weiss RB, Aisner J: Streptozotocin: An inactive agent in small cell carcinoma. Cancer Clin Trials 2:59–61, 1979

14. National Cancer Institute: Annual Report to the Food and Drug Administration: Chlorozotocin. Washington, DC, National Cancer Institute, 1980

15. National Cancer Institute: Annual Report to the Food and Drug Administration: AMSA. Washington, DC, National Cancer Institute, 1980

16. Hovstren H, Sorensen S, Rørth M, et al: 5-Fluorouracil in the treatment of small cell anaplastic carcinoma of the lung. A Phase II trial. Cancer Treat Rep (in press)

17. Wilson WL, VanRyzin J, Weiss AJ, et al: A phase III study on lung carcinoma comparing hexamethylmelamine (NSC 13875) to dibromodulcitol (NSC 104800). Oncology 31:293–309, 1975

18. Broder LE, Cohen MH, Salawry OS: Treatment of bronchogenic carcinoma. II. Small cell cancer. Cancer Treat Rep 4:219–260, 1977

19. Frei E, Blum RH, Pitman SW, et al: High dose methotrexate with leukovorin rescue. Rationale and spectrum of antitumor activity. Am J Med 68:370–376, 1980

20. Bunn PA: Personal communication

21. Skarin AT, Greene GP, Canellos R, et al: High dose methotrexate with citrovorum factor rescue (HD-MTX) alternating with combination chemotherapy (M-CAV-CMe) in small cell lung cancer. Proc Am Soc Clin Oncol 20:328, 1979

22. Hoth D, Loeky J, Baker J, et al: Limited small cell lung carcinoma:

Treatment with chemotherapy alone. Proc Am Soc Clin Oncol 21:455, 1980

23. Hande KR, Greco FA, Fer MF, et al: Combination chemotherapy plus high dose methotrexate for extensive stage small cell lung cancer. Proc Am Assoc Cancer Res 20:90, 1979

24. Neijstrom E, Capizzi R, Rudnick S, et al: High dose methotrexate with leukovorin rescue for CNS prophyllaxis in patients with small cell lung cancer. Proc Am Soc Clin Oncol 21:456, 1980

25. Neijstrom E: Personal communication

26. Killen J: Unpublished data, see ref. 22

27. Tattersall MHN, Fox RM, Woods RL, et al: A randomized study of high dose methotrexate and intrathecal methotrexate in small cell lung cancer treated by combination chemotherapy, in Second World Conference on Lung Cancer, Copenhagen, 1980

28. Salmon SE, Hamburger AW, Soehnlen B, et al: Quantitation of differential sensitivity of human tumor stem cells to anticancer drugs. New Engl J Med 298:1321–1328, 1978

18

RESULTS OF RECENT STUDIES IN SMALL CELL BRONCHOGENIC CARCINOMA AND PROSPECTS FOR FUTURE STUDIES

Paul A. Bunn, Jr.
Allen S. Lichter
Eli Glatstein
John D. Minna

Small cell lung cancer (SCC) is now recognized as a distinct clinical entity owing to its biologic and clinical differences from the other histologic types of lung cancer and particularly its sensitivity to chemotherapy and radiotherapy.[1,2] The differences in response to therapy are so striking that SCC has been contrasted with all other types, which are often termed "non-small cell lung cancer." During the past decade there has been an explosion of knowledge regarding the biology and therapy of SCC. Currently, a small minority of patients may be cured.[1] Unfortunately, however, the incidence of SCC is increasing, with 20,000–25,000 new cases per year, and its close association with cigarette smoking suggests there will be continued increases in the immediate future. Whereas the results of therapy may have reached a plateau during the last few years, new models providing insights into the biology of SCC open new areas for therapeutic studies. In this chapter, we review some of the important observations made during the past decade and consider some possibilities for studies during the next decade.

Pathology and Cellular Biology

The four major cell types of lung cancer and the light-microscopic criteria for their diagnosis are now well established (see Chapter 2, this monograph). Because SCC is more responsive to intensive chemotherapy, with or without radiotherapy, than the other histologic types, it is imperative that a correct histologic diagnosis be made. When using these criteria, expert pathologists can agree as to whether a tumor is small cell or non–small cell in 70–90 percent of instances. For any given patient, an adequate histologic or cytologic preparation must be available for review by a pathologist familiar with the current World Health Organization classification. If the specimen is inadequate, further tissue must be obtained. If there is debate over histologic interpretation, the material should be forwarded to an "expert" pathologist for review.

In contrast to the clinical significance of a histologic diagnosis of SCC, the subtypes of SCC appear to be clinically unimportant.[3–6] Several studies have shown that response rates to chemotherapy and survival are similar in the lymphocytelike and intermediate (fusiform, polygonal) forms of SCC.[3–5] In addition, in the NCI registry of long-term (over 30 mo) survivors, all the subtypes were equally represented (Table 18-1).[7] Finally, an agreement in subtyping among 3 "expert" pathologists, using the 1977 World Health Organization classification, was only 54 percent (see Chapter 2, this monograph).

A major problem in histologic diagnosis, accounting for much of the discrepancy among "expert" pathologists, is the occurrence of mixed tumors, particularly those with small cell elements mixed with elements of other cell types, most commonly large cell (see Chapter 2, this monograph). These mixed tumors account for 5 percent of all lung tumors at diagnosis in our experience at the NCI–VA Medical Oncology Branch.[8] In some instances, these mixed tumors are found within a single histologic specimen, while, in other instances, biopsy from one site reveals "pure" small cell and, from another site, "pure" non–small cell carcinoma. The biologic implications of these findings are discussed in Chapters 6, 7, and 10. There are insufficient clinical data at present to draw firm clinical conclusions. We have found that response rates to chemotherapy in these mixed tumors are high but not as high as in pure small cell tumors, and response duration and survival are shorter.[8] These observations, coupled with the finding of many mixed tumors in the NCI registry (Table 18-1), suggest that, at present, patients with mixed tumors should be treated with systemic chemotherapy and radiotherapy in the same manner as patients with pure small cell tumors.[7,8]

Mixed tumors and/or tumors of a different histologic type from that at

Table 18-1
Histologic Subtype of SCC in
NCI Registry of Long-Term
(30 mo Plus) Survivors*

Subtype	Percentage
Intermediate type	45
Lymphocyte-like	28
Intermediate/Lymphocyte	16
Intermediate/Large cell	10
Intermediate/Epidermoid	1

From Matthews et al.[7]
*N = 97.

diagnosis are even more frequent at autopsy or following relapse subsequent to a response to chemo- and/or radiotherapy (see Chapter 10, this monograph). It is by no means clear whether this represents the presence of two separate tumors, the presence of two clones of a single tumor, or the emergence of a new primary tumor. Some of the data derived from biochemical studies and from tissue-culture models suggest that all cell types are derived from a common precursor cell, much as all the hematopoietic cell types are felt to have a common cellular ancestor (see Chapters 6 and 7).

Biochemical Studies

During the 1960s Pearse identified a group of cells, present in many endocrine and nonendocrine organs, that stored amines and could take up precursor substances and decarboxylate them to amines.[9] The cells were called amine precursor uptake and decarboxylation (APUD) cells, after their principal features. Pearse initially felt that these cells were derived from the neural crest. In 1968 Hattori et al.[10] and Bensch et al.[11] described neurosecretory granules, characteristic of APUD cells, in SCC cells, providing an impetus for linking SCC with other APUD tumors. Reports of ectopic hormone syndromes, particularly ACTH, ADH, and calcitonin, suggested that many SCC cells had endocrine properties (see Chapter 8, this monograph). More recently, it has been demonstrated that SCC tumors and cultures have the APUD enzyme, dopa-decarboxylase, and have the ability to take up precursor amines, which confirms their APUD nature (see Chapters 3, 6, and 7, this monograph). There is evidence, however, as outlined in Chapters 6 and 7, that all types of lung cancer may display some of the APUD and endocrine properties of SCC cells, with some quantitative differences. In addition, Gazdar et al. (Chapter 7) have shown that conversion from one cell type to another can occur in vitro as well as in vivo. These data suggest that there may be a common origin of all bronchial mucosal cells and the tumors derived from them.

Model Systems

This monograph clearly defines the recently developed experimental model systems for SCC including (1) establishment of human tumors by heterotransplantation into athymic nude mice, (2) establishment of continuous cell lines in vitro, and (3) growth of tumor colony-forming cells in soft agar. Recent studies employing each of these models have demonstrated the SCC cells synthesize polypeptide hormones, possess biochemical and ultrastructural properties characteristic of APUD cells, have some kinetic similarities with the original SCC cells in the patient, and may undergo histologic changes similar to those seen in patients. Drug sensitivity studies in these model systems are also in progress. Thus, the development of these model systems should provide many new insights into the biology of SCC cells and assist in the development of improved therapeutic strategies.

Staging and Restaging

The TNM staging system for lung cancer adopted by the American Joint Committee on Staging and End Results Reporting has not proven useful in SCC, since prognosis is independent of stage in this system. The Veterans Administration Lung Cancer Study Group proposed separating inoperable patients into two groups—limited and extensive stages. This system has been adopted throughout the United States, although there are several problems in its use which have become apparent in the last few years and which are detailed in Chapter 11 of this monograph. The definition of limited disease has varied from center to center, particularly with respect to supraclavicular nodes and pleural effusions. In addition, the number and type of staging procedures influences the frequency of finding distant metastases. The currently recommended staging procedures are outlined in Table 11-2.

Recent studies have suggested that initial performance status may be a more reliable prognostic indicator than initial stage of disease. Several groups have shown that survival in patients with single sites of metastatic disease is no different from survival in patients with limited-stage disease. Patients with multiple metastases have a significantly poorer prognosis than those with single metastases and those with limited stage-disease. Liver and central nervous system metastases are associated with a particularly poor prognosis. Most groups have found that the presence or absence of supraclavicular nodes is prognostically unimportant. Several investigators have suggested that patients who undergo surgical resections with curative intent, particularly those with $T_1N_0M_0$ lesions, and who receive postoperative combination chemotherapy have a more favorable prognosis than other limited-stage patients. If these factors are confirmed in other studies, a new staging classification may become necessary.

Prognosis is also related to the response to therapy. Several recent studies have suggested that maintenance chemotherapy be continued for 1 yr or less in complete responders. Others have suggested that elective brain irradiation should be reserved for patients demonstrating an objective tumor response to therapy. For these reasons, it is important to repeat staging procedures after some initial period (usually 6–12 wk) and at the time that discontinuation of therapy is contemplated (usually 6–18 mo). Any study that was initially abnormal should be repeated. In addition, Ihde et al.[12] have shown that fiberoptic bronchoscopy is frequently useful, particularly in patients whose chest roentgenograms appear normal or are unevaluable.

New staging and restaging procedures need to be developed. Computer-assisted tomograms (CT) are being evaluated for their ability to detect central nervous system lesions in asymptomatic patients. Recent studies have suggested that CT scans of the abdomen are not more useful than other standard staging procedures in the detection of intra-abdominal metastases in SCC. CT scans of the chest can be useful in certain situations, particularly in radiotherapy planning (see section below on Radiation Therapy for SCC).

Chemotherapy

The major unresolved chemotherapeutic issues in SCC are shown in Table 18-2. Complete tumor responses are a prerequisite to prolonged disease-free survival in SCC, and treatment with single-agent chemotherapy only infrequently produces complete responses.[13] In contrast, combination chemotherapy yields complete responses in 20–50 percent of previously untreated patients, and 2-yr disease-free survival is found exclusively in patients treated with drug combinations. Thus, the first issue is the choice of drugs for a combination and the optimal number of drugs.

Table 18-2
Study Questions in Chemotherapy Trials

Induction therapy
  Number of drugs in a combination and most effective drugs
  Intensity of combination chemotherapy
    Dose of each drug
    Frequency of drug administration
  Schedule of drugs in combination
  Discovery of new agents
  Pretherapy selection of responsive agents

Maintenance
  Duration of therapy
  Alternation of non-cross-resistant combinations
  Early or late intensification

Induction Therapy

Optimal Drug Number

A summary of the reported results of drug combinations, segregated by the number of drugs, is shown in Table 18-3.[14] Each of the combinations in this table included cyclophosphamide. Both the overall and complete response rates increase as the number of drugs is increased from 2 to 3 and then from 3 to 4 drugs. There is no apparent improvement in results when the number of drugs given simultaneously is increased from 4 to 5 or more. Lengthening of survival with increasing numbers of drugs is more difficult to document in these nonrandomized trials, but 2-yr disease-free survival is found only in regimens containing 3 or more drugs.[14]

There are two randomized studies to determine the optimum number of agents. Hansen et al.[15,16] compared CTX + CCNU with CTX + MTX and also compared CTX + MTX + CCNU with CTX + MTX + CCNU + VCR. In the first study, the 3-drug regimen had a higher response rate than did the 2-drug regimen, with a 2-mo prolongation of median survival, although neither difference was statistically significant.[15] Response rates to the 3- and 4-drug regimens were similar, but the 4-drug regimen was associated with a 1.5-mo increase in median survival that was statistically significant.[16] However, even in the 4-drug combination, substantial myelosuppression was uncommon. It has been established that intensive 3-drug regimens are superior to less intensive regimens (see next section). It is possible that increasing the drug doses in 3-drug regimens is as effective as adding additional agents.

Table 18-3
Results with Chemotherapy Alone*

No. of Drugs†	No. of Patients	CR + PR (%)	CR (%)	MS	No. 2-yr DFS
2	193	50	21	4.5–14.5	0/52
3	452	63	30	5–12	3/162
4 or more	591	82	38	4–14.5	10/266

Adapted from Bunn and Ihde.[14]
*Abbreviations: CR, complete response; PR, partial response; MS, range in median survival; DFS, disease-free survival.
†All regimens contain cyclophosphamide.

Optimal Drug Dose

In a randomized study, Cohen et al.[17] compared the results of a 3-drug regimen, CTX + MTX + CCNU, in standard outpatient doses with those achieved by doubling the doses during the first 6-wk induction period. Overall response rate and median survival were significantly superior in the high-dose chemotherapy group. More importantly, complete response and 2-yr disease-free survival were noted only in the high-dose regimen. The concept of the importance of high-dose induction therapy with con-comitant moderate degrees of myelosuppression has been confirmed in many other trials employing this and other 3- and 4-drug regimens.

The finding of a steep dose–response curve led several groups to in-vestigate even higher doses of induction therapy, which have generally been achieved by increasing the induction dose of cyclophosphamide. Ta-ble 18-4 summarizes the results of increasing induction doses of cy-clophosphamide in 3-drug regimens at 3 institutions.[17–22] It is clear from these studies that the dose–response curve reaches a plateau at 1500 mg/m² every 3 wk, or 3000 mg/m² in the first 6 wk. Further increases in induc-

Table 18-4
Effect of Induction CTX Dose in First 6–8 wk of Extensive-Stage Disease (CMC or CAVP16 ± VCR)

Cytoxan (mg/m²)	No. of Patients	CR* (%)
2000	60	22
3000	42	29
4000	33	27
4800–6000	26	23

Adapted from ref. 17–22.
*CR, complete response.

tion therapy were associated with increased toxicity but were not associated with increased response rates or 2-yr disease-free survival.

Increased intensity of induction therapy can be achieved by increasing the frequency of induction cycles as well as by increasing the dosage of one or more drugs. Table 18-5 illustrates the results of a trial using various numbers of induction cycles.[20] This study, designed to give a 4-drug regimen in frequencies greater than every 3 wk, showed that higher response rates could be achieved with more frequent drug administration. Unfortunately, there was increased toxicity, without survival benefit, associated with the increased number of drug cycles.

It thus appears that the best therapeutic results can be achieved by 3- or 4-drug regimens with a 6–8 wk induction utilizing cyclophosphamide in a dose of 1500 mg/m² given every 3–4 wk. The cyclophosphamide dose can be reduced subsequent to induction. Increasing the dose or frequency of cyclophosphamide administration does not appear to enhance results. Whether procedures to ameliorate toxicity from increased intensity (i.e., autologous bone marrow transfusions) would allow us to see some therapeutic benefit from intensive induction therapies has not been tested to date.

Optimal Drug Schedule

The scheduling of drug administration has been shown to be of critical importance in experimental model systems. Little is known, however, about the proper timing and sequencing of cytotoxic drug therapy in human tumors, including SCC. Burke and co-workers[21] and Vindelov and co-workers[23] have demonstrated sequential changes in the tumor cell-cycle distributions following chemotherapy. Both groups are currently evaluating "timed sequential" drug combinations designed to take advantage of the cell-cycle changes induced by the initial therapy. It is clearly too soon to determine whether these approaches will improve therapeutic results. Nevertheless, such studies can increase out understanding of how to schedule drugs and this may lead to improvements, particularly over drug combinations currently designed without any such rationale.

New Agents

Even with 3- and 4-drug combinations of the most active drugs (with or without chest irradiation), only a small minority of patients survive 2 yr. There is some evidence that a plateau in the improvements in therapeutic results has occurred during the last several years.[14] Myelosuppres-

Table 18-5
Effect of Increased Number of Induction Cycles*

No. of Cycles	No. of Patients	CR[†] (%)	CR + PR[†] (%)
2	16	13	63
3–4	23	26	100
5–6	11	27	100

From Minna et al.[20]
*CTX, ADRIA, VP-16, VCR.
[†]CR, complete response; PR, partial response.

sion is the dose-limiting toxicity of most of the drugs active in SCC. Thus, the discovery of new active agents, particularly nonmyelosuppressive agents, is as important as ever. Clearly, the continued search for new agents is imperative. Perhaps the use of new model systems (*vide infra*) will improve our ability to screen for new active agents.

Model Systems for the Selection of Active Agents

The model systems recently developed and discussed in Chapters 3, 4, 5, and 7 of this monograph have at least two important potential therapeutic uses. The first is in the development of new active agents, and the second is for tailoring drug therapy in an individual patient. The screening system currently used for new drug development is a long, time-consuming process. Most of the models use animal tumors, which are biologically quite different from human tumors. In addition, they tend to select agents which are effective against relatively rapidly proliferating tissues. Thus, most of the agents effective in these models have considerable myelosuppressive activity. The ability to screen large numbers of drugs using human SCC tumors grown in vitro may aid considerably in the detection of new active agents.

We know that 3- and 4-drug combinations of agents active against SCC will produce objective remissions in about 90 percent of patients with SCC, yet only about 30–40 percent have complete remissions and all but 5–10 percent relapse within 2 yr. The ability to combine only those agents most active against the tumor of a particular patient could increase the complete response rate and decrease the fraction of patients who relapse. Preliminary studies suggest that the soft-agar colony systems can detect agents effective against a particular tumor. Methods for obtaining soft-agar growth of SSC in up to 90 percent of positive specimens are described in Chapter 4 of this monograph. This model system now needs to be evaluated for its ability to predict drug response in patients.

Maintenance Therapy

Altering Drug Combinations

The development of large numbers of agents active against SCC allowed the development of second-drug combinations which were active after failure in a primary drug combination (i.e., non-cross-resistant). Several groups then attempted to prevent drug resistance and prolong remission duration and survival by the early introduction of second non-cross-resistant drug combination after initial response to a first combination. The two combinations were subsequently alternated. Cohen et al. (Table 18-6) found that the complete response rate increased from 30 to 48 percent when a primary 6-wk combination of CTX + MTX + CCNU was followed by a 6-wk cycle of the non-cross-resistant regimen VCR + ADR + PCZ.[18] Unfortunately the introduction of a third regimen of VP16 + IFOS at week 13 produced no further increase in complete response rate. Furthermore, despite the increased complete response rate, median survival and 2-yr disease-free survival were not significantly improved by the addition of the second and/or third regimen. This was explained by a longer survival for patients achieving a complete response during the first 6 wk compared to those achieving complete response later.

At least five groups have ongoing or recently completed studies of alternating drug combinations, and the preliminary results are summarized in Table 18-7.[24-28] There is evidence for a slight improvement in response duration with alternating drug combinations, but differences in survival are not present or are of modest degree. Thus, it appears unlikely that this approach will add significantly to the fraction of patients disease free for 2 yr or more.

Duration of Maintenance Chemotherapy

Based on results in childhood acute lymphocyte leukemia, most studies have continued maintenance chemotherapy for periods of 2 yr or more. Recent evidence has suggested that shorter periods of therapy may be preferred, particularly in responding patients with adult solid tumors. There is circumstantial evidence that shorter periods of maintenance therapy may be preferred in SCC as well (Table 18-8).

In the nonrandomized studies listed in Table 18-7, very similar therapies were given for variable periods.[29-31] There are no obvious differences in therapeutic results, suggesting that short periods of intensive therapies may be as good as longer periods of therapy. Clearly randomized studies addressing this issue are needed.

Table 18-6
Effect of Adding Non-Cross-Resistant Combinations

Combination(s)*	No. of Patients	CR[†] (%)	2-yr DFS[†] (%)
CMC	23	30	9
CMC–VAP ± VPIF	61	48	7

From Cohen et al.[18]
*CMC, CTX + MTX + CCNU; VAP, VCR + ADR + PCZ; VPIF, VP16-213 + IFOS.
[†]CR, complete response; DFS, disease-free survival.

Table 18-7
Randomized Trials of Alternating Non-Cross-Resistant Combinations*

SECSG[24]	Prolonged time to disease progression
FINSEN[25]	Improved response duration
BCRC[26]	No difference
SWOG[27]	? Improves duration complete response
NCOG[28]	Improved response duration and survival in extensive disease

*Abbreviations: SECSG, Southeast Cancer Study Group; FINSEN, Finsen Institute, Copenhagen, Denmark; BCRC, Baltimore Cancer Research Center; SWOG, Southwest Oncology Group; NCOG, Northern California Oncology Group.

Table 18-8
Effect of Duration of Maintenance Therapy in Limited Disease*

Duration[†] (months)	No. of Patients	Survival Median (months)	2-yr DFS[‡] (%)
3–4 (NCI–ROB)	36	18.5	28
14 (Vanderbilt)	32	14+	25
24 (Indiana)	19	17	26

From refs. 29–31.
*All patients received VCR + ADR + CTX, with chest RT.
[†]Duration of chemotherapy.
[‡]DFS, disease-free survival.

"Late" Intensification

There is some similarity between the therapeutic results of acute myelogenous leukemia (AML) and those of SCC, in that both have high initial response rates but low rates of long-term disease-free survival. Recent studies in AML have suggested that intensive therapy (with or without bone marrow transplantation), given after an initial response has been achieved, can prolong remission duration and increase the fraction of patients "cured" by cytotoxic chemotherapy.[32] Similar strategies need to be tested in SCC. Recent studies from the M. D. Anderson Hospital have demonstrated that high response rates can be achieved in SCC patients who have failed initial cytotoxic therapy with the use of high dose chemotherapy and autologous bone marrow support.[33,34] Unfortunately, the duration of these remissions was short. Nonetheless, these approaches need to be evaluated in patients during initial remission. Such an approach is currently under investigation at the National Cancer Institute.

Radiation Therapy for SCC

SCC is one of the most sensitive of all solid neoplasms to the effects of ionizing irradiation. Rarely does SCC fail to regress when irradiated, and often a complete disappearance of local tumor is achieved.[35] However, owing to the systemic nature of SCC, measures that treat only the local lung mass seldom lead to long-term survival in this disease.[36] With the high rate of response seen with chemotherapy for SCC and the establishment of the apparent curability of the disease through the use of drug treatment, the role of irradiation in the treatment of SCC has come under serious scrutiny and represents one of the major therapeutic controversies in SCC management.

Limited (Intrathoracic) Disease

The primary intrathoracic tumor represents by far the most common site of failure in SCC patients with limited-stage disease treated with chemotherapy alone.[18] With the high response rate shown by SCC to irradiation, it is logical to combine the two therapies in an effort to reduce the local failure rate and possibly enhance long-term survival. When the results of all nonrandomized series employing chemotherapy alone or both chemotherapy and radiation therapy are compiled (Table 18-9), the potential benefit of combined modality treatment over chemotherapy

Table 18-9
Results in Limited Disease*

Treatment	No. of Patients	CR (%)	2-yr DFS (%)
CT alone	246	52	7
CT + RT	492	50	17

From ref. 14.
*Abbreviations: CT, chemotherapy; RT, radiotherapy; CR, complete response; DFS, disease-free survival.

alone is seen as an increase in long-term survivors, although the complete response rates and median survivals are similar. On the other side of the coin, it is apparent that the addition of irradiation to chemotherapy increases the toxicity of treatment considerably. Esophagitis, pneumonitis, and enhanced myelotoxicity have been reported with combined modality treatment.[31,37] Thus, the current major questions in limited-stage disease are whether combined modality therapy significantly increases the fraction of long-term disease-free survivors, and whether it can be given with acceptable toxicity. These questions must be answered in controlled, randomized trials.

Two randomized, controlled trials have been reported in limited-stage SCC.[38,39] In both studies, patients randomized to receive chemotherapy alone did just as well in terms of median survival as patients who received the addition of radiation therapy to the local disease. Further follow-up is necessary to assess whether there are long-term differences in the plateau phase of the survival curve. The radiation given in these two randomized trials was split-course treatment, with 3500–4000 rads given in 2 1-wk courses beginning 3 to 7 wk after the onset of systemic chemotherapy. It is far from obvious that this method of using irradiation is to be preferred in treating SCC. In fact, the use of split-course treatment for SCC can be criticized on theoretical grounds.[40] It is unlikely that a benefit from the addition of irradiation will be noted if the irradiation is applied in a suboptimal fashion. In addition, efforts to achieve long-term local control will probably require a radiation dose to the tumor in excess of 3000 rad, as late recurrence in the chest after small doses is often seen when chemotherapy controls distant tumor for periods of 10 mo or more.[31]

There are few data to guide oncologists in selecting the best method of combining irradiation and chemotherapy in the treatment of SCC. Between 1974 and 1977 the National Cancer Institute treated a group of 71 consecutive SCC cases (42 limited) with combined modality therapy.[31,41] What is unique about this experience is that the short, intensive chemo-

Table 18-10
Radiation Therapy Schemas, 1974–1977

Group	No. of Patients	Rad per Fraction	No. of Fractions per Day	Planned Split	Total Dose/Weeks*	No. Weeks Concurrent Radiation–Chemotherapy
1	10	200	1	No	3000/3 weeks	3
2	11	200	3	No	3000/1 weeks	0
3	12	100	1	No	3000/6 weeks	6
4	9	200	3	Yes[t]	3000/11 weeks	0
5 and 6	15	150	1	Yes[‡]	4500/8 weeks	0
7	14	100	1	No	4500/9 weeks	9

*Includes split.
[t]600 rad after each drug cycle.
[‡]2250 rad, then 2-week split, then 2250 rad.

therapy (vincristine, adriamycin, cyclophosphamide) was virtually identical from patient to patient, while the irradiation schedule varied such that six different schedules were employed (Table 18-10). Groups 1, 3, and 7 received 3, 6, and 9 wk of concurrent combined modality therapy, while groups 5 and 6 received no concurrent therapy, but rather sequential treatment in which split-course irradiation followed 4 complete cycles of chemotherapy. No maintenance therapy was given to any patient.

An analysis of the results in groups 1, 3, 5 plus 6, and 7 is presented in Table 18-11. Groups 2 and 4 are excluded due to their highly unusual radiation fractionation. The rate of complete response was essentially the same from group to group and clustered about the overall complete response rate for the entire series (72 percent). However, local control after complete response increased with the length of concurrent treatment. Treatment-induced death also increased markedly as one progressed from no concurrent treatment up to 9 wk of concurrent therapy, where an unacceptable frequency of treatment-related deaths occurred (50 percent). When one plots the composite effect of these variables on 2-yr survival, 3 wk of concurrent treatment appears to be more effective than sequential treatment and produces a much more acceptable rate of treatment toxicity.

In addition to restricting the length of time over which the two modalities are applied concurrently, the toxicity of combined modality therapy can be reduced by employing sophisticated treatment planning techniques to minimize the volume of tissue taken to full dose. The poor prognosis associated with patients suffering from non-small cell lung cancer has mitigated against complex and sophisticated radiotherapeutic techniques. Yet, the prospect of curative treatment in SCC has caused us to

Table 18-11
Response, Local Control, Toxicity, Survival in SCC Patients, 1974–1977

Group*	No. of Weeks Concurrent Treatment	No. of Patients	Complete Response (%)	No. of Complete Responders with Local Control (%)	No. of Deaths from Toxicity (%)	No. of 2 yr Survivals (%)
5 and 6	0	15	10 (67)	4 (40)	1 (7)	3 (20)
1	3	10	8 (80)	6 (75)	1 (10)	5 (50)
3	6	12	8 (67)	5 (63)	3 (25)	4 (33)
7	9	14	10 (71)	9 (90)	7 (50)	4 (29)

*From Table 18-10.

427

think how we might individualize and customize the target volume to be irradiated to high dose. Over a 3-wk course of treatment (15 fractions), we will almost always reduce the size of the portal at least once, and more often twice, to account for the response of the tumor to the therapy. Rather than use unblocked rectangular or square fields, we extensively shield normal-appearing lung by individually constructing shaped portals similar to the mediastinal component of a mantle field in the treatment of Hodgkin's disease. The best method we have found for normal-tissue shielding is through the use of custom-shaped focused blocks that can be produced in a short time using a low-melting-point alloy such as cerrubend. On the fifth or sixth treatment day, the patient is routinely resimulated, and a new set of blocks can be fabricated and employed for the following day's treatment. These blocks correspond to the individual patient's anatomy far better than straight-line blocks (Figs. 18-1 to 18-4). The tumor-bearing areas receive 4000 rad in 3 wk, while the dose to the spinal cord is limited to 3000 rad in 3 wk by shielding the spinal cord in the posterior field for several treatments. This posterior block also partially shields the esophagus from excessive irradiation and minimizes the severity of radiation esophagitis (Fig. 18-5).

Further reductions in treatment volume can be accomplished using CT visualization of tumor. In the case illustrated, a 39-yr-old woman had regrowth of local tumor following a complete response to chemotherapy. In the PA chest film (Fig. 18-6), the disease is seen projected over the hilum of the lung, but CT scanning showed that this residual tumor, confirmed by the fine needle aspiration, was actually posteriorly located (Fig. 18-7). By combining a pair of right-angle fields modified by wedge filters, the tumor volume could be encompassed in the high-dose region, while the maximum amount of normal lung tissue could be spared (Fig. 18-8).

There are many ways to combine irradiation and chemotherapy in the treatment of SCC, as outlined in Table 18-12. Carefully designed clinical trials are necessary to determine the optimum sequencing of irradiation and chemotherapy and then to compare this best method to chemotherapy alone. Careful attention to detail must be paid in the radiation treatment planning so as to minimize undesirable complications. It is only through this type of effort that the role of combined modality treatment can be fully and objectively evaluated.

Extensive Disease

Most centers treat extensive SCC with chemotherapy alone. Since the disease is already grossly disseminated, control of the local lesion is, in theory, unlikely to spell the difference between success and failure. If the chemotherapy can control the disseminated deposits, it should, theoretically, be able to control the pulmonary component as well. One small randomized series of extensive SCC patients treated with chemotherapy alone versus chemotherapy plus irradiation to the lung, liver, and brain failed to show a difference of median survival between the two treatments.[42] Four important points need to be made concerning this study. Firstly, the number of patients included was so few that, even if there were a true difference between the two treatments, this study would have been unlikely to detect such a difference.[43] Secondly, the same discussion concerning the optimal method of combining irradiation and chemotherapy pertaining to limited disease also holds for extensive disease—we simply do not know the best technique at present. In the above mentioned study, the irradiation was similar to that given in the previously cited limited trials, that is, split-course therapy sandwiched between several cycles of chemotherapy. Thirdly, the extrapulmonary sites were irradiated sequentially, such that patients in the radiation side of the study were taken off chemotherapy for a mean of 66 days while radiation was administered. Fourthly, failure to detect differences in *median* survival does not preclude the possibility of long-term differences of the plateau phase of the survival curves.

It would be prudent to repeat this trial employing a different schedule of irradiation, possibly 3 wk of concurrent therapy as outlined in the preceding section. It could be argued that several or all known sites of metastatic spread (excluding marrow) should be treated. There is a wide spectrum of cases in the extensive disease category, ranging from patients with multiple tumor foci and marked symptoms on one extreme, to patients who would be classified as limited-disease patients, were it not for a solitary bone deposit. If combined modality therapy is restudied, it should be with large enough numbers of patients so that differences between therapeutic outcome, if not identifiable for the group at large, may, at least, be identifiable for subgroups with varying amounts of tumor burden. It should not be forgotten that, today, 97 percent of all patients with extensive-stage SCC at presentation ultimately succumb to their disease, despite intensive multiagent chemotherapy. New and innovative approaches to this clinical entity are clearly warranted.

Prophylactic Cranial Irradiation

Central nervous system metastases have been recognized as a frequent complication of SCC since 1973 (see Chapters 12 and 15, which address the problem). Both randomized and nonrandomized studies suggest that the frequency of recurrence can be reduced dramatically by prophy-

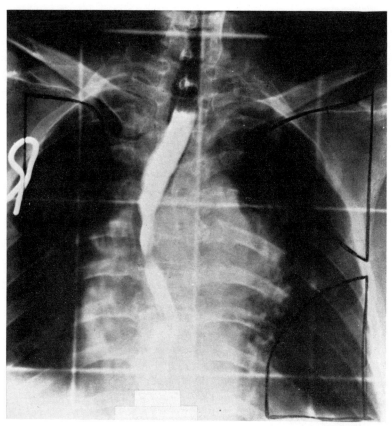

Figure 18-1. *Simulator film for planning radiation treatment in a patient (59-yr-old male) with SCC. Areas outlined in dark crayon are to be shielded with custom-shaped blocks.*

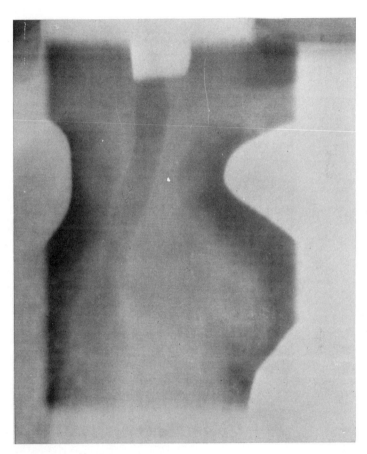

Figure 18-2. *Portal film taken under therapy to verify that the treatment indicated by the simulator film is being accurately carried out.*

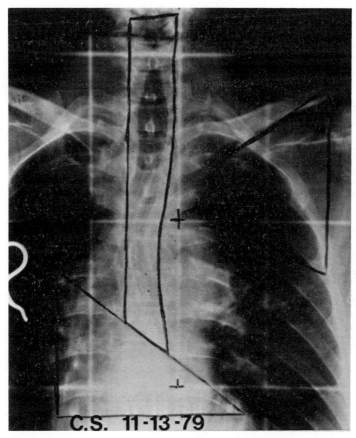

Figure 18-3. *After seven treatments, the simulation is repeated and the field reduced to allow for the marked tumor response.*

432

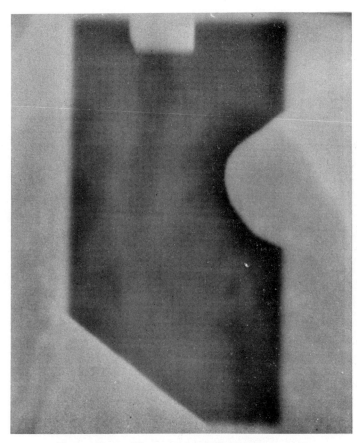

Figure 18-4. *Therapy portal film of Figure 18-5.*

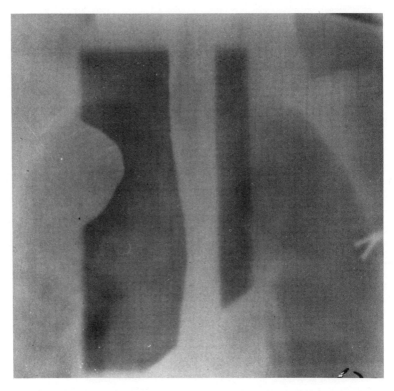

Figure 18-5. *A posterior spinal cord block protects the spinal cord and also the esophagus for the last several treatments.*

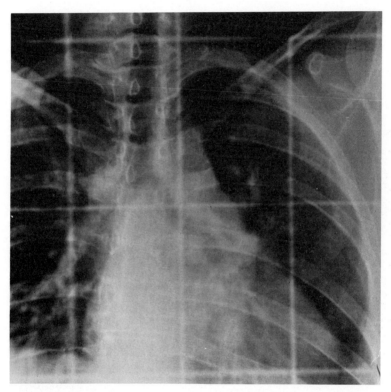

Figure 18-6. *Right hilar SCC on an anterior simulator film in a patient (37-yr-old female) with SCC.*

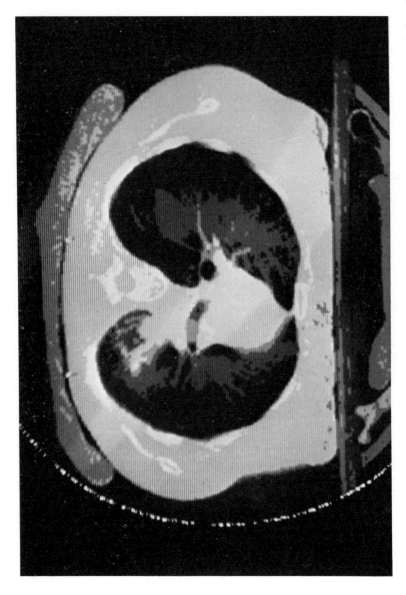

Figure 18-7. *Computerized tomogram (CT scan) of patient in Figure 18-8 showed her lesion to be posterior in location.*

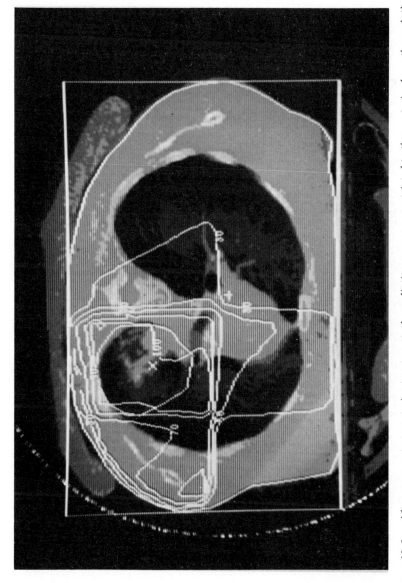

Figure 18-8. *After some anteroposterior treatment, the radiation area was restricted to the posterior lung through the use of right-angled fields. The anterior right lung was spared the high dose of radiation, as indicated in the treatment plan. Circular area surrounding tumor received full dose (100 percent), while the anterior lung received only 30 percent of this dose.*

Table 18-12
Methods of Combining Irradiation
and Chemotherapy in
the Treatment of SCC

Concurrent starting day 1
    Continuous
    Split course

Concurrent after initial chemotherapy
    Continuous
    Split course

Sequential
    Irradiation first
    Chemotherapy first
    Continuous or split course

Sandwich
    Chemotherapy–irradiation–chemotherapy
    Continuous or split course

lactic cranial irradiation (PCI) (Table 18-13). Unfortunately, no increase in survival has been demonstrated for patients treated with PCI. This may be due in part to our inability to control local or systemic disease, or both. Nonetheless, a central nervous system metastasis can be a catastrophic event and should be prevented if possible. A number of fractionation schemas are effective; we prefer 2400 rad in 8 300-rad fractions. The therapy should be given no later than week 12 of therapy, since brain metastases become more frequent after this date.[49] Arguments have been made that treatment of symptomatic brain metastases accomplishes as much benefit as PCI; the problem with such an argument is that the median survival after any relapse of this disease is only 2 mo. The maximum benefit could probably be better assessed by confining discussion of the merits of PCI to only those patients who achieve a complete response to their treatment, since patients with only a partial response remain at risk for further seeding of their central nervous system.

New Directions in Radiotherapy in Small Cell Lung Cancer

As noted in the discussion on limited disease, we must learn how best to integrate irradiation and chemotherapy for maximal benefit in SCC. Furthermore, more attention should be paid to treatment planning

Table 18-13
Prophylactic Cranial Irradiation in SCC—Results of
Randomized Trials

Author	Reference	CNS Radiation		No CNS Radiation		Relapse Signif- icance	Survival Signif- icance
		No. of Patients	No. of CNS Relapses	No. of Patients	No. of CNS Relapses		
Jackson	44	14	0	15	4	0.05	NS
Maurer	45	79	3	84	15	0.01	NS
Hirsch	46	55	5	56	7	NS	NS
Beiler	47	23	0	31	5	0.05	NS
Cox	48	24	4	21	5	NS	—
Total		195	12 (6%)	207	36 (17%)		

NS, Not significant.

and to limiting the normal tissue volume exposed to irradiation. With the advent of highly effective multiagent chemotherapy in SCC, it may not be necessary to irradiate large volumes always in an anterior–posterior approach, as one normally does in routine non-small cell lung cancer treatment. Irradiation may be required in the truly "bulk" tumor, with chemotherapy eradicating microscopic pulmonary and mediastinal extensions, as we trust it to eradicate systemic micrometastatic disease. With CT scanning and computerized treatment planning employing custom-shaped blocks and frequent cone-down field modifications, it may be possible to deliver effective, high-dose irradiation to intrathoracic SCC with success, safety, and minimal toxicity.

Hypoxic cell radiosensitizers are undergoing evaluation in a variety of neoplasms.[50] With the volume of necrosis often seen in SCC biopsy specimens, it appears that hypoxic cells are present in this tumor. Local tumor control is still a problem in SCC, even with combined modality therapy, and hypoxic cell radiosensitizers may deserve a trial in this setting.

Finally, total-body irradiation (TBI) may have a role to play in the treatment of SCC. Although small-fraction, low-dose treatment has not proven effective, high-dose TBI along with intensive chemotherapy has been reported to induce responses (one complete response) in relapsed SCC in the setting of bone marrow transplantation.[33,34] Autologous marrow reconstitution could be considered for marrow-negative patients as a means whereby high-dose chemotherapy and high-dose TBI could be safely combined in an "intensification" regimen.

Table 18-14
Long-Term Results of NCI SCC Trials*

	Long-term Survivors (%)
CT + RT† (16/85)	19‡
CT (4/83)	5

*$N = 168$.
†CT, chemotherapy; RT, radiotherapy.
‡$p < 0.02$; $p < 0.05$ for limited stage.

Long-Term Survivors: Results at the National Cancer Institute (NCI)

Since the early 1970s, when trials employing intensive combination chemotherapy regimens were instituted, it has been appreciated that a small minority of patients will survive without evidence of lung cancer for periods of 2½ or more years. Reports of such patients from several institutions have appeared in the literature,[51,52] and a registry has been formed at the National Cancer Institute.[7] Analysis of these long-term survivors can provide some insights into our current treatment approaches.

Between March 1973 and July 1977, 168 SCC patients were entered on the therapeutic protocols of the Radiation Oncology Branch or the NCI–VA Medical Oncology Branch.[52] Twenty of these 168 patients (12 percent) were alive and without clinical evidence of SCC 30 mo or more from the onset of therapy. After extensive pretherapy staging procedures, the patients were treated on protocols employing intensive combination chemotherapy, with or without chest irradiation.[17,18,31] Twenty-five percent of all patients with limited-stage disease became long-term survivors, compared to only 3 percent of patients with extensive-stage disease. No patient with multiple sites of extensive disease was a long-term survivor. While none of these trials involved a randomized comparison between chemotherapy and with chemotherapy without chest radiotherapy, there were significantly more long-term survivors in patients receiving combined modality treatment (Table 18-14), even when the initial stage of the patients was considered.

The long-term toxicity for patients surviving intensive therapies has received little attention in the past (see Chapter 16). Not unexpectedly, there is considerable late toxicity associated with these treatments. Table 18-15 shows the current status of the 20 NCI long-term survivors.[52] Seventeen of the 20 patients are alive, and only one relapsed with SCC at month

Table 18-15
Current Status of Long-Term Survivors in NCI Trials*

Alive	17†	PS 1‡	4
SCC relapse (PS 2)	1	PS2	2
Asymptomatic	10	Pulmonary fibrosis	7

*N = 20.
†The 3 deaths were from gastic carcinoma (month 53), erythroleukemia (month 40) and sudden death of unknown cause (month 48, clinically free of SCC at month 47).
‡PS, Performance status.

53. Of the 16 living patients without relapse of SCC, 10 are asymptomatic, 4 have symptoms but are fully ambulatory, and 2 have symptoms with some restrictions of activity. These symptoms are related to chronic cardiopulmonary disease and treatment-related toxicities. A total of 7 patients, including 6 who are symptomatic, have evidence of pulmonary fibrosis. Two of the 3 patients who died had developed second malignancies 40–53 mo after the onset of therapy, including one who had developed erythroleukemia.[53]

In addition to late complications of treatment, we must consider the acute, early toxicity that occurs during the early induction therapy. In the acute nonlymphocytic leukemias this induction mortality may be as high as 25 percent. In SCC there is considerably less acute morbidity. As shown in Table 18-16, 4–7 percent of patients die during induction in most series, although up to 20 percent of patients have died in some studies.[17,18,20,22,26,28,54]

Analysis of long-term survivals thus shows that intensive therapies employing combination chemotherapy can yield long-term survival in as many as 12 percent of patients, including 25 percent of patients with limited disease. This intensive therapy has a significant 5–10 percent early

Table 18-16
Treatment-Related Mortality During Induction Therapy for SCC

Institution*	No. of Patients	Treatment-Related Deaths (%)
NCI–VA[17,18,20]	106	7
NCOG[28]	154	4
SWOG[54]	138	4
BCRC[22,26]	85	4

*NCI–VA, National Cancer Institute–Veterans Administration Medical Oncology Branch; NCOG, North California Oncology Group; SWOG, Southwest Oncology Group; BCRC, Baltimore Cancer Research Center.

mortality rate and some chronic treatment-related complications, including pulmonary fibrosis and, possibly, the development of second malignancies. However, at present we believe the therapeutic results to be sufficiently promising to justify risking these toxicities. Future studies must, of course, consider means of reducing the toxicity.

Conclusions

Pathologic, biologic, and therapeutic advances in SCC during the past decade have been vast and are well summarized in this monograph. By refinement of present knowledge, with cross-fertilization of the results from each of these disciplines, there is good reason to expect that further progress in the management of SCC will be made during the ensuing decade.

References

1. Bunn PA, Cohen MH, Ihde DC, et al: Advances in small cell bronchogenic carcinoma. Cancer Treat Rep 61:333–342, 1977
2. Cohen MH, Matthews MJ: Small cell bronchogenic carcinoma: A distinct clinicopathologic entity. Sem Oncol 5:234–243, 1978
3. Burdon JGW, Sinclair RA, Henderson MM: Small cell carcinoma of the lung. Prognosis in relation to histologic subtypes. Chest 76:302–304, 1979
4. Hirsch F, Hansen HH, Dombernowsky P, et al: Bone marrow examination in the staging of small cell anaplastic carcinoma of the lung with special reference to subtyping. Cancer 30:2563–2567, 1977
5. Nixon DW, Murphy GF, Sewell CW, et al.: Relationship between survival and histologic type in small cell anaplastic carcinoma of the lung. Cancer 44:1045–1049, 1979
6. Carney DN, Matthews MJ, Ihde DC, et al: Influence of histologic subtype of small cell carcinoma of the lung on clinical presentation, response to therapy and survival. J Natl Cancer Instit 65:1225–1230, 1980
7. Matthews MJ, Rozencweig M, Staquet MJ, et al: Long-term survivors with small cell carcinoma of the lung. Eur J Cancer 16:527–531, 1980
8. Radice P, Matthews MJ, Ihde DC, et al: Characterization of mixed histology large cell/small cell lung cancer and its response to combination chemotherapy. Proc AACR/ASCO 20:409, 1979

9. Pearse AGE: The cytochemistry and ultrastructure of polypeptide hormone-producing cells of the APUD series and the embryologic, physiologic and pathologic implications of the concept. J Histochem Cytochem 17:303–313, 1969

10. Bensch KG, Corrin B, Parriente R, et al: Oat cell carcinoma of the lung—Its relationship to bronchial carcinoid. Cancer 22:1163–1172, 1968

11. Hattori S, Matsuda M, Tateishi R, et al: Oat cell carcinoma of the lung: clinical and morphologic studies in relation to its histiogenesis. Cancer 30:1014–1024, 1972

12. Ihde DC, Cohen MH, Bernath AM, et al: Serial fiberoptic bronchoscopy during chemotherapy for small cell carcinoma of the lung: Early detection of patients at high risk of relapse. Chest 74:531–536, 1978

13. Broder LE, Cohen MH, Selawry OS: Treatment of bronchogenic carcinoma. II. Small Cell Cancer Treat Rev 4:219–260, 1977

14. Bunn PA Jr, Ihde DC: Small cell lung cancer: Review of therapeutic studies, in McGuire (ed): Lung Cancer: Advances in Research and Treatment. Boston, Martins Nijhoff, 1981

15. Hansen HH, Selawry OS, Simon R, et al: Combination chemotherapy of advanced lung cancer: A randomized trial. Cancer 38:2201–2207, 1976

16. Hansen HH, Dombernowsky P, Hansen M, et al: Chemotherapy of advanced small cell anaplastic carcinoma: Superiority of a four-drug combination to a three-drug combination. Ann Intern Med 89:177–181, 1978

17. Cohen MH, Creaven PJ, Fossieck BE, et al: Intensive chemotherapy of small cell bronchogenic carcinoma. Cancer Treat Rep 61:349–354, 1977

18. Cohen MH, Ihde DC, Bunn PA, et al: Cyclic alternating chemotherapy for small cell bronchogenic carcinoma. Cancer Treat Rep 63:163–170, 1979

19. Abeloff MD, Ettinger DS, Khouri N, et al: Intensive induction therapy for small cell carcinoma of the lung. Cancer Treat Rep 63:519–524, 1979

20. Minna JD, Ihde DC, Bunn PA, et al: Extensive stage small cell carcinoma of the lung (SSCL): Effect of increasing intensity of induction chemotherapy. Proc AACR/ASCO 21:448, 1980

21. Pendergass KB, Abeloff MD, Ettinger DS, et al: Intensive timed sequential combination chemotherapy and adjunctive radiotherapy in extensive stage small cell carcinoma of the lung (SCC). Proc AACR/ASCO 21:447, 1980

22. Aisner J, Wiernik PH, Esterbay RJ: Treatment of small cell carcinoma of the lung with cyclophosphamide, adriamycin, and VP16-213 with or without MER, in Salmon SE, Jones SE (eds): Adjuvant Therapy of Cancer. New York, Elsevier-North Holland Biomedical Press, 1977, pp 245–250

23. Vindelov L, Hansen HH, Christensen IJ, et al: Treatment of small cell carcinoma of the lung monitored by sequential flow cytometric DNA analysis. Abstracts of II World Conference on Lung Cancer, 1980, p 274

24. Lowenbraun S, Bertolucci A, Smalley RV, et al: The superiority of combination chemotherapy over single agent chemotherapy in small cell lung carcinoma. Cancer 44:406–413, 1979

25. Dombernowsky P, Hansen HH, Sorenson S, et al: Sequential versus non-sequential combination chemotherapy in advanced small cell carcinoma: A comparative trial including 146 patients. Proc AACR/ASCO 20:277, 1979

26. Aisner J, Whitacre M, Van Echo DA, et al: Alternating non–cross resistant combination chemotherapy for small cell carcinoma of the lung (SSCL). Proc AACR/ASCO 21:453, 1980

27. Livingston R, Mira J: Non-cross resistant combinations in patients with extensive small cell lung cancer. Proc AACR/ASCO 21:449, 1980

28. Daniels JR, Chak L, Alexander M, et al: Oat cell carcinoma. Alternating compared with sequential combination chemotherapy. Proc AACR/ASCO 21:346, 1980

29. Greco FA, Richardson RL, Snell JD, et al: Small cell lung cancer: Complete remission and improved survival. Am J Med 66:625–630, 1979

30. Einhorn LH, Bond WH, Hornback W, et al: Long term results in combined modality treatment of small cell carcinoma of the lung. Sem Oncol 5:309–313, 1978

31. Johnson RE, Brereton HD, Kent CH: "Total" therapy for small cell carcinoma of the lung. Ann Thorac Surg 25:509–515, 1978

32. Thomas ED, Buchner CD, Fefer A, et al: Marrow transplantation for acute nonlymphocytic leukemia in first remission. N Engl J Med 301:597–599, 1979

33. Spitzer G, Dicke KA, Litam J, et al: High-dose combination chemotherapy with autologous bone marrow transplantation in adult solid tumors. Cancer 45:3075–3085, 1980

34. Gale RP: Autologous marrow transplantation in patients wtih cancer. JAMA 243:540–542, 1980

35. Salazar, OM, Rubin P, Brown JC, et al: Predictors of radiation re-

sponse in lung cancer—A clinico-pathological analysis. Cancer 37:2636–2650, 1976

36. Fox W, Scadding, TG: Medical Research Council comparative trial of surgery and radiotherapy for primary treatment of small cell or oat-celled carcinoma of the bronchus. Ten year follow-up. Lancet 2:63–65, 1973

37. Seydel HG, Creech RH, Mietlowski W, et al: Preliminary Report of a Cooperative Randomized Study for the Treatment of Localized Small Cell Lung Carcinoma. Int J Radiat Oncol Biol Phys 5:1445–1447, 1979

38. Hansen HH, Bombernowsky P, Hansen HS, et al: Chemotherapy versus chemotherapy plus radiotherapy in regional small-cell carcinoma of the lung. Proc AACR/ASCO 20:277, 1979

39. Stevens E, Einhorn L, Rohn R: Treatment of Limited Small Cell Lung Cancer. Proc AACR/ASCO 20:435, 1979

40. Ajaikumar BS, Barkley T: The role of radiation therapy in the treatment of small cell undifferentiated bronchogenic cancer. Int J Radiat Oncol Biol Phys 5:977–982, 1979

41. Catane R, Lichter A, Lee YS, et al: Small cell lung cancer: Analysis of treatment factors contributing to prolong survival. Cancer (in press)

42. Williams C, Alexander M, Glatstein EJ, et al: The role of radiation therapy in combination with chemotherapy in extensive oat cell cancer of the lung. A randomized study. Cancer Treat Rep 61:1427–1431, 1977

43. Haybittle JL, Fowler JF, Emery EW: The number of patients required in a clinical trial. Br J Radiol 44:122–125, 1971

44. Jackson DV, Richards F, Cooper MR, et al: Prophylactic cranial irradiation in small cell carcinoma of the lung. A randomized study. JAMA 237:2730–2733, 1977

45. Maurer LH, Tulloh M, Weiss RB, et al: A randomized combined modality trial in small cell carcinoma of the lung: Comparison of combination chemotherapy-radiation therapy versus cyclophosphamide-radiation therapy, effects of maintenance chemotherapy and prophylactic whole brain irradiation. Cancer 45:30–39, 1980

46. Hirsch FR, Hansen HH, Paulson OB, et al: Development of brain metastases in small cell anaplastic carcinoma of the lung, in Kay J, Whitehouse J (eds): CNS Complications of Malignant Disease. New York, Macmillan, 1979, pp 175–184

47. Beiler DD, Kane RC, Bernath AM, and Cashdollar MR: Low dose elective brain irradiation in small cell carcinoma of the lung. Int J Radiat Oncol Biol Phys 5:941–945, 1979

48. Cox JD, Petrovich Z, Paig C, et al: Prophylactic cranial irradiation in patients with inoperable carcinoma of the lung. Cancer 42:1135–1140, 1978

49. Nugent JL, Bunn PA, Matthews MJ, et al: CNS metastases in small cell bronchogenic carcinoma. Cancer 44:1885–1893, 1979

50. Chapman JD: Current concepts in cancer: Hypoxic sensitizers—Implications for radiation therapy. N Engl J Med 301:1429–1432, 1979

51. Ginsburg SJ, Comis RL, Gottlieb AJ, et al: Long term survivorship in small cell anaplastic lung carcinoma. Cancer Treat Rep 63:1347–1349, 1979

52. Minna J, Lichter A, Brereton H, et al: Small cell lung cancer. Long term, potentially cured survivors in National Cancer Institute trials. Clin Res 28:419A, 1980

53. Bradley E, Matthews MJ, Cohen M, et al: Erythroleukemia, pancytopenia, and peripheral blood aneuploidy as complications of therapy in long term survivors of small cell carcinoma of the lung. Proc AACR/ASCO 21:321, 1980

54. Livingston RB, Moore TN, Heilbrun L, et al: Small cell carcinoma of the lung: Combined chemotherapy and radiation. Ann Int Med 88:194–199, 1978

INDEX

a
b
c
d
e
f
g
h
1 i
8 2 j